B

Beauty and the Brain
Biological Aspects of Aesthetics

Edited by
Ingo Rentschler
Barbara Herzberger
David Epstein

Birkhäuser Verlag, Basel · Boston · Berlin

Library of Congress Cataloging in Publication Data

Beauty and the Brain.
   Bibliography: p.
   Includes index.
   1. Aesthetics--Physiological aspects. I. Rentschler, I. (Ingo), 1940-   II. Herzberger,
B. (Barbara) III. Epstein, David.
BH301.P45B43 1988   11'.85   88-26249

CIP-Kurztitelaufnahme der Deutschen Bibliothek

Beauty and the Brain : biolog. aspects of aesthetics / I. Rentschler ... (ed.). - Basel ;
Boston ; Berlin : Birkhäuser, 1988
   ISBN 3-7643-1924-0 (Basel) Gb.
   ISBN 0-8176-1924-0 (Boston) Gb.
NE: Rentschler, Ingo [Hrsg.]

This work is subject to copyright. All rights are reserved, whether the whole or part of the
material is concerned, specifically those of translation, reprinting, re-use of illustrations,
broadcasting, reproduction by photocopying machine or similar means, and storage in data
banks. Under § 54 of the German Copyright Law where copies are made for other than
private use a fee is payable to "Verwertungsgesellschaft Wort", Munich.

© 1988 Birkhäuser Verlag, Basel
Book and jacket design: Justin Messmer, Basel
Printed in Germany on acid-free paper
ISBN 3-7643-1924-0
ISBN 0-8176-1924-0

Table of Contents:

7 **Acknowledgments**
9 **Introduction**
  Ingo Rentschler, Barbara Herzberger, and David Epstein

Part I:
Aesthetics – Personal or Universal?

Chap. 1.
15 Gregor Paul: **Philosophical Theories of Beauty and Scientific Research on the Brain**
Chap. 2.
29 Irenäus Eibl-Eibesfeldt: **The Biological Foundation of Aesthetics**

Part II:
Three Enduring Pleasures

Chap. 3.
71 Frederick Turner and Ernst Pöppel: **Metered Poetry, the Brain, and Time**
Chap. 4.
91 David Epstein: **Tempo Relations in Music: A Universal?**
Chap. 5.
117 Walter Siegfried: **Dance, the Fugitive Form of Art – Aesthetics as Behavior**

Part III:
The Eye of the Beholder

Chap. 6.
149 Heinrich Zollinger: **Biological Aspects of Color Naming**
Chap. 7.
165 Günter Baumgartner: **Physiological Constraints of the Visual Aesthetic Response**

Chap. 8.
181 Ingo Rentschler, Terry Caelli, and Lamberto Maffei: **Focusing in on Art**

Part IV:
Two Brains – One Mind?

Chap. 9.
219 Jerre Levy: **Cerebral Asymmetry and Aesthetic Experience**
Chap. 10.
243 Marianne Regard and Theodor Landis: **Beauty May Differ in Each Half of the Eye of the Beholder**
Chap. 11.
257 Otto-Joachim Grüsser, Thomas Selke, and Barbara Zynda: **Cerebral Lateralization and Some Implications for Art, Aesthetic Perception, and Artistic Creativity**

Part V:
The Essence and the Appearance

Chap. 12.
297 Andrew Strathern: **The Aesthetic Significance of Display**
Chap. 13.
315 Elizabeth Rozin: **Aesthetics and Cuisine – Mind over Matter**

327 **Index**

Acknowledgments

The chapters of this volume evolved from seven meetings of the "Studiengruppe Biologische Grundlagen der Aesthetik" held at the Werner-Reimers-Stiftung, Bad Homburg vor der Höhe, West Germany. Authors and editors are grateful to this foundation and especially to Herr Konrad von Krosigk and Frau Gertrud Söntgen for supporting their work. They are equally indebted to all participants of these meetings whose contributions made it possible to write this book.

The original suggestion to pursue the problems at issue came from Professor Ernst Pöppel, who later generously supported the editorial process. Very important for the project was the continuous interest and encouragement received from Professor Jürgen Aschoff.

The editors further wish to acknowledge the help afforded to them by Ms. Haide Ansari, Dipl.-Biol. Ute Engler, Ms. Monika Herzog, Ms. Joyce Nevis-Olesen, Mr. Takao Maruyama, Dr. Marianne Regard, Dr. Petra Stoerig, Dr. Christa Sütterlin, Dipl.-Phys. Bernhard Treutwein, Dr. Hans Brettel, Mr. Matthias Pflieger, Dr. Wulf Schiefenhövel, and Mr. Mahmoud Zuberi.

Introduction

Ingo Rentschler and Barbara Herzberger
Institute of Medical Psychology, University of Munich, Munich, Federal Republic of Germany

David Epstein
Department of Music, Massachusetts Institute of Technology, Boston, Mass., USA

"Beauty in things exists in the mind which contemplates them." This statement made by the English philosopher, David Hume, in his work *On Tragedy* may seem strange to some and obvious to others. How is it possible for beauty not to be intrinsic to the object itself but dependent upon the observer? Or, who can expect the beauty of an object not to be the result of our observation – to be dependent upon the structure and function of our sensory experience?

By Hume's statement we are necessarily steered to the question of how body and mind, or the material and the psychic, are connected. We are required to state our position regarding the haunting problem that has occupied philosophers for more than 2000 years. If one advocates the so-called dualistic position (that body and mind are two separate, independent entities), as do many, like Sir Karl Popper and Sir John Eccles[1], then David Hume's comment concerning beauty implies that aesthetics is a philosophical discipline whose truths are inaccessible to empirical methods. The question of the biological foundations of human experience would, then, be irrelevant to the consideration and evaluation of beauty.

One of the main postulates of Schopenhauer, the German philosopher, was (in agreement with Kant) that the world, as it appears on the surface, is the world of our subjective imagination: We can *know* neither a sun nor an earth but only an eye that sees the sun and a hand that feels the earth.[2] The world surrounding us only exists in relation to the perceiving individual.

In modern physics[3] and also in modern brain research[4] one classical question of philosophy keeps reappearing: What, actually, is *reality*? We have become accustomed to considering reality as that which is made available to us by sensory input from our surroundings. We tend, however, to forget the extraordinary plasticity and learning ability of the human brain – a fact emphasized by modern brain research. Reality is, then, a construct – the validation or rejection of hypotheses that we have established concerning the so-called objective world.[5] We create this reality not only by using our senses; we create a *new* reality in art. Cultural history is characterized by the continuing development of new artistic styles. These are necessarily contained by biological boundaries; however, the human mind attempts to produce new art forms. These are initially found disturbing, but, with the passage of time, they become accepted. New realities are created that surpass the sensory impressions we receive from the outside world. In this way, art serves to extend our concepts of reality – within the limits of sensory perception and the processing abilities of the brain – and to incorporate new realms of experience.

As the neurosciences reveal more about the functional organization of the brain, philosophical problems about the mind have become the subject of combined efforts within the areas of neurobiological, psychological, and computational research. This has resulted in a view of the mind that is, like science, open to revision as a consequence of empirical findings and theoretical insight. Consequently, many researchers who have studied the fundamentals of subjective processes, for example Watanabe,[6] Bunge,[7] Churchland,[8] and Pöppel,[4] have explained the physical and the psychic by the same principle, thus confirming the so-called monistic position assumed earlier by Ernst Mach.[9] This position becomes clearer if one observes the evolution of brains of various creatures up to the human level. One can see that each psychic function or every type of behavior is dependent upon the existence of certain neuronal structures and the related algorithms. As scientists we are, therefore, obliged to investigate neuronal processes to achieve an understanding of mental activity.

With these developments in mind, a group of neuroscientists, psychologists, anthropologists, philosophers, artists, musicians, and a poet met seven times between July 1979 and January 1983 at the Werner Reimers Foundation, Bad Homburg vor der Höhe, West Germany, to discuss the question of whether there are biological aspects of aesthetic judgement and creativity. None of the participants was a recognized specialist in the field of art history or aesthetics. Instead, it was the expectation that scientists and performing artists who are concerned with the biological foundations of mental processes may have something valid to say about the biological basis of aesthetics. As a result of these meetings, the group succeeded in establishing some concepts and elucidating some problems in the emerging field of *neuroaesthetics*, which are documented in the contributions of this book.

For the members of the group, another experience was equally important. New perspectives – a heightened awareness of hitherto ignored features, forms, colors, and combinations – were presented. The contributions made during the meetings deepened the participants' appreciation of certain aspects of human behavior that belong to the essential pursuit of self-expression, exaltation, and enlightenment. The compulsion to create something of beauty or significance of oneself and one's surroundings revealed itself as a universal human quality, uniting mankind vertically throughout history and horizontally across the most diverse of cultures. Aesthetic behavior (rhyming, dancing, making music, painting, self-decoration, cooking) was found to be not only a socializing process but also a vent for frustrations and hostility, serving to contain conflict. Thus, it was recognized as a communicative process providing a universally understandable bond to reaffirm the humanness and nobility of each individual in his/her culture.

References

1. Popper KR, Eccles JC (1977) The self and its brain. An argument for interactionism. Springer International, Berlin
2. Schopenhauer A (1883) The world as will and idea. Routledge and Kegan Paul, London. Translation of: Die Welt als Wille und Vorstellung, 1818
3. Rohrlich F (1987) From paradox to reality. Our basic concepts of the physical world. Cambridge University Press, Cambridge
4. Pöppel E (1988) Mindworks. Time and conscious experience. Harcourt Brace Jovanovich, Boston. Translation of: Grenzen des Bewusstseins. Über Wirklichkeit und Welterfahrung. Deutsche Verlagsanstalt, Stuttgart, 1985
5. Gregory RL (1987) Perception as hypotheses. In: Gregory RL (ed) The Oxford companion to the mind. Oxford University Press, Oxford, pp 406–408
6. Watanabe S (1985) Pattern recognition. Human and mechanical. John Wiley, New York
7. Bunge M (1985) Treatise on basic philosophy. Epistemology and methodology III: Philosophy of science and technology. Part II: Life science, social science and technology. D. Reidel, Dordrecht
8. Churchland PS (1986) Neurophilosophy. Toward a unified science of the mind-brain. MIT Press, Cambridge
9. Mach E (1914) The analysis of sensation and the relation of the physical to the psychical. The Open Court, Chicago. Translation of: Die Analyse der Empfindungen – und das Verhältnis des Physischen zum Psychischen, 6th edn. G. Fischer, Jena, 1911

Part I
Aesthetics – Personal or Universal?

Philosophical Theories of Beauty and Scientific Research on the Brain

Gregor Paul
*Osaka City University, Department of German, Sugimoto 3-3-138,
558 Sumiyoshi-Ku, Osaka, Japan*

Beauty and the Aesthetic Judgement of Beauty

> "This *is* a beautiful sculpture!"
> "Beautiful?! It's simply obscene!"
> "You are utterly puritanical. You haven't even got the slightest idea of the distinctions between aesthetics and moral ..."

Such disputes are common among people who live under conditions which leave time for aesthetic consideration. Their mere frequency shows that questions of beauty are thought important, and this becomes even more obvious from the fact that dissent may lead to servere discord and spoil whole evenings.

What is beauty? What do we mean, when we call an object "beautiful?" Are there any characteristics of beauty? What are they? Are there even universally valid characteristics? How can they be described? Are there any characteristics of universally valid aesthetic judgements on beauty? These questions, which belong to the main topics of philosophical aesthetics, are not merely academic exercises.

The term "philosophical aesthetics" refers to aesthetic theories, such as those of Plato, Aristotle, Leibniz, Kant, Hegel, Nietzsche, Adorno, and Marcuse, but also includes, among others, teachings of Indian, Chinese, and Japanese aesthetics. Most of these theories, Western as well as non-Western, answer the above questions in a similar way: they share the same general concepts of beauty and/or the aesthetic judgement of beauty.[1] Beauty is conceived of as something harmonious, as an organic or quasi organic whole, as a gestalt rather than a mere addition of separate parts and, hence, as an object of pleasure. That is to say, according to philosphical aesthetics, there exists a universally valid concept of beauty, and there are respective criteria.

Plato, in one of the most emphatic statements ever made about concepts of beauty, claimed that real beauty does not depend on time, place, and personal judgement but has a purely intrinsic value.[2] Beautiful things are characterized by features such as harmonious shape, orderliness, "good" and "shapely grace," "fit proportion," and "pliancy of form."[3] However, according to Plato's idealism, only the most general and abstract, immaterial idea of beauty is real and perfect beauty. From a logical point of view, this idea cannot have any gestalt at all. On the other hand, spatio-temporal objects are beautiful only in so far as they "partake" of the idea of beauty. We recognize their beauty by comparing them with the *idea* and realizing an agreement with the idea. Apparently, Plato's notion that the beauty of things is defined by gestalt properties is not easily reconciled with his idealism.

Departing from idealism, Aristotle could accentuate the gestalt character of beauty. He demanded that, for instance, a tragedy should be a whole, comparable to an organic being, composed in a way that makes it impossible to change or omit a part without changing the whole tragedy.[4] Following suit, many later aestheticians also emphasized the gestalt qualities of beauty. Leibniz considered beauty a distinct whole which includes parts that cannot be clearly distinguished from each other. Accordingly, beauty differs from mere agglomerates, such as a heap of stones, which do not constitute a distinct whole at all.[5] Burke put emphasis on such criteria of beauty as "smoothness" and "gradual variation." His examples, mostly animals and plants, also show that he conceived of beautiful things as gestalts.[6] According to Kant, only art which looks as if it were nature is beautiful.[7] Hegel maintained that a beautiful work of art depicts things in the form of natural phenomena.[8] Nietzsche, in his criticism of Wagner, equates beauty with a kind of organic wholeness.[9]

Beginning with Burke, these concepts were worked out even more fully. Burke suggested that mathematical proportion, usefulness, and perfection are no general attributes of beauty.[10] Kant and most later aestheticians agreed with Burke. In a pronouncedly empirical approach, the latter argued against the confusion of practical, moral, and mathematical questions with aesthetic issues, thus refuting views common to most European philosophers, particularly the Platonists.

Adorno, often misunderstood and considered a radical opponent of traditional aesthetics, emphasized that even today (i.e., with respect to modern art) the traditional category of beauty is indispensable. He also said: "Categories such as unity, and even harmony are not gone without traces...," adding that works of art must be "coherent."[11] Marcuse, who was influenced by Kant even more strongly than Adorno, also claimed the indispensability of the traditional concept of beauty.[12]

All these philosophers agreed that the pleasure arising from the contemplation of beauty differs from erotic or sexual pleasure and interest. Leibniz introduced the term "uninterested love".[13] Burke spoke of "love... different from desire."[14] Kant coined the famous and still influencial expression "uninterested pleasure," by this meaning a pleasure unrelated even to such a desire as the wish to possess the beautiful object in question.[15]

Examples from Indian, Chinese, and Japanese aesthetics, which indicate that beauty is characterized in the same way as in Western aesthetics, i.e., as a gestalt, which, in principle, causes pleasure in every contemplator, abound. The Chinese philosopher, Zhuang Zi (fourth century B.C.), told of a woodcarver who had created a work of heavenly beauty, which was generally admired. Asked about his methods, he explained that he started carving only after having found the right tree, i.e., a tree which, in its natural shape, already contained a preformation of the sculpture. The principle of artistic creation expressed in this anecdote could be called the "harmonious interpretation of the natural material" or the "principle of natural preformation." This principle has been put forward and applied by numerous aestheticians and artists, among them Leonardo da Vinci, Michelangelo, Max Ernst, and Adorno.[16] The Chinese painter, Song Di (12th century),[17] and Xiao Tong (501–531)[18] in his poetics demanded that beautiful pictures or literature should constitute a harmonious whole. Such outstanding Japanese writers as Murasaki Shikibu (about 1000), Seami (1363–1443), Chikamatsu (1653–1725), and Soseki (1867–1916) all claimed that beautiful literature is characterized by its natural structure.

All philosophers and artists referred to, Western as well as non-Western, were among the most influential theoreticians of their cultures. Of course, philosophical aesthetics not only deals with questions of beauty. It also explores other topics, for instance, how to formulate a convincing concept of the sublime (Burke, Kant) or of the aesthetic object in general (Kant). Often, the social relevance of aesthetic values is investigated (Plato, Aristotle, Kant, and Adorno, among others).

More recently, some scholars voiced the opinion that the philosophy of beauty is obsolete since modern art does not aim at beauty and/or is not beautiful. The related idea that a "new" aesthetics is needed results from the confusion of aesthetics with the specific disciplines of art theory and art criticism. Moreover, it is empirically wrong. For example, most of the famous works from van Gogh to Max Ernst are, indeed, beautiful and are recognized as such. Moreover, one must distinguish between the words and works of modern artists. While criticizing ideas of beauty, they actually often painstakingly strove to realize them. This, for instance, was the case with Max Ernst.[19]

However, even if one rejects the distinction between philosophical aesthetics and art theory and art criticism and does not consider modern art to be beautiful, this would not lessen the actual importance of philosophical aesthetics. We still prefer what is beautiful to what is not beautiful, and so-called modern art is only one period and/or kind of art among numerous others, many of which are considered to belong to the traditions of beautiful arts. Hence, the mysteries of beauty and the philosophical attempts to solve them certainly deserve enduring interest.

As indicated, the different schools of philosophical aesthetics agree that universally valid aesthetic judgements about beauty are possible. By a "universally valid aesthetic judgement," I mean an evaluation which, in principle, could and should be shared by everyone. Among other things, such judgements express pleasure, displeasure, or indifference. "X is beautiful," implies the expression of a pleasant emotion. However, in spite of the mentioned concurrence, philosophical concepts of more particular characteristics of beauty and/or aesthetic judgement may differ widely. Broadly speaking, most of these differences are due to differences in epistemology (theory of knowledge), ontology (theory of the conditions and the attributes of being), and anthropology (theory of human nature). Actually, the various schools of philosophical aesthetics can be classified according to these distinctions. As to epistemology, the most important theories are empiricism (Burke), rationalism (Plato, Leibniz), and transcendentalism (Kant). According to empiricism, knowledge must be empirically based. The only exceptions some empiricists admit are mathematics and logic. Empiricism emphasizes the importance of the senses as faculties of knowledge. Rationalism claims that man can attain knowledge by mere thought or reason. Transcendentalism maintains that human knowledge is limited to the realm of experience but depends on and is structured by the human mind, or, if one takes the term "transcendental" in a broader sense, by all the human functions that come into play when knowledge is gained. "Transcendental" means the human conditions of the possibility of knowledge.

Today probably no philosophical scholar advocates pure empiricism. Discussions within the philosophy of science and epistemology have invalidated the concept of pure empirical knowledge. Knowledge is not possible without a predetermined frame. Traditional empiricism was often connected with the view that the mind is a "tabula rasa," a more or less passive mirror or reproduction of the outside world (like a camera). This approach led to the conviction that aesthetic judgements are statements a posteriori. "Nihil est in intellectu quod non prius fuerit in sensu." (Nothing is in the mind which has not been in the senses.)[20] Consensus among observers of aesthetic objects was attributed to inherent characteristics of the respective objects. Such an approach, however, makes it difficult to understand why objects of art from different cultures lead to a common aesthetic evaluation, as the acculturation within such cultures differs widely.

Classical rationalism permits a priori aesthetic judgements to be made but underrates the importance of experience. As Kant pointed out, the logically possible is often incorrectly equated with the actually possible. This is especially evident in the so-called ontological proof of god, which deduces the existence of god from the mere concept of a perfect being.[21] Concerning the character and functions attributed to the human mind, rationalist schools differ. In Platonism, the mind merely passively recognizes ideas, while philosophers such as Leibniz tend to regard the human mind as being active and, in a certain sense, creative. These differences notwithstanding, agreement in judgements is explained as a result of the nature of the respective objects and the human mind, with its universally common attributes, although in Platonism, the emphasis is undoubtedly on the objects, that is, ultimately on the ideas. Thus, we may note that rationalist epistemology leads to a strong concept of judgement validity but is also not very convincing. This particularly applies to Platonism, where the neglect of spatio-temporal reality is evident from the radically idealistic ontology (according to which only ideas "truly" or "really" exist).

Transcendentalism, as first developed by Kant, conceives of the human mind and the senses as necessary preconditions for the possibility of human experience. Thus, transcendentalism recognizes both, the mind and the spatio-temporal objects. To be more precise, according to transcendentalism, only that which is subjected to the mind and the senses is an object. The object is constituted by the very act of subjection. If the mind, in its activities, leaves the spatio-temporal frame within which objects are constituted, its concepts will be "empty" or, at most, merely logically possible notions. According to Kant, preexisting epistemology postulated that knowledge is determined by objects; Kant maintained that it is determined by the human mind.

The points relevant to the question at issue should be clear. According to transcendentalism, the mind is active and creative. It enables and limits human knowledge, experience, and aesthetic judgement. Hence, the mind comprises conditions of validity of human judgements. As with rationalism, universally valid aesthetic judgements are possible because the relevant mental faculties are the same in all human beings. However, transcendentalism differs from rationalism in that the mind's perceptions and concepts are perceptions and concepts of spatio-temporal phenomena. This fundamental idea of transcendental epistemology is still acceptable,[22] and this is the basis for considering aesthetic judgements to be valid. Long before twentieth-century ideological disputes about the possible impacts that innate characteristics and/or the environment have on gaining knowledge (and learning in general), Kant offered a convincing solution.

The other hypotheses that seem plausible emphasize the transcendental character of the human *body* as a whole and especially of its instincts and drives (e.g. libido). One of the most influential is Nietzsche's hypothesis of a biological foundation of our ideas of beauty.[23] This hypothesis comes close to the modern idea that aesthetic evaluations are functions and/or means of evolutionary adaptation. Kantian transcendentalism and what I should like to call phenomenological and/or anthropological transcendentalism (Nietzsche) are not mutually exclusive. The former is mainly concerned with logical questions and explanations, while the latter often concentrates on biological ones. From a pragmatic point of view, a kind of comprehensive transcendentalism is the best means to understand and explain our experience of beauty.

While different epistemological views imply different concepts of the mind and its epistemological functions and lead to different validity concepts of aesthetic judgement, differences in ontology lead to different notions of the aesthetic object. Idealism favors the development of an aesthetic theory which emphasizes content, i.e., conceives of beauty as a function of content rather than form. This is evident from the history of idealist aesthetics, as exemplified by Plato, Plotinus, Augustine, or Hegel. For these authors, it is primarily (the depiction of) the idea, god, the sacred, or the absolute which is beautiful. There is even a tendency to claim that only these ideas and their correlates can be beautiful. Apparently, this is empirically wrong. Contrary to idealism, a transcendental ontology favors so-called formal aesthetics, i.e., aesthetic theories which consider beauty a function of form rather than content. Radical materialism (the view that there is nothing but matter) is almost extinct in philosophy. Aesthetically, it is unconvincing to conceive of beautiful objects, say a drawing, as consisting purely of matter. Such a drawing also expresses a meaning or an intention. The term "intention" designates a kind of deliberate orientation, direction and/or purposiveness of the mind or the mind's ideas. Even the beauty of nature is conceived of as if it expressed a purpose. Kant, in this connection, spoke of "purposeless purposiveness" and "formal purposiveness" (as contrasted to the ideas of the "purposiveness" of beauty so common prior to Burke).[24] The now prevalent philosophical view seems to be that beauty is "nondualistically and nonreductively affiliated" with and, thereby, "embodied" in matter.[25]

At this stage, some important conclusions can be drawn. According to philosophical aesthetics, universally valid aesthetic judgements of beauty are possible. This view implies that aesthetic judgements are different from what is commonly called a comprehensive interpretation of a work of art. Such an interpretation presupposes information which is usually available only to specialists. At least to a certain extent, aesthetic judgements of beauty are independent of an understanding of the respective object.[26] This conclusion is further substantiated by the insight that it is the gestalt, i.e., form rather than content and/or matter that determines beauty. As to a more detailed description of the characteristics of beauty and aesthetic judgement, transcendental approaches seem most convincing. They also explain best the possibility of universally valid aesthetic judgements. This being the case, studying biological hypotheses possibly related to transcendentalism, among them the hypotheses on the human brain, is imperative.

The Universal Validity of Aesthetic Judgements on Beauty

Having argued that universally valid aesthetic judgements on beauty are possible, I would like to present a few examples. There are many different works of art that have been considered beautiful throughout their history by the overwhelming majority of the people whose judgements are known. Belonging to widely different cultures, these individuals have nothing in common other than their knowledge of the works of art. Examples of such masterpieces are the pyramids, the Taj Mahal, old Chinese palaces, the Buddhist temple Toodai in Nara, the Katsura-villa in Kyoto, Michelangelo's sculptures, Leonardo da Vinci's drawings, Dürer's etchings, Utamaro's wood-block prints, Shakespeare's tragedies, Goethe's *Faust*, the Chinese novel *A Dream of Red Mansions*, Murasaki Shikibu's *Tale of Genji*, and Beethoven's symphonies. Since all these works have proved objects of concurring (affirmative) aesthetic judgements, there seems to be no satisfactory explanation for this fact but to postulate universal aesthetic rules.

Accordingly, a judgement, such as that the pyramids are ugly, could be called wrong, and its wrongness would be considered a result of failing to recognize the adequate rules. The character of aesthetic rules must be general, for all the works mentioned above are strikingly different. This suggests that these are rules of *form* rather than rules of *content*.

There are numerous treatises on rules of beauty and, especially, rules of beautiful art, evidently governed by the firm conviction that there exist such rules and that they should be known and followed without exception. Apart from the works of philosphical aesthetics, there are countless theories concerning beautiful art. I need only mention the poetics of Horace, Goethe, the Indian writer Dandin (about 700), the Chinese writer Li Yu (1611–1680), and the Japanese writers Ki no Tsurayuki (882–945), Chikamatsu, Soseki, and such theories of visual arts as put forward by Leonardo da Vinci, Kandinski, and Mondrian.

There has been art criticism almost as long as there has been script. Perhaps the most impressive example is the "Doctrine" of Ptahhotep, an Egyptian poem from about 2200 B.C., which, among other topics, deals with the beauty of speech.[27] In many cultures, there exists a long history of different kinds of beauty contests and art contests. Well-known examples are the ancient Greek theater contests and the Chinese and Japanese poetry contests. The rituals Strathern describes in chapter 12 are also beauty contests. The existence of art criticism and beauty contests would be a ridiculous error unless the phenomena and objects judged can be evaluated in a universally accepted way.

The numerous translations of poetry and fiction, the countless exhibitions of Japanese art in Europe and of European art in Japan, the performances of the Beijing Opera or of Noh in the United States, of a Russian ballet or the Viennese Philharmony in China and Japan would have been impossible without the fundamental belief that, in principle, everyone can aesthetically appreciate all kinds of art in the same or at least in a similar manner.

The history of art has always displayed converging tendencies and/or tendencies to accept an increasing plurality of arts. Today, these tendencies are worldwide. Between 13000 und 6000 B.C., the "X-ray style," i.e., the depiction of the inner organs and bones of animals in hunters' animal drawings and paintings, spread from Europe to Asia and further to Australia and South America. The arts of the nomads who lived in the Pamirs and Carpathians about 3000 B.C. influenced the arts of Central Asia, China, Indonesia, and, during the migration of nations, of Western Europe. While modern European painting was influenced by the Japanese "ukio-e," modern Japanese painting has been influenced by cubism, surrealism, or pop art. Some contemporary Thai paintings could be displayed in European museums without anyone recognizing that they are works of Asian artists. However, if a Japanese print were distinctively "Japanese," it would not be difficult to convince an "average" European that it is as beautiful as a painting by van Gogh. One can also find famous works of Western art in Japanese museums. Japanese literature was influenced almost too strongly by its Western counterparts during the Meiji period (1868–1912). But to recall an example probably even more illustrative than all the others, the history of the Silk Road is a paradigm of the phenomenon that I want to point out here. If works of art of a culture c_1 and a time t_1 are of aesthetic value and are shown to artists of a culture c_2 and a different historical time t_2, these works may well influence the artists' later creations. For artists, taking over and/or accepting aesthetic ideas originating in different cultural settings and historical epochs apparently poses no serious problems. As to nonartists, the situation is basically the same, although they usually need more time and often artistic guidance until they accept the new ideas. The history of art presupposes a universally acceptable basis for the judgements of beauty.

There are also many beautiful creations that display strikingly similar and even congruent structural qualities, although they originated completely independently. This is particularly true of architecture and ornamentation. Such similarities and congruencies are partly due to the similarities of the employed materials and tools and of general environmental conditions. This explains such terms as "style of the hunters," which aim at expressing the uniformity of the arts of hunters as well as the uniformity of their respective environments. However, references to similar materials, tools, and environmental conditions cannot sufficiently explain the similarities and congruencies of the above-mentioned beautiful products. Existing environmental differences were much too great, and the relevant empirical data, which might have influenced the production of these beautiful objects, much too incomplete and vague. Accordingly, this discussion leads to the conclusion that there must be a universally common ground for the aesthetic evaluation of beauty apart from environmental congruencies.

The well-known political obstacles novelists, dramatists, and even poets have faced in many countries can be interpreted as an expression of the belief in a general understanding of so-called subversive or "dangerously" critical features of literature, and, accordingly, of the respective functions of literary beauty and of literary beauty per se. Although reliable statements are difficult to make, there are cases in which it would be reasonable to assume that the works at issue were attacked particularly fervently because of a supposed general appeal of their beauty. Examples are Molière's *Tartuffe*, Heine's "political" poems, and the *Dream of Red Mansions* (which was forbidden during the so-called Cultural Revolution).

Most of what I have said about the beauty of arts also applies to the beauty of nature. Some natural objects, like roses, are generally considered extremely beautiful, as are certain landscapes, many of which have become favorite tourist spots. Perhaps there exist additional and more convincing indices that universally valid judgements on beauty are, indeed, possible, that there exist respective rules and/or that there is a universally acceptable common ground for these judgements and rules. But the given indices appear to be sufficient. To doubt this would amount to declaring a considerable part of human behavior and almost the whole world history of art to be but a grotesque and ridiculous error. Although this is logically possible, from an empirical point of view, it is reasonable to accept and defend the conclusion. Universally valid judgements of beauty do, indeed, exist.

Philosophical and Scientific Explantations of the Universal Validity of Aesthetic Judgements on Beauty

If universally valid aesthetic judgements about beauty are, indeed, possible, the old Kantian question arises again: how can this be? The answer, implied in the above discussion, is that there are universally valid *rules* of how to judge beauty aesthetically. Such rules must be based on fundamentals which are common to all human beings or are intrinsic, common properties of the beautiful objects. The emphasis of the explanation should be placed on the first aspect, especially on the universal properties of human perception: the perceived object is constituted by an active and creative human mind, including what Kant calls the "faculty of imagination."

The very view that transcendental methods are the best means to explain our experience of beauty favors an approach which concentrates on an investigation of the faculties of human perception: the objects per se cannot be known anyway, and every description of an object is necessarily one of a mental construction. Hence, it seems appropriate to first study the mechanisms involved in the construction of beauty rather than to deal with the infinite variety of beautiful objects. If beauty is, as suggested above, a function of form rather than content and matter, this approach is further justified, since it is primarily form that is constructed. Further, if Chomsky's hypothesis that there exists a universal grammar[28] is acceptable, then a similar hypothesis concerning universal aesthetic rules is even more convincing. Chomsky justifies his hypothesis by pointing out the misproportion between language input and output. The empirical data available, when we (learn how to) judge aesthetically, are even more uncertain, ambiguous, incomplete, and much fewer in number than the respective linguistic inputs. Nevertheless, the processing of these data results in an astonishingly regular output: the very fact that different cultures arrive at corresponding conclusions concerning the beauty of a given object implies similar or identical controlling and organizing mechanisms. There must exist a universal aesthetic grammar, as there presumably exists an universal linguistic grammar, both based on the neuronal organization of the human brain.

This again leads to and further substantiates the above conclusion: when explaining the possibility of universally valid aesthetic judgements of beauty, philosophy must consult the sciences of the brain. It must take into account the results of such disciplines as biology, ethology, and neuroscience. This does not imply that philosophical theories of beauty must be reduced to biology. Universal aesthetic rules cannot be equated with their biological basis. Aesthetic rules are *normative principles*, while their biological bases are a set of *empirical facts*. Since what *is* does not determine what *should be*, the universal rules and their biological bases are different categories. Moreover, the biological basis is often a purely material one, as dictated by the aims and methods of biology. Aesthetic rules, however, cannot be merely material entities. It might be helpful to add that the distinctions between norm and fact reflect aspects of the distinction between mind and brain.

These distinctions not only point to a philosophical realm different from the field of biological research, but also imply philosophical questions: How are the neurobiological bases of perception and the normative rules of aesthetic judgement interrelated? What is the relationship between brain and mind? These questions must be approached from causal, logical, and ontological points of view. While they cannot be answered without taking into account respective hypotheses from sciences such as biology, they remain philosophical problems. We might even say that they are modern versions of classic philosophical problems, i.e., modern versions of the fact-and-norm problem and the mind-body problem. Biology contributes to their solution in that it supports what I have called the general transcendental approach.

Scientific findings about the laterality of the brain proved that perception and cognition are, indeed, *functions* of the brain. Consequently, this also applies to aesthetic perception and evaluation. Since brain damage can alter perception and cognition, these faculties must depend on neurobiological functions. (See chapters 7, 9, and 10.) Since in visual illusions identical objective data are perceived as a particular illusion by all observers, this must depend on neuronal mechanisms that are common to all observers. A similar point is made by Rentschler, Caelli, and Maffei, who argue that differences in styles of painting can be related to shifts in the activity of different brain functions (chapter 8).

Contemporary philosophical aesthetics, which aims at explaining concepts of beauty without relating them to brain function, is unrealistic. Similarly, materialist aesthetics, based solely on environmental impacts, is also unsatisfactory.

Biological research during the past decades has resulted in a detailed model of the human brain. According to this model, the human brain and cerebral information processing are: a) active, b) restrictive, c) determinative, d) habituative (with a bias towards processing new stimuli), e) synthetic (seeking gestalt, even when none is present), f) predictive, g) hierarchical, h) hemispherically specialized, i) rhythmic, j) self-rewarding, k) reflexive, and l) social (see chapter 3). Most of these characteristics or seemingly equivalent properties were attributed to the human mind by Kant! How are these astonishing parallels to be explained? What are the possible reasons for the striking correlations between the assumed functions of the brain and the mind? As to our concepts and evaluations of beauty, almost all these characteristics come into play. For instance, it is a particularly self-rewarding cerebral information processing which constitutes our experience of beauty. Again, this is strongly reminiscent of a Kantian hypothesis. He assumed that the experience of beauty is constituted by a self-rewarding interplay of faculties and powers of the human mind. He also spoke about a pleasure which is, itself, a motive to preserve the prevailing state of mind. Yet the similarities go further. According to scientific research, an optimally self-rewarding cooperation between right-hemispheric and left-hemispheric functions constitutes our experience of beauty (chapters 9, 10, and 11). Kant maintained that it is the harmonious (inter)play between the faculty of knowledge and the power of imagination that is constitutive of this experience. He also spoke of a "harmony between concept and sensual perception." From the standpoint of contemporary scientific brain research, the Kantian concepts are mainly left-hemispherically determined perceptions, while his sensual perceptions are mainly right-hemispherically determined.[29]

Since philosophical aesthetics and sciences use different methods, such concurring results are particularly significant. They might be considered strongly validated and hence deserve particular interest. However, because of the existence of such concurrent results, divergences also gain in importance. Indeed, contemporary philosophical aesthetics must consider the fundamental scientific results on how humans perceive the world, how they see pictures, how they hear music, how they express themselves, and how they eat or dance. Transcendental philosophy provides a framework within which these results can be discussed. Our perception and behavior reflect human nature. A philosophy which does not pay due attention to this fact is, literally, groundless.

Notes and References

1. For a detailed discussion on the basic congruencies of Western and Eastern aesthetics, see: Paul G (1985) Der Mythos von der modernen Kunst und die Frage nach der Beschaffenheit einer zeitgemäßen Ästhetik. Steiner, Wiesbaden
2. Plato (1953) Lysis, Symposium, Gorgias. William Heinemann, London, 210E ff
3. Plato, ibid. 195Eff, and Plato (1969) The republic. William Heinemann, London, 400C–403C
4. Aristotle (1965) Poetics. William Heinemann, London, 1450B, 1459A
5. Leibniz GW (1972) New essays on human understanding. Cambridge University Press, Cambridge
6. Burke E (1968) A philosophical enquiry into the origin of our ideas of the sublime and beautiful. University of Notre Dame Press, London, pp 91–125
7. Kant I (1952) The critique of judgement. Oxford
8. Hegel GWF (1979) Hegel's introduction to aesthetics. Oxford University Press, Oxford, pp 69 ff
9. Nietzsche F (1966) The case of Wagner. In: Basic writings of Nietzsche. New York
10. Burke, op. cit. 5
11. Adorno TW (1970) Ästhetische Theorie. Suhrkamp, Frankfurt a. M., p 80, p 82
12. Marcuse H (1978) Die Permanenz der Kunst, 2nd edn. Hanser, München
13. Leibniz, op. cit. 5, book 2, chap XX, 4, 5
14. Burke, op. cit. 6, p 91
15. Kant, op. cit. 7, pp 5 ff
16. Paul op. cit. 1, pp 129–135

17. Gombrich EH (1978) Kunst und Illusion. Belser, Stuttgart, p 212
18. Wong, Siu-kit (1983) Early Chinese literary critisism. Joint Publishing Company, Hong Kong
19. Paul, op. cit. 1, pp 142–159
20. Locke, J (1690) Essay concerning human understanding. London
21. Kant I (1929) Critique of pure reason. McMillan, London
22. Paul G (1976) Die kantische Geschmacksästhetik als Philosophie der Kunst. Dargestellt und erörtert insbesondere in einer Anwendung auf surrealistische Malerei. PhD dissertation, University of Mannheim, pp 109–118
23. Nietzsche F (1968) Twilight of the idols and the anti-Christ. Penguin Books, Harmondsworth, pp 78 ff
24. Kant op. cit. 7, pp 32–61
25. Paul, op. cit. 1, p 36
26. Paul G (1983) Literaturverständnis und die Gültigkeit ästhetischer literarischer Wertung. Kumamoto Journal of Culture and Humanities 11:87–118
27. Hornung E (1973) Ancient and Egyptian literature, vol 1. Burkeley, pp 62–76
28. Chomsky N (1965) Knowledge of language: Its nature, origin and use. New York
29. Paul G (1984) Gehirn, Sprache und Verslänge. The Japanese Journal of Constitutional Medicine 48 (2):111–130

The Biological Foundation of Aesthetics

Irenäus Eibl-Eibesfeldt
Forschungsstelle für Humanethologie in der Max-Planck-Gesellschaft, 8138 Andechs, Federal Republic of Germany

Our perception is biased in specific ways so that not everything appeals equally to our senses and cognition. To explore this bias is one of the aims of research in aesthetics. In considering aesthetics, one should not, however, explore the perceptual bias alone but also consider art, which entails the skill to manipulate the mechanisms which underly our perceptual bias to trigger aesthetic experiences.

To begin this investigation, I shall discuss perceptual biases, which occur at three different levels: first, our basic biases, which we share with the higher vertebrates; next, our species-specific biases; and, finally, our specifically cultural, perceptual biases. I shall then explore in which ways and contexts art exploits these biases to examine how it contributes to reproductive success. I propose that art functions within communication systems to convey messages by means of social releasers and cultural symbols encoded in aesthetically appealing ways, and that outstanding among these messages are ones supporting cultural values and ethics.

Why do we perceive things as beautiful, for example a sunset, a flower or the portrait of a maiden? Furthermore, why do we create objects or patterns with aesthetic appeal?

If we are to take a biological approach to the above problems, we want to find out about both proximate and ultimate causes.[1] We need to learn what triggers certain behavior and what motivates an individual to act in a particular way. But we not only need to know how the organism functions, but also the specific functions involved and what selection pressures shaped its present form. For this, we need to gain some understanding of what functions a structure or a system fulfills.

Princples of Aesthetic Perception and Production

To produce objects of aesthetic appeal, the artist has to follow some basic propensities of perceptive physiology, which did not evolve in the service of social communication but, at a more basic level, to serve pattern recognition, perceptual constancy, spatial orientation, etc. The principles underlying such natural inclinations have been best explored in the visual realm.[2-6]

Of particular importance are the contributions of Gestalt psychology. Several principles have been elaborated, which demonstrate a clear bias in our perception. First, it has been found that perception is an active process of searching for order, categorizing, and interpreting. This can be demonstrated by simple experiments. Babies strive towards visual clarity when lines out of focus are projected to them. They learn to operate switches in their pillows by head movements to put the lines in focus. The Necker cube (see chapter 8) illustrates another perceptual activity. When we look at an image of this cube, we initially see either the lower left or the upper right square as the front of the cube. Regardless of what we see first, after approximately 3 seconds, we suddenly perceive the other square in front. It is as if our attention, once having recognized one feature, detaches in order to be free to see what else is to be seen. In Rubin's cup, we experience the same phenomenon of ambiguity. We see either two human profiles or the cup in the center first (Fig. 1).

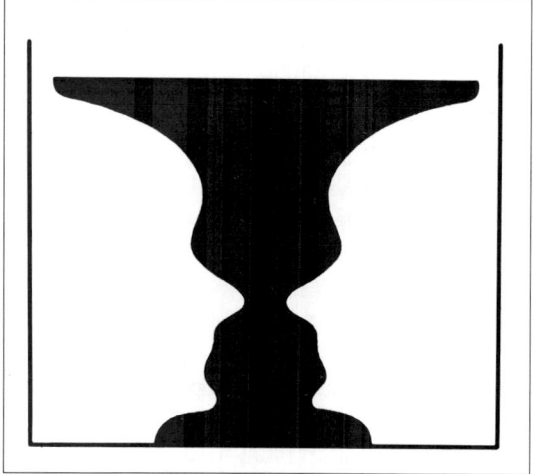

Fig. 1. Rubin's cup. In this case, the dark cup contrasts against the background and, thus, is perceived first. The profiles are discovered later. If they, however, were black, they would catch our attention first.

However, if we instruct the observer that a cup can be seen, then he will be biased and see the cup first. Furthermore, if the cup and the general background around the figures are white, then he or she sees the dark profiles first. Apparently, we have a tendency to see a figure in contrast against a lighter background (Prägnanztendenz). Our perception actively constructs contrast by emphasizing certain characteristics upon repeated presentation while eliminating others considered as unimportant. This tendency does not characterize visual perception alone but perception in general, as reflected in man's tendency to express his views in a polarized, dogmatic way (to "state his point clearly").[7]

We also are biased to see *gute Gestalten* (distinct forms) when we briefly observe geometrical figures, squares, triangles, and circles that show light irregularities or asymmetries. Even then, we perceive a complete or a symmetrical figure. We also generalize and repress the irregularities. In this context, experiments performed by Wertheimer[8] with children are noteworthy. He presented children with simple symmetrical figures, from which parts were cut out. If the experimenter tried to place the piece cut from a square onto the missing part of a circle, the children protested and became emotionally upset. They wanted the gestalt to appear perfect. Our perception thus strives to perceive regularity and symmetry and, accordingly, tends to project the latter onto observed objects.

In 1931, Sander[9] (and Fechner already in the nineteenth century) found that people experience as aesthetically appealing squares and also rectangles with the ratio of the sides corresponding to the golden section (1:1.63). Rectangles that deviate slightly from a square shape are experienced as "bad squares," and larger deviations in the rectangle are considered to result in a "bad rectangle." Sander argues that this principle of "gute Gestalt" explains the appeal of different architectural styles. Renaissance architecture, in essence, has a quiet beauty that makes the observer feel comfortable. The architectural principles by which this effect is achieved include the dominance of squares and rectangles in the above-mentioned proportions. Furthermore, right angles and circular arches are used in preference to other forms; windows are placed in metrically regular rows, and horizontal structures are symmetrical.

In contrast, Baroque architecture induces awe and unrest to the extent of ecstasy and transmits a dynamic experience. The stylistic means by which this is achieved are imperfect squares and rectangles, which are exaggerated in width and length. Arches are elliptical and wide, acute angles are used instead of right angles, the axis of symmetry is not in the middle, etc. Slight irregularities and deviation from the perfect create tension and unrest. Baroque thus overcomes the perfect form of the Renaissance by creating forms which stop just before perfection and which stimulate corrective activity on the part of the observer.[5]

Our perception seeks and enjoys order,[4] and this quest seems to be a general principle which derives, in part, from the limited capacity of our brain to process information. Our short-term memory seems to have the capacity to process 16 bits per second; less is perceived as boring, and more is stressful. In patterns, we attempt to discover regularities that allow us to form "supersigns" to reduce the amount of information confronting us.[10]

In 1936, Metzger[11] suggested that there is a tendency of senses towards order which creates order even where it does not exist. Schuster and Beisl[5] also point out the need for pattern recognition to facilitate information processing in the following quote: "...man is dependent on finding regularity in his environment because he can thereby perceive his surroundings better and with less difficulty of retention. Therefore, finding such patterns or supersigns is rewarding." That regularity, as opposed to irregularity, is perceived as beautiful was also experimentally demonstrated by Dörner and Vehrs[12], who asked persons to place red and green colored squares onto a grid to produce in one case a beautiful and, in another, an unattractive arrangement. Designs intended to be beautiful allowed the observer to perceive crosses and rows, i.e., presented supersigns. Unity is another characteristic listed by Hospers[13] as an element of aesthetic perception.

If it is too easy for the observer to discover order, then the object lacks aesthetic appeal, as it also does if one cannot discover relational regularities. Thus, an aesthetic object must have a certain amount of order that should be neither too complex nor too simple. It must allow processes of reduction of information to occur, i.e., permit the discovery of supersigns.[5]

Of course, our effort to see regularities and to categorize does not find its origin in our limited capacity to process information only. It is economical and also highly adaptive to recognize categories of animals, plants, etc. and to attribute certain characteristics to them.

A remarkable experiment (first conducted by Francis Galton in the nineteenth century[14]) by Daucher (H.Daucher 1979, unpublished work) suggests how templates are formed by means of a "statistical learning process." He superimposed the photographs of 20 female faces upon one another. Facial features then created an image in which the individuals' outstanding features became absorbed and the typical or characteristic ones preserved (Fig. 2). The resulting composite face was considered "beautiful" to observers, suggesting the existence of innate reference patterns (templates) that set a standard against which the perceived is evaluated. Daucher's experiment demonstrates how many fleeting experiences are abstracted and compiled in one's memory to create schemata or templates. This indicates that our perception is basically categorical or typological.

Children begin to categorize at an early age. For example, when they address a dog, a cat, and a cow as "wau wau," they apparently refer to shared characteristics. The tendency to categorize is innate, and educational efforts aimed at correcting the child by teaching it that a cat is not a wau wau and must be distinguished from a dog only serve to refine categories. Categorial schematic perception is one of the prerequisites for language, and it predominates in childrens' drawings (Fig. 3).[15]

Visual art makes use of the basic characteristics of our perceptive

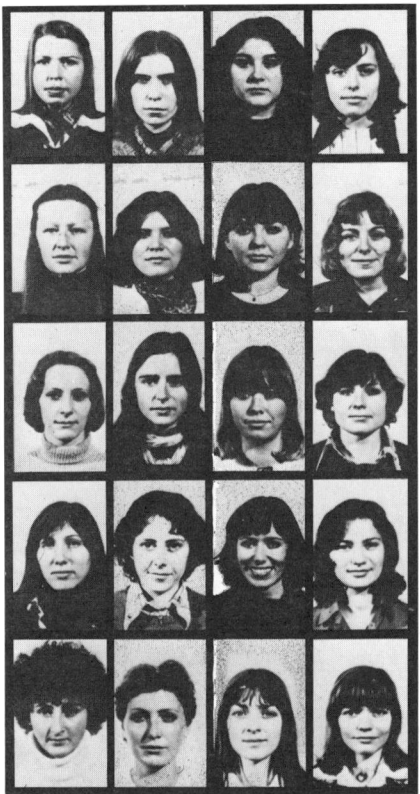
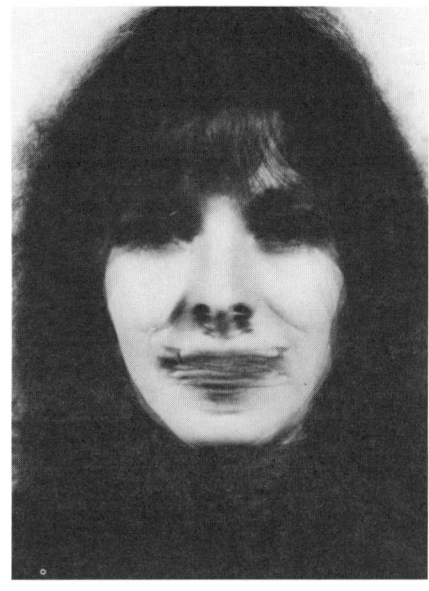

Fig. 2. Templates are formed by "statistical learning." The superimposed exposure of the twenty photographs *(left)* results in a typological presentation *(right)* since the individual features are superseded by the shared "typical" ones. Photo: H. Daucher 1979, unpublished manuscript

mechanisms, as is impressively illustrated by the Dutch artist M.C. Escher, who experiments playfully with our perceptive biases.

In other products of art, the basic characteristics of aesthetic perception are used as a means to catch and retain the attention of the observer to convey encoded messages by means of pictorial description, allegories, and symbols. Our urge to recognize order is of great importance in this context, since it leads to the active discovery of a message that is accompanied by a highly rewarding experience (flash of recognition). Through this experience, the message is reinforced. In my opinion, this is the basic function of art. It is not surprising, then, that primitive art takes advantage of our perceptual biases. For example, the prows of the canoes of the Trobriand Islanders have intricately carved boards. The designs have symbolic meaning, and they are composed in such a way that one first sees a dominant human figure, but, after a few seconds, one perceives the two eyes of the figure as the eyes of birds shown in profile. And on still another level, one suddenly realizes that the entire board is designed to show a face. This form of coding seems fairly widespread in the aboriginal art of New Guinea (Fig. 4).

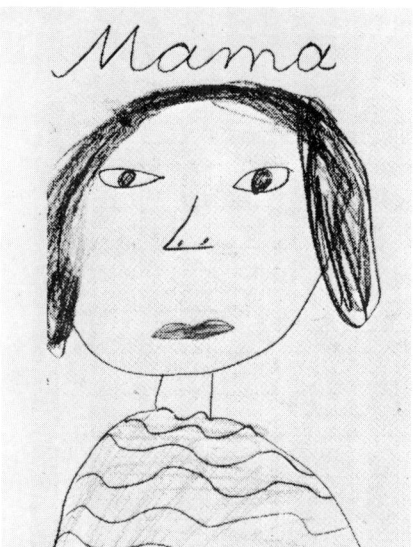 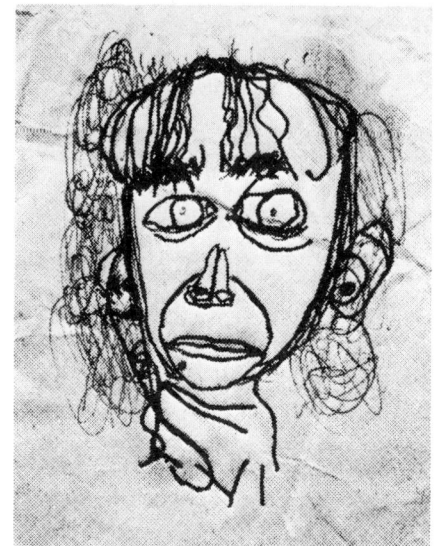

Fig. 3. In children's drawings, the tendency for schematic presentation predominates. Asked to draw her mother, a girl (age 7) first created a highly stereotyped, schematic woman's face *(left)*. Only after the mother insisted that her daughter draw her as she saw her, did she create a face with the individual features of her mother *(right)*.   Photos: Nguyen-Clausen.[15]

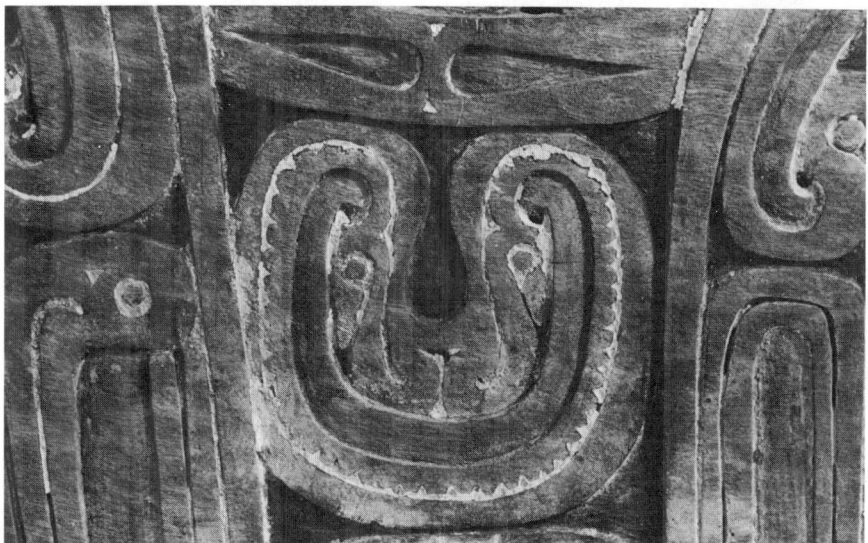

Fig. 4. The closure boards (Lagim) are carved with an apotropaic design. As a supersign, it portrays a face. But this is composed of a number of ornamentally intertwined heads of ritually important mythical birds. In the center of the board, four birds are joined into a human figure, reminiscent of a Polynesian tiki. The figures' eyes are also the eyes of two birds viewed laterally. The mouth of the figure, with many small teeth, surrounds the head in a fashion similar to that found in Hawaiian figures.   Photo: I. Eibl-Eibesfeldt

Interestingly, aesthetic biases of the basic type are not unique to man. Through choice experiments with monkeys, raccoons, and birds, Rensch[16,17] demonstrated that animals show aesthetic preferences in that regularity, symmetry, and order are preferred to asymmetry and irregularity. In a series of imaginative experiments, Desmond Morris[18] had chimpanzees paint. The resulting paintings had aesthetic appeal. Aside from this appeal to humans, he found the following interesting regularities: The animals filled the sheet symmetrically, staying within the given frame. Had Morris already painted a square or a spot on one side, then the animals painted on the opposite side of the sheet, later connecting the two structures with a few strokes. One individual produced fan patterns again and again, filling the sheet harmoniously. The patterns were far from simple scribblings. If different colors were given to the chimpanzees, they avoided smearing the colors on top of each other. Had a chimpanzee produced a fan pattern in one color, then it continued by placing the other colors between the existing strokes, thus producing another fan within the fan. Individuals developed individual styles, which they varied in a playful manner. Thus, the activities were performed for amusement. They demonstrated control of composition, the existence of individual style, and thematic variations. They reflected general principles of aesthetics and the achievement of an optimal balance of tensions, since the animals often refused to continue painting when they appeared to have finished.

When I heard about Morris' fascinating findings, I took paint, brushes, and sheets to the Hellabrunn Zoo in Munich and had two chimpanzee females paint for me. The dominant one produced rainbow structures filling the whole sheet. The subordinate one, however, used only the lower part of the sheet and painted a spot. Given the next color, she just painted within the spot, continuing to paint there until the sheet became waterlogged. She behaved as if she did not dare to enter the free space. This strongly reminds me of certain projection tests used by psychologists to ascertain latent problems. I continued my experiments for several weeks, and, surprisingly, the individuals maintained their own styles of painting, which seemed to express certain consistent personality traits (Fig. 5).

Morris exhibited his chimpanzee paintings in an art gallery among paintings of modern artists – without telling who had painted them. Some experts praised them as particularly vital and important works of art, especially those with a tachist (action art) orientation. However, other abstract paintings can also be reduced to those basics of aesthetics like balance, rhythmicity, opposition, and linkage. The motivation of the chimpanzees, as can be derived from their behavior, was playful experimentation. This is probably the primary motivation of human tachists too – experimenting with their skills and with their spectators as well.

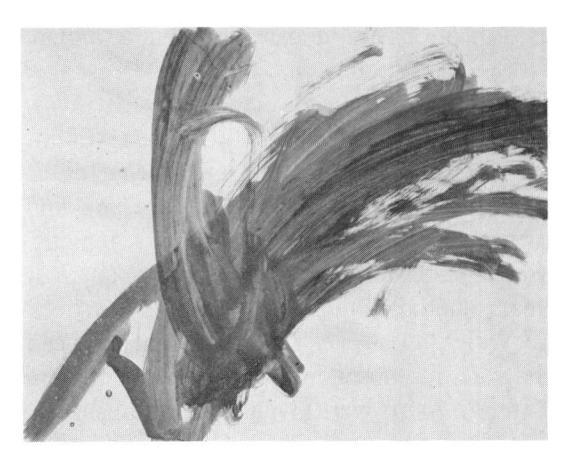

Fig. 5. Chimpanzee painting: The painting of a high-ranking female fills the sheet in a rainbow-like pattern.

The low-ranking female painted one color over the other. Both individuals stuck to their individual styles of painting.
Photos: I. Eibl-Eibesfeldt

Since the Romantic epoch, originality and uniqueness have become criteria for evaluating an object of art. Although they provide a measure of the artist's ingenuity, they do not constitute aesthetic criteria per se but have gained importance with increasing competition among artists. The creation of something new stimulates our perception and is also an expression of our urge for creative experimentation.

Species-Specific Biases and their Expressions in Art

So far, we have dealt with very general principles that determine aesthetic perception, most of which we share at least with higher mammals and birds with, perhaps, the exception of preferences for certain proportions for which our "ideal" body proportions might have set the scale. I shall now discuss some more specific phylogenetic adaptations that determine aesthetic perception and production which bias human perception. To do this, it will be necessary to backtrack and briefly discuss the ethological[19] concept of key stimuli.

It has been demonstrated that animals respond to certain features of their environment in an adaptive way, often without previous exposure. In doing this, they respond to certain sign stimuli toward which their receptors have been tuned in the process of phylogenetic adaptations. Such sign stimuli may indicate that an animal is in its right habitat; others signal the presence of prey or predator and, correspondingly, trigger responses of prey pursuit or flight and defense. For such adaptive responses to occur, the animals must be outfitted with detecting devices tuned toward the perception of such stimuli and linked with data-processing mechanisms, which allow the adaptive response to occur. The perceptual mechanisms involved have been called innate releasing mechanisms by Tinbergen[20] and innate template by Lorenz.[21]

The adaptation in many cases takes place on the side of the perceiver only, who attributes value to some feature or event of importance to him. In the case of intraspecific communication, receiver and sender developed mutual adaptations in the form of appropriate signals and innate releasing mechanisms. Stimuli that have developed in the service of signaling are called releasers or social releasers, and they are adequate to trigger responses. Sometimes they are very simple – just a colored patch – while at other times, they are configurations, e.g., two spots alligned horizontally with a third centered below to characterize the mouth of mouth-breeding cichlids. Here the hatchlings seek shelter in flight. Not only visual signals, but also acoustic, olfactory, and tactile signals may act as releasers. For instance, newborn babies respond to tape recordings of crying with crying. Such a response is not elicited by tapes with other noises of the same loudness. This early response to specific auditory stimuli may be considered as a basic unconditioned response of empathy, crying being a social releaser.[22] Moreover, experiments with decoys (dummies) revealed that innate releasing mechanisms are responsive to exaggeration: it is possible to artificially create objects that surpass the natural releasing object in its releasing quality.

Designs with child appeal, which serve the functions of bonding and appeasing, are widely used. This is motivated by the fact that certain child features release nurturant behavior as demonstrated by Konrad Lorenz'[23] *Kindchenschema* (baby schema), which is characterized by conspicuous size relations. For instance, a baby's head is very large in relation to its body, and, by exaggerating this feature, it is possible to create objects that are particularly cute (Fig. 6). Cartoonists exploit this feature to infantilize animals in cartoons. Other features, such as the relationship of a small face to round puffy cheeks and a large skull, are also employed.

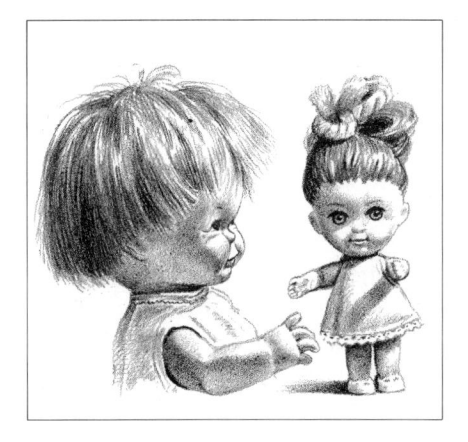

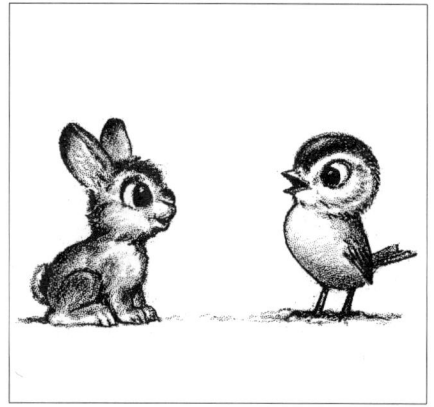

Fig. 6. The "infant schema": The attributes of the small child (big head in relation to the body, high prominent forehead, chubby cheeks, short limbs with rounded contours, small mouth) are often greatly exaggerated in dolls and other products of commercial art meant to be cute. Drawing: H. Kacher, from I. Eibl-Eibesfeldt[31]

Many primitive artifacts serve to communicate with spirits and other imaginary beings, who are attributed with human characteristics. One threatens them with fierce displays and often, in antithesis, appeases them at the same time with signals and behaviors conceived of as friendly by man. The messages often are presented directly without further encoding and by applying the principle of the supernormal object presentation, i.e., by presenting the stimuli in an exaggerated manner. Let me present some examples. In scare devils and amulets serving the function of warding off evil, we often find certain key characteristics in combination, sometimes alone, and usually in exaggerated presentation. Eye patterns are of particular importance. Conspicuous eyespots and bulging, staring eyes in figurines are universally found in designs meant to ward off evil (apotropaic). We find eye patterns painted on the bows of ships in Greece as well as in Bali (Fig. 7a), and staring eyes are found in masks or scare devils in a variety of cultures. Eye patterns can be found on amulets and curtains, or they may be used to guard the entrance of a house (Fig. 7b and c). Koenig[23] devoted a special monograph to the eye pattern in art, demonstrating its universal as well as its individual cultural uses.

In social interactions, we perceive eye contact with ambivalence. On the one hand, we must look at our partner in order to communicate. But we dare not look too long, otherwise we will be perceived as staring and, thus, as dominating or threatening. Eye contact arouses us and, to prevent escalation, we have to interrupt eye contact periodically. We do this automatically in conversation. The speaker regularly shifts his gaze, while the listener may continuously look at the speaker until his turn to speak. If we want to threaten a

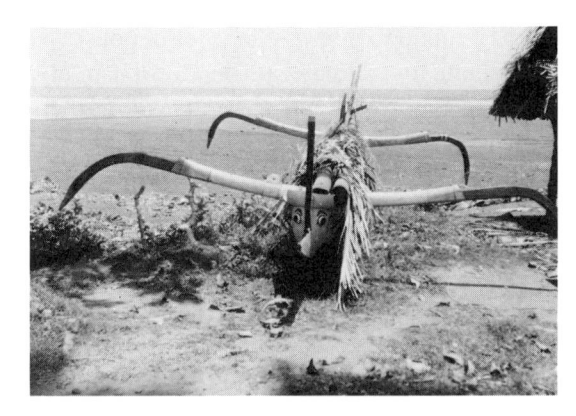

Fig. 7. Protective eyes on the bow of Balinese ships *(left)*

Protective eyes guarding the entrance of a house in Kathmandu (Nepal) *(below left)*

Fighting shield with bulging eyes and mocking tongue display. Middle Sepik (Simar), Völkerkunde Museum, Berlin *(below right)*
Photos: I. Eibl-Eibesfeldt

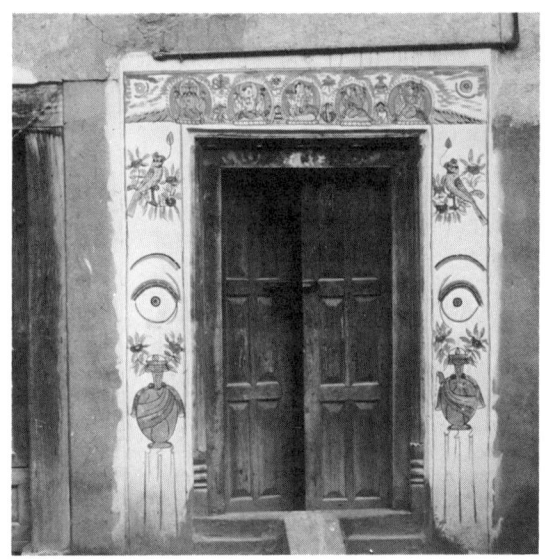

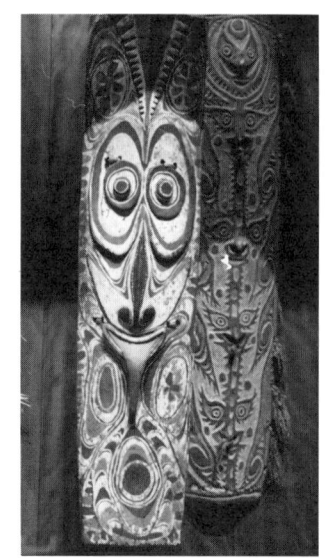

person, we may stare. I found staring to be a strategy employed in aggressive encounters by Europeans as well as by Yanomami, Bushmen, and Balinese children.[24-26] Our particular receptiveness to eye patterns could have very ancient roots. There are indications that many mammals and birds become irritated when stared at – a response probably related to the fact that predators fixate their prey before attacking.

In an experimental investigation by Coss[27], the brow raising, which indicates interest and arousal, was strongest for paired eyespots presented in a horizontal position as opposed to eyespots placed vertically or obliquely. In friendly face-to-face interactions, we tilt our heads sideways to dampen the arousal brought about by eye contact.

We tend to physiognomize and anthropomorphize our nonhuman environment. Lorenz[22] pointed out that we tend to interpret facades of houses as if they were faces. We may perceive them, for example, as friendly or haughty, the little roofs above them resembling eyebrows, and so forth. We, furthermore, evaluate animals by human standards as noble and elegant if they are muscular and slender or as plump and ugly if their proportions approximate those of a hippo. Remarkable also is the idealized presentation of the human body. The male "partner schema" is characterized by broad shoulders, narrow hips, and a strong, muscular but slender body. The emphasizing of a man's shoulders can be found in portraits, sculptures, and fashion in a wide range of cultures (Fig. 8). In this context, it is interesting to note that the body hairline pattern is reminiscent of our hairy ancestors, who had tufts emphasizing shoulder breadth,[18] suggesting a phylogenetic bias to an aesthetic evaluation.

Concerning ideals of beauty for the female body, there seem to exist two ideals in homo sapiens (Fig. 9). One is the well-known ideal of the Greek Venus, which is predominant in modern man, and the other can be characterized by the paleolithic Venus of Willendorf, a plump figure with pronounced buttocks and large breasts. In the Bushmen and Hottentots, these features are racial characteristics of the adult woman and considered as beautiful. The ideal figure for a young girl, however, coincides more with the classical European ideal of female beauty. It may well be that, in human evolution, our bias increasingly shifted toward a preference for the features of youth, in accordance

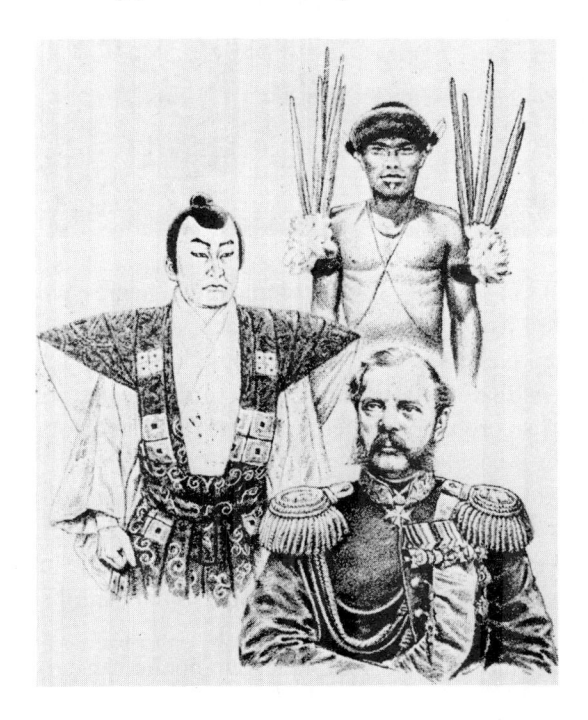

Fig. 8. In the most varied cultures, the human male emphasizes his shoulders in dress. Above: Yanomami Indian; center: Kabuki actor (Japan); below: Alexander II of Russia.
From: I. Eibl-Eibesfeldt[31]

The Biological Foundation of Aesthetics

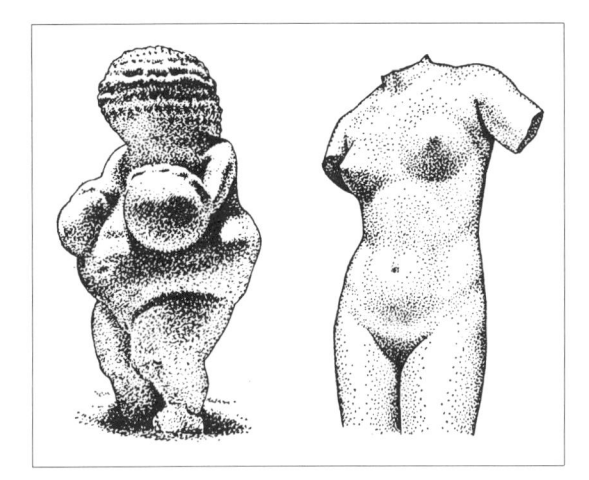

Fig. 9. *Left:* Venus von Willendorf (Austria, Museum of Natural History); *right:* Aphrodite of Cyrene (Thereme Museum, Rome)

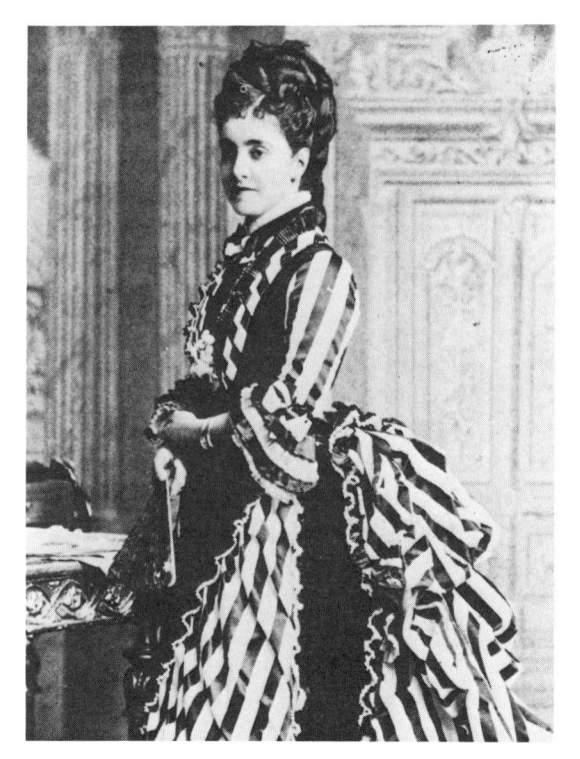

Fig. 10. The emphasis of the buttocks in women's fashion: Pauline Lucca, photograph taken around 1870.
From: von Boehn M (1976) Die Mode. Eine Kultur-geschichte von Barock bis zum Jugendstil. Bruckmann, München

with Bolk's theory of the general fetalization of man.[28] Certain features in fashion, such as emphasizing the buttocks (bustle), indicate that a rudimentary bias toward the archaic Venus type survived in Europe, too (Fig. 10).

The "ideal" human faces share some universal features. Regardless of race, in China, Europe, and Africa a fine nasal bridge is considered attractive.

This is the case even in cultures in which the majority of individuals do not conform to this ideal. Schiefenhövel[29] questioned members of the Eipo of New Guinea about the complex theme of marriage, love, and beauty. He was often told, "X is a handsome man; he has a beautiful nose ('u yal')." Furthermore, less prognathic faces are given preference. Since the Eipo had no European contacts prior to the time of investigation, we can assume that these ideals are, indeed, their own. It is, furthermore, important to realize that only a small fraction of the population actually conforms with this ideal of beauty. But this is also true in our culture with the Greek ideal of beauty, which we, nonetheless, praise. An investigation by Rensch[30] revealed that the ideal type of European face is characterized by delicate features, in particular one with a small nose and no beard. These are features of juveniles.

I hypothesized[31,32] that the preadaptations for this preferential bias are partially founded in those perceptual adaptations that evolved in connection with parental behavior. A child appeals to us due to its delicate features, predominant forehead, and other characteristics already discussed in connection with the *Kindchenschema*. Males, indeed, consider as attractive those females who have features that combine infantile facial characteristics with the typical sex characteristics of the mature female (Fig. 11). In quite a number of races, females exhibit strong paedomorphic traits. It is also apparent that this feature, in combination with the aesthetic appeal, releases protective, caretaking behavior. A recent investigation by Cunningham[33] revealed a posi-

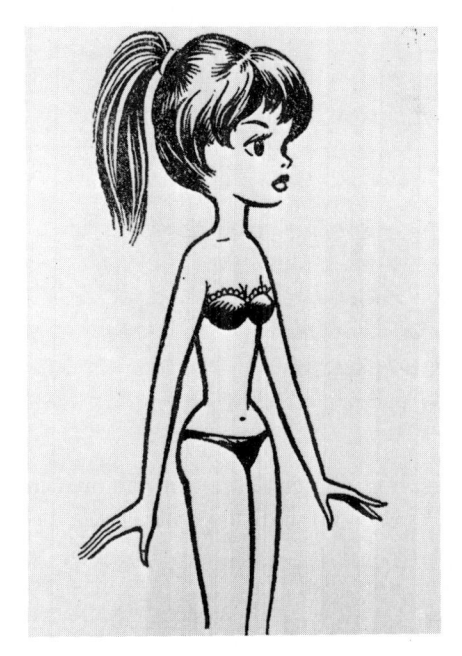

Fig. 11. The paedomorphic features of women appeal to men. In commercial art, the infantile attributes as well as the sexual attributes are frequently exaggerated.
Drawing: H. Kacher, from I.Eibl-Eibesfeldt[31]

tive correlation between the neonate's features (large eyes, small nose, and small chin) and female attractiveness. Fauss[34] found that a small baby's mouth is considered beautiful by males and females alike. Should cross-cultural investigations support my theory of a universal paedomorphic beauty ideal for human facial characteristics, we would have an aesthetic preference which, by mate selection, favors the selection of modern hominoid traits over archaic paleohominoid features (Fig. 12). In this context, a study by Langlois et al.[35] deserves attention, since it challenges the commonly held assumption that physical attractiveness is solely culturally defined and gradually learned. Even small babies watch photographs of attractive faces with delicate and regular features longer.

Patterns of movement that serve as visual signals are called expressive movements. They originate by a process called ritualization, which can take place during phylogeny or during cultural evolution.[36] Even though man is unique in his cultural capacities and his capacity for learning, there is no longer any doubt that he is preprogrammed in many ways and is not born into the world as a "tabula rasa." Among other things, his data- processing mechanisms are tuned to perceive specific stimuli and stimuli configurations and are constructed to release specific responses to these. No prior knowledge of the releasing stimulus situation is required for the appropriate response to occur, although individual learning may modify responsiveness in certain ways. Fourteen-day-old babies respond to the projection of dark, symmetrically ex-

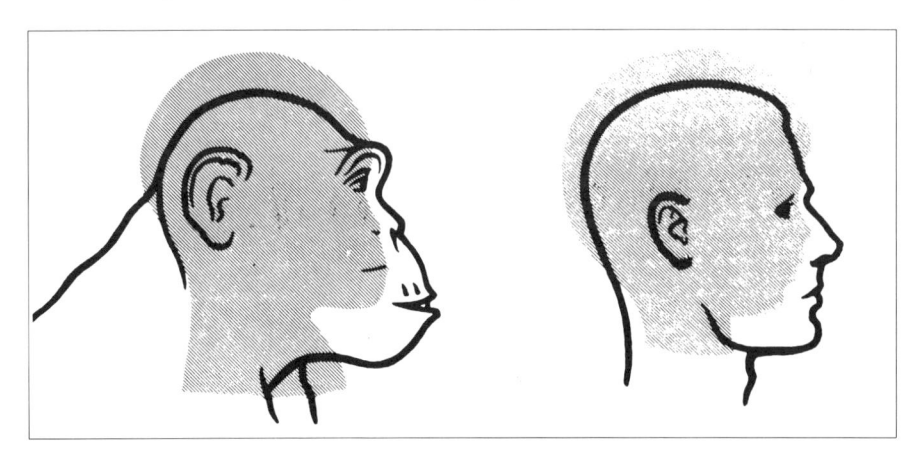

Fig. 12. Even among the great apes, the infantile face and skull is characterized by more delicate features, a less prognathic face, and a relatively large cranium. I hypothesize that the "infant schema" adapted to these features causes an aesthetic bias which influences the choice of sexual partners, selecting against certain protohominoid features.
From: Osche G (1979) Kulturelle Evolution: Biologische Wurzeln, Vergleich ihrer Mechanismen mit denen des biologischen Evolutionsgeschehens. In: Hassenstein B, Mohr H, Osche G, Sander K, Wülker W (eds) Freiburger Vorlesungen zur Biologie des Menschen. Quelle und Meyer, Heidelberg, pp 33–50

panding blotches with clear avoidance responses, as if an object were approaching them on collision course.[37] Thus, visual stimuli trigger tactile expectations (hit, collision, and, in response, avoidance). Here, our data-processing mechanisms are programmed to deal with events in the outer world that are of significance for the individual's well-being.

Certain gestural elements also appear cross-culturally in art, such as the presentation of a vertical open palm, which occurs in many cultures as a symbol of warding off evil, either in figurines or simply as an isolated hand in the form of an amulet or door painting. I filmed this gesture in a girl born deaf and blind, who was trying to ward off evil. A series of exposed teeth with the mouth gaping and threatening to bite is another widespread feature of apotropaic designs, and, if the face is human, a vertical frown is often added.

For a long time, the phallic displays of apotropaic figurines have been misinterpreted as fertility gods. However, a more plausible interpretation for this phallic symbol derived from a threat to mount, which is widely used to demonstrate dominance in mammals. In many nonhuman primates, males sit and guard their group against intruders from other groups. They place themselves with their backs to their groups and display their genitalia at the sight of strangers. To enhance their signaling functions, the penis and scrotum are often brilliantly colored. Should a stranger approach, erection may take place.

Phallic displays are also used as dominance displays in encounters between male group members.[38–40] In man, phallic displays occur in aggressive encounters, including mounting and rape. The Eipo of New Guinea, for example, loosen the tip of their penis gourd and jump up and down to make the gourd swing conspicuously while yelling curses at the enemy. Often, phallic threats are only verbalized, although they may also be expressed in carvings and paintings intended to guard houses and territorial boundaries or be carried as amulets to protect the bearer from the evil of malicious spirits (Fig. 13).[31,41,42] We find such symbolic phallic displays on all continents. In our culture, they are found both in amulets and in the gargoyles on cathedrals. They have not been given adequate attention so far, and, unfortunately, their decay is often not prevented by restoration, which concentrates on the sacred symbolism of Christianity.

The fending off of evil may also be performed by a combination of appeasement and threat displays. For instance, if an Eipo woman is startled, she grasps her breast with her hands, lifts them, and squeezes them – an action which results in milk squirting if the woman is lactating (Fig. 14). At the same time, she utters "basam kalje" (referring to the fat of the pig), a sacred utterance to ban the danger. Alternatively, "wanje" may be used, referring to a sacred plant used in initiation. We also use similar sacred words like "Jesus" in startling situations. In curses, the utterance becomes profane.[26] Eipo women thus

The Biological Foundation of Aesthetics

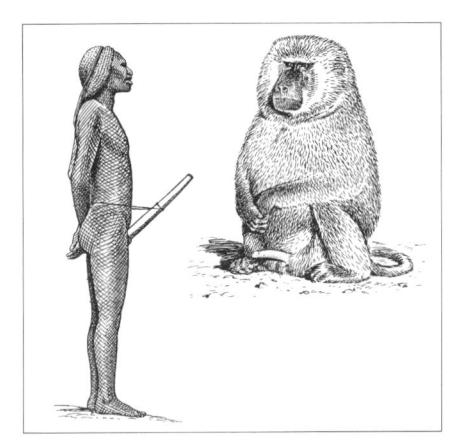

Fig. 13. Phallic displays in primates:
a) *left:* Papuan with penis sheath; *right:* Hamadryas baboon sitting on guard

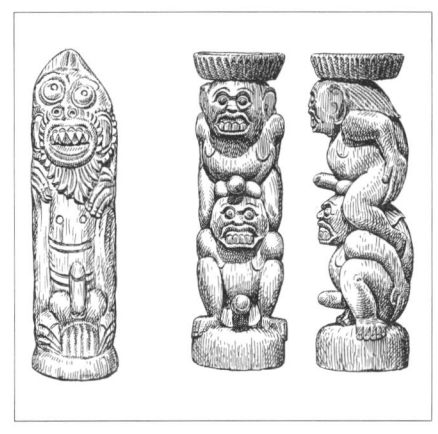

b) Two wooden guardian figures from Bali (the one on the right in frontal and side view)

use a verbal utterance to ward off danger in combination with gestures of appeasement, the squirting of milk. The milk squirting can be interpreted as a placating appeal, as suggested in Basedow's report[43] on how an Australian patrol surprised two aboriginal women, who were cooking a snake. One ran away, while the other squirted milk at the men. Later, when asked why she did so, she replied that, in this way, she could show that she was a nursing mother, hoping to arouse mercy.

I have also found this appeal combined with a threatening face in a Balinese figure, which was considered to be a guardian figure (Fig. 15a). In Ecuador, I acquired a pre-Columbian figurine from the Manteno culture (Fig. 15b), showing a similar display, and I discoverd this gesture in apotropaic stone sculptures on European churches. Finally, a highly stylized version of this gesture can be found on the carvings of the Maori in New Zealand. The maternal appeal, thus, seems to have a very widespread use. This, of course, is not to imply that the gesture is inborn in man, but rather that our inborn attitudes toward mothers probably gave rise to the independent development of similar appeals.

One puzzling gesture often seen in Romanesque and Gothic grotesques is the presenting of the beard. Ethological studies link it to a male threat display.[44] In New Guinea, angry males grasp the ends of their beard with their hands and pull them apart. The display was also found in some African ancestral sculptures (Fig. 16). In apotropaic art, the cultural and the innate intertwine in a fascinating way. For pioneering studies in this field, see Hansmann and Kriss-Rettenbeck;[45] for further information in an ethological context, see Sütterlin[46] and Eibl-Eibesfeldt.[32]

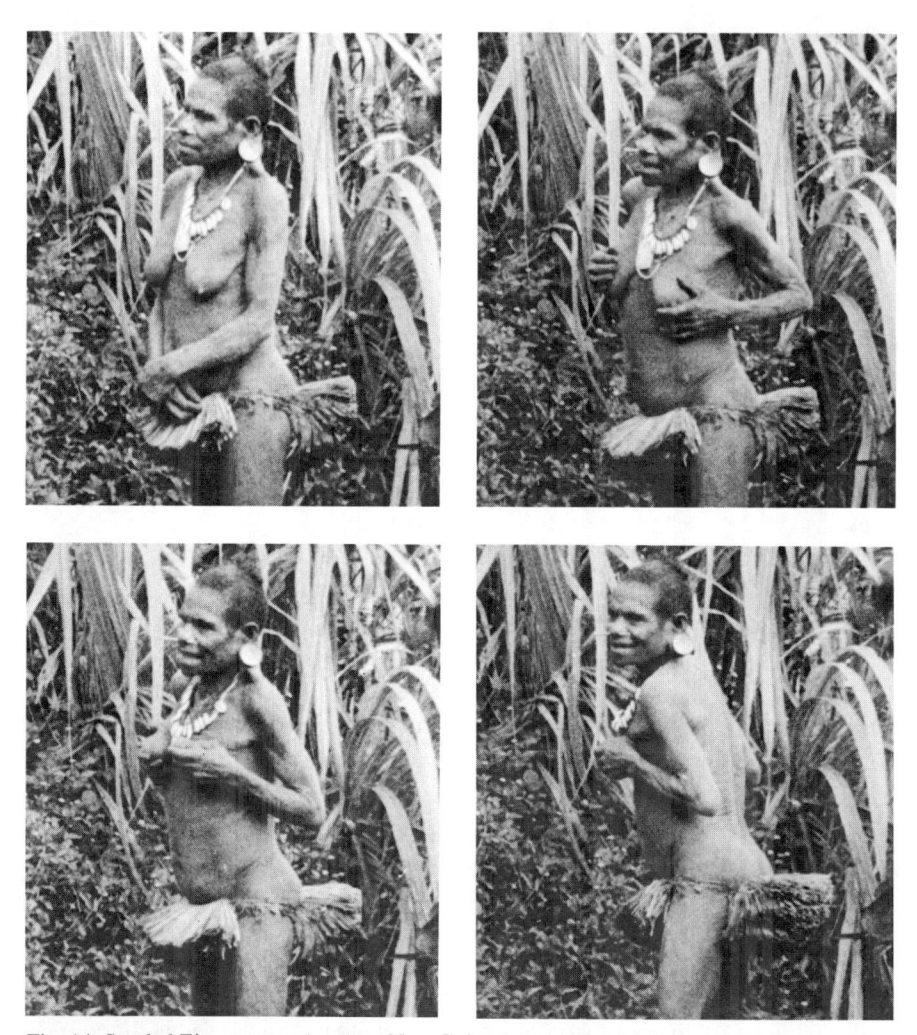

Fig. 14. Startled Eipo woman (western New Guinea) presenting her breasts
From a film sequence taken by I. Eibl-Eibesfeldt

Thus, the perception of certain stimuli or stimulus configurations activates emotion and/or satisfies appetitive behaviors and needs. Since man is capable of creating the releasing or comforting stimuli artificially, he is able to play with them, comforting or arousing himself and others at will. Man has a great variety of appetites, which he seeks to satisfy. At one time, he may seek quiescence and comfort and at other times, sensory stimulation, excitement, or satisfaction of curiosity.

Fehling[47] investigated the conditions under which we experience comfort in a home. He found that the ideal home has, among other things, to offer

The Biological Foundation of Aesthetics

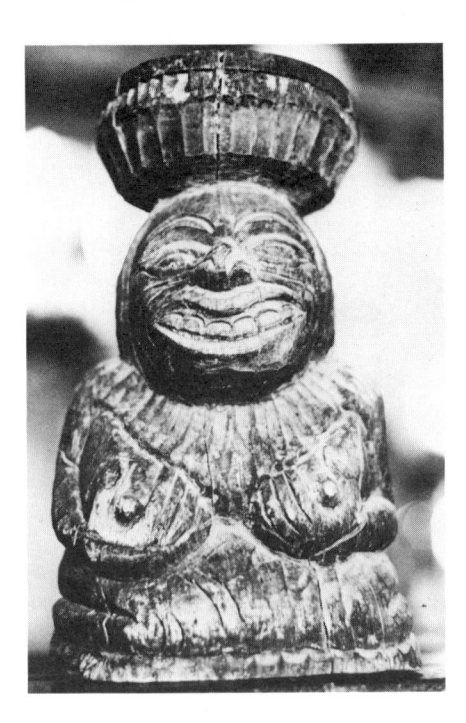

Fig. 15. The presenting of the breast as a protective gesture

Balinese guardian figure *(left)*

Pre-Columbian Ecuadorian ceramic (Manteno culture) *(below left)*

Sherborn/Dorset (England) St. John's Almshouse *(below right)*
Photos: I. Eibl-Eibesfeldt

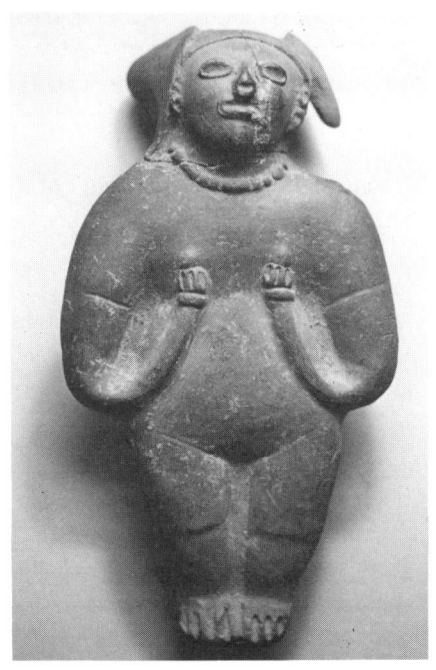

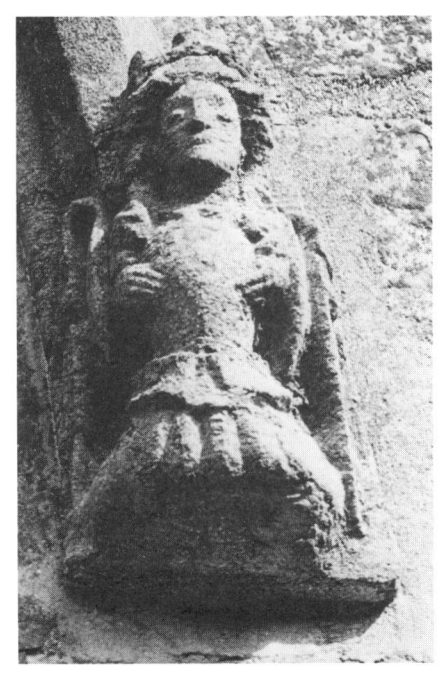

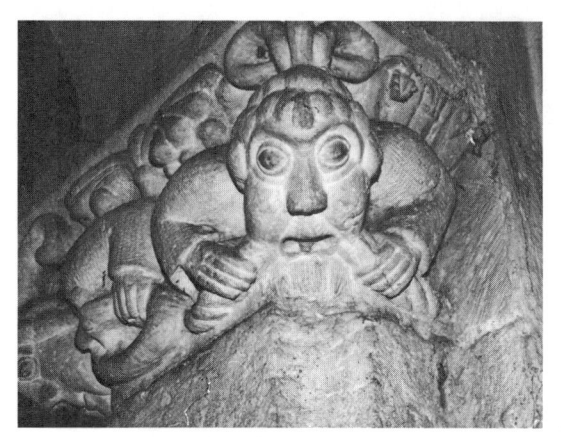

Fig. 16. The presenting of the beard:
Sculpture from a capital in the crypt of the cathedral in Freising, Bavaria

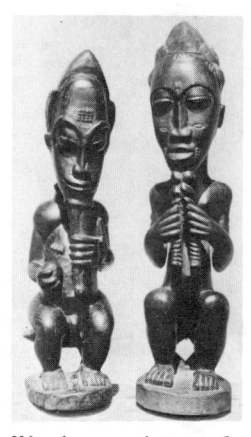

Wooden sculpture from the Baule, Ivory coast, Africa
Photo: I. Eibl-Eibesfeldt

protection. For example, a feeling of security is achieved by the thick walls of old farm houses. As for seating, we prefer niches that offer protection. It has been found in restaurants that the tables in corners or other nooks are occupied first, and, only after these are filled up, will people sit at tables which stand free. People also prefer seats allowing them to sit with their backs to the walls or other structures providing protection. In this context, man is constantly on the alert, subconsciously scanning his environment.[48] Housing sites are chosen with unobstructed views. These preferences evolved in the service of predator and enemy avoidance.

Another environment-dependent preference concerns our diurnal habit. We tend to attach positive value to brightness and negative value to darkness. We fear the night, where dangers lurk unseen, and this seems to be the basis of our negative evaluation. This bright/dark symbolism is not restricted to Europe. We found that the Eipo in West Irian attach similar values to bright and dark. In affectionate greeting, they address a person with "nani korunje" – "you my fair fellow." Since they are not fair, but dark, there is no ethnocentric reference to skin color implied.

There is also agreement that basic colors are perceived in a similar way cross culturally.[49,50] Yellow and red are considered to be warm colors and red especially attention attracting, although sometimes alarming, thus having an ambivalent quality. It is intriguing to speculate that red, on the one hand, is the color of many consumable fruits, but also the color of blood. I remember that my son, Bernolf, at the age of three got very upset when he saw on color television two iguanas fighting with interlocked jaws, one drawing blood. It was a very spontaneous, sympathetic response to the sight of blood. In contrast, blue is considered as calm. Itten[51] reports that rooms painted red-orange are perceived as 3°–4°C warmer than rooms painted blue-green, when both were, in fact, 15°C. "Warm" colors activate our autonomous nervous system, raising our pulse rates and blood pressure.[52]

If we observe the decorations in our homes, we are struck by the richness of the plant decor. Curtains, carpets, wallpaper, and cushions as well as objects like porcelain are decorated with plant designs, flowers, fruits, and leaves (Fig. 17). Furthermore, we cultivate a rich variety of plants in our rooms or on our balconies for pure aesthetic pleasure. Evidently, the city dweller provides himself with vegetation, which he misses in his urban environment.

We thus exhibit, as a phylogenetic bias, a clear "phytophilia."[32] It can be interpreted as an adaptation to a habitat in which our ancestors were sure to find food. The perceptual bias ensures that man will select the right habitat, and when he has removed himself from such a habitat, he artfully creates substitute nature. In this context, it is also noteworthy that gardens and parks are designed to imitate a savannah habitat. Scattered trees and bushes and lots of open space are characteristic of parks in Japan and Europe alike. Orians[53] hypothesized that this, indeed, reflects an inherited habitat preference, the savannah being the habitat in which hominization took place. We could term this aesthetic preference a primary, habitat-related preference in contrast to

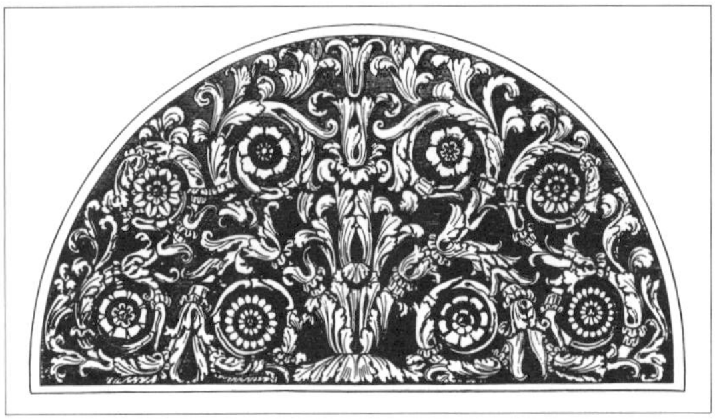

Fig. 17. Man's phytophilia as expressed in decorative art: Fragment in white marble from the Mattei Palace, Rome. From: Vulliamy L (1838) Examples of ornamental sculpture in architecture. Museo Bresciano, Brescia

secondary, culturally imprinted preferences, such as Dutch landscape paintings with dominating skies and heavy clouds above flat land or the romantic mountainscapes of painters in Bavaria, Switzerland, and Austria.

Culture-Specific Biases: A Look at Style

The foregoing discussion demonstrated that our perception is biased on two levels. The first is on a very basic and general level of seeking order, regularity, and patterns in the world around us. We share these tendencies with other mammals and with birds. The second level of perceptual biases are species-specific ones which, in some cases, have phylogenetic roots and, in others, are found in a wide variety of cultures because of universal attitudes. Inborn attitudes, such as nurturant tendencies towards children or nonaggressive attitudes toward mothers, give rise to the use of appeals associated with these categories of persons.

Now, I would like to mention a final perceptual bias, a culturally specific one that is learned in early childhood and later used by the culture as a whole to evoke emotions in the service of group bonding, separating it from others, manipulating individual actions, or reinforcing social norms and values. To do this, I would like to briefly examine style as a means of encoding these culture-specific messages and thus communicating the spirit of a time or a specific weltanschauung. Let me start with some familiar examples.

In European history, style in art was and still is a strong factor promoting European unity and bridging national and ethnic borders. The epochs of style (Romanesque, Gothic, etc.) united Europe from the Atlantic east as far as Russia and from southern Scandinavia to the Mediterranian Sea. Considering the diversity of European cultures, the basic stylistic unity reflected in architecture, music, and painting during specific eras is astounding and, certainly, has facilitated communication. Style in art continues to play an important role in reinforcing intra- and intercultural bonds. Cultural values and norms are often passed on via aesthetic mediums. Historic paintings provide a good example. The portraits of important men inspire the viewers with awe and encourage identification with their good and/or brave ideas. Historical events may thereby be justified and the way paved for similar events to occur in the future. Political and religious attitudes are formed and imprinted upon the viewer. Here, art becomes a medium of indoctrination.

In this context, the idealized presentation of the human image is remarkable and of great interest. The virtues of bravery, honesty, generosity, and charity are depicted and reinforced. Furthermore, models for group loyalty are set, many of which conflict with individual interests. Abraham's sacrifice can be seen as an allegory for a new virtue, which demands that group interests – as presented by the ruler – should have priority over the individual's interest and that of his family. This indoctrinability and openness to accept group values is highly characteristic of man. It paved the way for group selection.[54]

On other levels, style is used to emphasize international distinctions within Europe, as well as to mark regional and ethnic differences within countries, as illustrated by Wobst's[55] study on dress as a marker of ethnic distinction within Yugoslavia. For this reason, art has often been considered to be the instrument of politics. Although there is some truth in this statement, this does not diminish the aesthetic value of Angkor Wat or the cathedral of

Strasbourg. The worldwide styles of modern times in fashion and youth culture could exert a unifying influence on a global level, even though the moving force behind them is business. The artistic level of pop art, rock music, and the like usually is simplified to appeal to many and not to just a sophisticated elite or one specific culture.

It is interesting to note that style also serves ideological functions, such as those of bonding, in both hunting and gathering societies and in tribal societies. Wiessner,[56] studying the relationship between style in artefacts and social factors among the !kung, G/wi, and !ko Bushmen of the Kalahari, has found that style operates at a number of levels and serves numerous functions. On the group level, certain stylistic features found in arrows, which serve as emblems of linguistic group membership, "... help overcome discrimination which might result from residential arrangements and unites the larger population, which pools risk." These emblems allow bushmen to tell at a glance whether an arrow comes from their group or from a foreign one and consequently enables them to predict whether the maker adheres to similar values and practices or not. If the groups are known to each other, the stylistic differences signal different values and practices, making interaction more predictable and, thus, less stressful. Arrows coming from unknown foreign groups, in contrast, release spontaneous, violent reactions of fear, awe, and anxiety among !kung Bushmen, and conversations which ensued contained horror stories about murders or strange events in the past. Emblemic messages of identity were also found in other artefacts, body markings, clothing, and decorative items.

Style was also used daily by individuals to express features of individual identity and worth, which separated them from similar group members and demonstrated individual interpretations of affiliation with certain groups or other individuals. In the latter case, it reinforced bonds and, in the former, projected an aesthetic experience to others, which served to create a positive self-image and to achieve social recognition. Reasons given by the !kung for investing effort in decorating objects and clothing were to make themselves appear to be "one who knows things and does things" and to appear attractive to members of the opposite sex.[56]

Both of these motivations for creating and possessing items of aesthetic value are common. Aesthetic appeal is decisive in courtship and sexual relations, and sexual selection enhances aesthetic features and appeals, birds of paradise and bower birds being outstanding examples. Chiefs, nobles, heads of states, etc. display wealth by means of art, since objects of art are the product of an extraordinary investment of working time and skill, and this is the essence of value. The principle is an old one, which is also encountered in tribal societies. The Eipo in western New Guinea produce nets, which they trade in exchange for stone axeheads, which come from quarries outside their area. Nets represent an investment of work and are, therefore, valuable. Some are decorated with fibers of orchids woven into the fabric to produce color patterns. They are decorative and even more highly valued during dances. Men decorate themselves with particularly well-made and large nets, sometimes enbellished with feathers, which they carry on their backs (Fig. 18). Among the neighboring In, who speak another language of the same language group, the dance nets have become even more elaborate to the extent that they have lost their capacity as a carrying container and function only to support an elaborate pattern of feathers, which in themselves signify value, since they are difficult to obtain (Fig. 19).

Similar developments can be seen in New Guinea with stone axes, which, in many cases, have lost their functional value by the investment of extra work and have become decorative axes with highly polished blades and/or intricately carved handles, which serve as "money." The investment of extra work in all of these cases adds aesthetic appeal. Through this investment, the objects take on a different function. In this context, I would also like to refer to the very stimulating works of Otto Koenig[57,58] on the "biology of uniforms," in which he demonstrates how functional parts of uniforms in time change into decor when much working time is invested in them, making them too valuable to serve their previous functions.

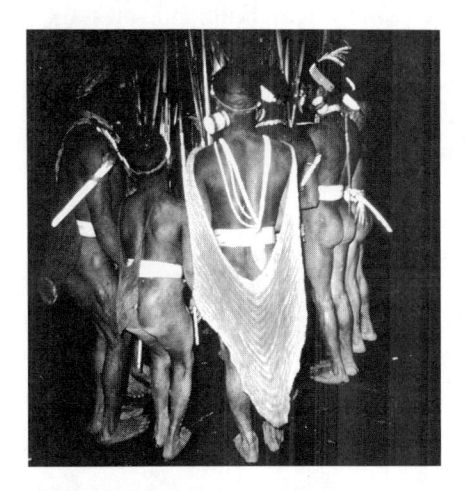

Fig. 18. *(left)* Eipo dance net

(right) Decorative net of Eipo neighbors (Irian Jaya) Photos taken in Irian Jaya, western New Guinea by: I. Eibl-Eibesfeldt *(left)* and V. Heeschen *(right)*

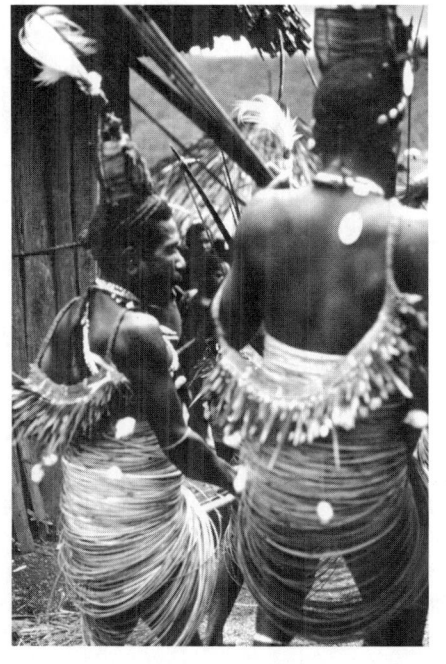

The Biological Foundation of Aesthetics

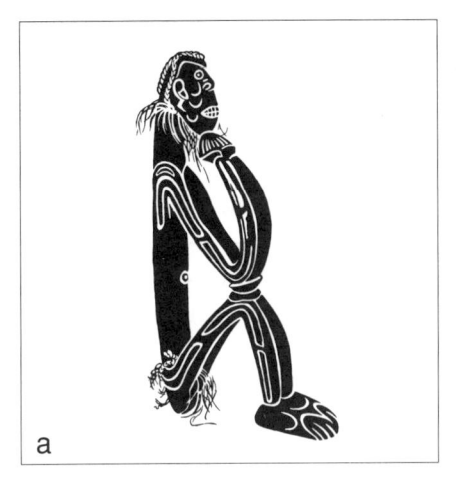

Fig. 19. Examples for the stylization of human figures in New Guinean art:

a) Ancestral figure (profil), Lorenz River, Asmat

b) Shield with a strongly abstracted depiction of a human figure seen from the side (Asmat)

c) Shield with simple depictions of human figures in frontal and lateral view presentation, North-west River

d) Highly stylized human figures on a shield from western New Guinea, Utumba River, Asmat

e) Human figures changed into signs on a shield from western New Guinea, Oba River

All examples from Lommel[60]

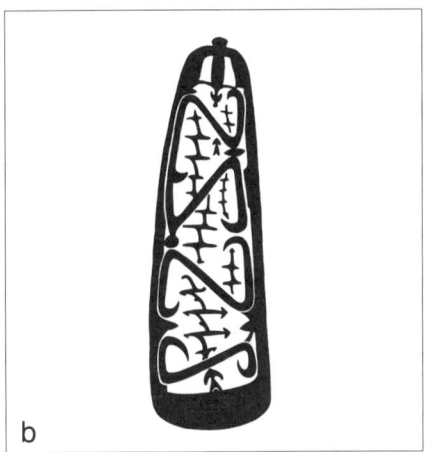

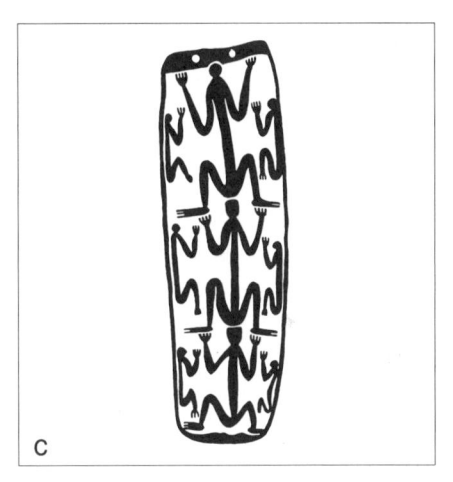

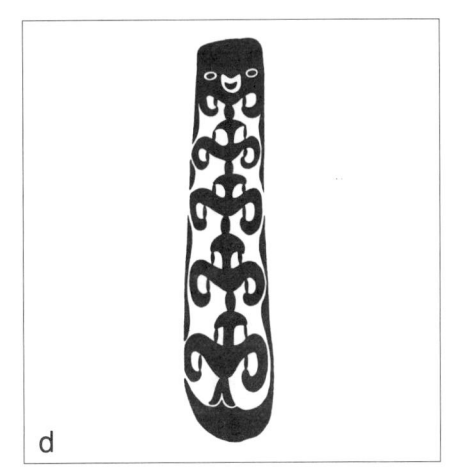

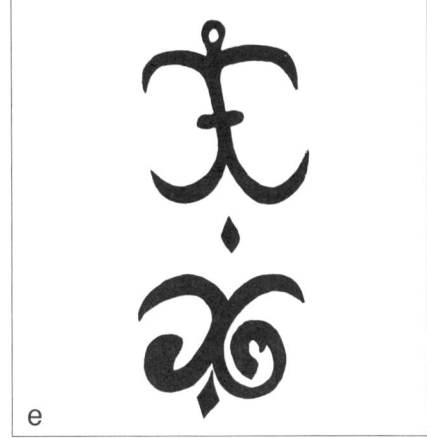

Besides achieving status, display of individual style helps an individual to be recognized as an industrious exchange partner in trade relationships, due once again to an investment of labor.[56] Every bank facade also follows this principle, displaying wealth to create trust. There are many other related functions of individual style. Yanomami, for example, mark their arrow heads individually. This allows the enemy to recognize who shot the arrow in case of a raid. Whether this is intended by the maker of the arrow or not, we do not know yet. In Biocca's[59] interview of Helena Valera (who was kidnapped by the Yanomami as a child and remained their captive for 30 years), the fact was merely reported without being discussed further.

Bamboo arrow heads are also an important token of exchange among men, and Yanomami always carry a number of arrows from other men in their containers as tokens of alliance. During a recent visit, I found that a young man of the Hasubuweteri displayed the content of his container to a visitor, telling him from where each arrow came. By doing so, he was displaying his network of friendship ties and, consequently, his social standing. This reminded me of a custom in central Europe, where visitors placed their visiting cards in a plate in the hall, where others already lay. Nowadays, guestbooks, in addition to containing personal messages, serve this purpose. Finally, style is a way to culturally encode messages in an artistic way. I mentioned earlier that this is the case in the carved canoe prows of the Trobriand Islanders. Here, the aesthetic experience, in addition to its emblemic display function, is used to attract and keep the attention of humans and spirits, which are considered to perceive like man and to pass on more specific messages of appeasement and threat. On this level of communication, sign stimuli and releasers enter the design, skillfully woven into a cultural code.

During the process of stylization, schematization takes place: Certain features of the objects become emphasized, and less important characteristics are left out. Thus, by gradual abstraction, an object may even change into a sign. The process in many ways resembles the ritualization of behavior, by which animal and human behavior patterns change into signals through phylogenetic and cultural evolution.[24,32] That signs develop similarly in phylogenetic and cultural evolution is not particularly surprising since, in both cases, the selecting agent is the perceiver of the signal. The signals must be conspicuous, easily perceived, and unmistakably characteristic. The process of stylization is dictated by the laws governing abstractive (typological) visual perception. By gradual schematization, Papuans artistically change human figures or faces in sculptures and on carved shields into signs. All transitions from recognizable human figures to abstract signs are found (Fig. 19).[60] Another example of how naturalistic depictions become stylized is pre-Columbian whorl patterns (Fig. 20).[61]

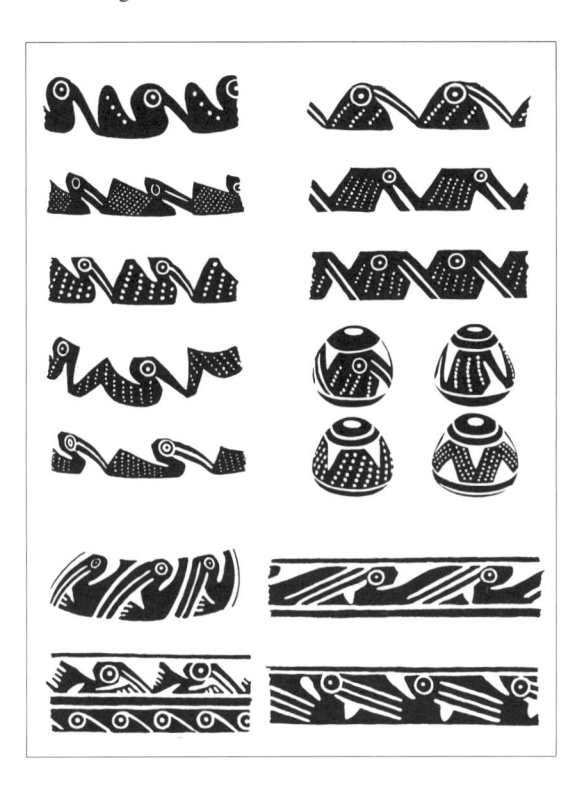

Fig. 20. The stylization of pelican ornaments on Ecuadorian whorls (pre-Columbian, Manteno culture). Note the reduction of the birds' images into a geometrical pattern. Without the transitional stages, one would not recognize the derivation of the sign.
From: Wickler and Seibt[61]

Ethological Aspects of Music, Dance, and Poetry

Music

Rhythm exerts puzzling physiological effects upon man. It tends to synchronize behaviors within certain limits. Thus, breathing can be slowed down or speeded up. And this seems to be a basic response, which has already been found among lower vertebrates: Fish synchronize their breathing movements (opercula movement) with the accuracy of a metronome. In a similar way, it is possible to influence the locomotory activity of squirrels.[62]

The neurophysiological effects of rhythm have not been studied so far, but the investigations of David Epstein (chapter 4) indicate that the stable phase relationships in meter (beats) are the same as those found by Erich von Holst[56,63,64] in his studies on the central coordination of automatisms. We may postulate that there are basic rhythms, probably universal, which have a characteristic soothing or arousing influence on human behavior. We still do not know whether the nature of arousal is a general one or whether some basic rhythms act as releasers for specific emotions, such as aggression. The question whether basic rhythmic units serve as specific releasers to trigger certain emotions or whether they control emotions through more general arousal or sedation must be left open to future investigation. Certainly, rhythms exert a coordinating effect on a crowd and, thereby promote bonding via concerted action or coaction. This is explicit, for example, in march music, as well as in choral singing. For melodies, I propose that there exist basic themes. Kneutgen[65] played lullabies from different cultures to Europeans and found that they exerted a comforting, consoling influence, regardless of their origins. Listeners' breathing became more flat and regular, and, as their breathing rhythms followed the melody, the phase of inhalation coincided with the ascending phase of the melody and expiration with the slow descent of the melody. The listeners felt relaxed, and the frequency of their heart beats dropped. In contrast, jazz had the opposite physiological and emotional effects. Of course, melody and rhythm, in this case, formed a functional unit.

The concept of basic universal themes also derives from the study of the vocal behavior of man. Bolinger[66], among others, has pointed out a number of universals in speech intonation. Sedláček and Sychra[67] had the Czechish sentence "Tož už mám ustlané", "...the bed is prepared," a sentence from Leoš Janáček's *Diary of a Missing Person*, in which the gypsy Zefka seduces the boy Janáček, spoken by various actors with different emotional loading. Tapes of these sentences were then presented to persons who did not speak Czech. They were able to guess the underlying emotional content with a high degree of success. Emotions of happiness and love are characterized by a higher voice and vivid melodic course, erotic emotions by a slightly lower pitch, and emotions of sadness by a tone lower than that used for emotionless statements.

During my film documentation of unstaged social interactions, I found that, in all cultures studied by us so far, babies are addressed in a higher pitch than normal. The cross-cultural similarity of the pattern is striking. Eggebrecht[68] and Schröder[69] found that different types of well-defined songs – war songs, love songs, and wailing songs, for example – coming from different cultures were recognized by listeners and put into the right category with a statistically significant degree of success. Thus, objective studies as well as subjective impressions teach us that music has a particularly penetrating and arousing effect, with much more urgency than the visual arts, which invite one to contemplate the object and only gradually arouse the viewer.

By using primary and secondary themes, man is in a position rapidly to arouse emotions in himself, as well as in others – to the extent of introducing altered states of consciousness, such as trance. Furthermore, by playing different emotive melodies in succession, changes in the degree of emotional arousal are produced that surpass the experience of daily life. A symphony can carry us through all the peaks of happiness, sadness, triumph, and despair imaginable within an hour's time. The heightening of emotional experience is one important aspect of music that can function in a variety of ways, ranging from entertainment to the reinforcement of group bonding and adherence to mutual values and ideals (e.g., hymns and marches).

It has struck me that, in a number of societies where I have lived for extensive periods, certain melodies are constantly hummed and sung by children and adults alike. Certain melodies can, therefore, be characteristic of a community, creating a feeling of identity. In a !ko Bushmen group, one repeatedly hears the same melodies that accompany the women's melon ball dance. In Bali, Legong melodies provide the background for everyday life. This means that cultural encoding promotes a feeling of group membership and separates a group from others.

However, at a higher level, the primary themes or releaser melodies appear to be universal. As in visual arts, musical encoding falls within limits set by our perceptual biases, since it activates and challenges the listener and provides him with the pleasure of unravelling the hidden information.

Dance

Music invites action; dance is music in action. The same principles and functions apply to both music and dance. Dance can be performed in front of spectators, often in the form of a structured ritual, as is the case in the dance performances at a temple feast in Bali. These usually start with a baris and a pendet, the former being a ritualized war dance and the latter, a dance in which girls present flowers to greet the spectators. Display and appeasement are thereby combined in antithesis, as is the case in rituals opening a friendly encounter in many cultures (Fig.21).[70]

Some of the patterns of male and female display in dance appear to be universally present. Thus, male display dances are characterized by abrupt motions, mainly oriented toward the spectator by demonstrations of power in jumping, by frontal orientation of the body, and legs spread apart with arms held so as to enlarge the frontal appearance. The body is presented as a powerful unit. Women present their bodies in a very different way. Their movements are graceful, their bodies moving to present themselves from a variety of angles. Coquetry plays an important role, as expressed by movements of approach and withdrawal, either in alternation or in simultaneous superposition, expressing the ambivalence of interpersonal relationships. Female sexual releasers are presented either in an encoded, subtle form or more directly in "flash presentation," as is the case in the French cancan, where, with a sudden turn, the skirts fly high and a leg is suddenly raised. Frontal and dorsal sexual presentations occur.

Dance, as an interaction between dancers, takes many forms and serves

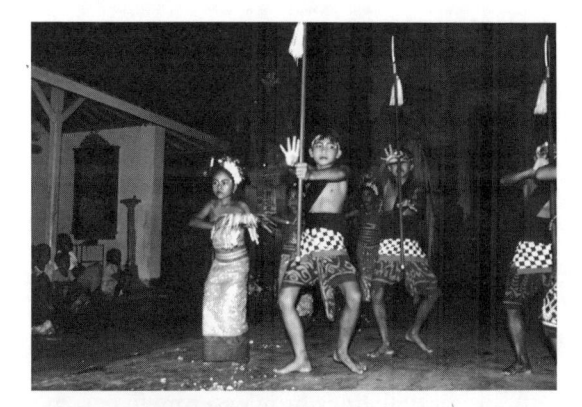

Fig. 21. The Balinese greeting dance "puspa wresti" combines in antithesis the flower-offering dance (pendet) with a war dance (baris).

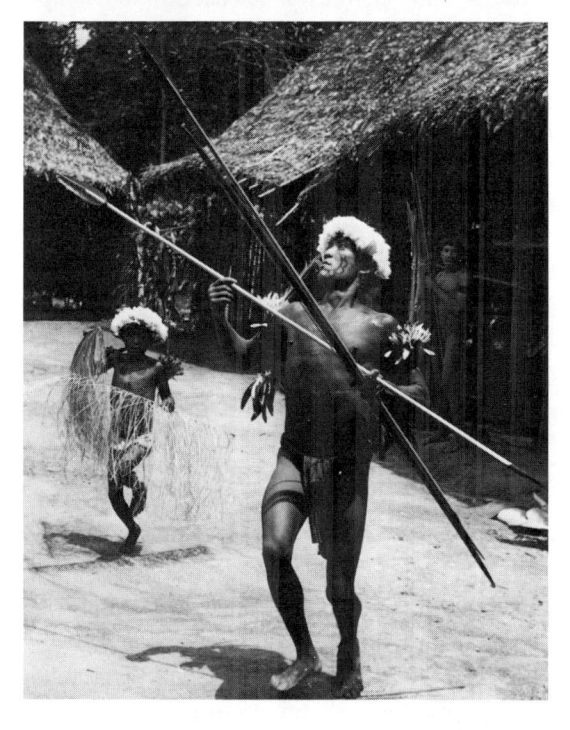

The same combination of aggressive display and friendly appeal is encountered in the greeting dance, which Yanomami men perform when they enter a village as guests for a feast. While the man performs a war dance, a child dances with him waving green palm fronds.
Photos: I. Eibl-Eibesfeldt

a variety of functions. Courtship and pair-bonding is achieved by heterosexual pair dancing and group dancing. During dancing, the partners find out whether they are in harmony through the ease in which they can synchronize their actions.[71]

Group dances also serve to demonstrate group unity and enhance group identity and cohesion. When the group presents itself to others, synchronization of action (coaction) prevails. A very impressive image is presented when a hundred warriors stamp the ground in union, when they turn simultaneously or stand in rows, jumping for minutes in perfect synchronization, as do the Medlpa to the beat of their drums during feasts when different villages meet. Thus, a group presents itself as a closed unit. The inner cohesion becomes additonally reinforced by dances in which the members of a group smoothly integrate their actions to present a functioning whole as, for example, in the melon ball dance of the San women. The essence of this dance is that the group acts as a unit, and the dance functions only when every member of the group is familiar with the rules of the game. Otherwise, she steps out of the line and excludes herself from the group.[72,73]

Through dance, altered states of consciousness can be achieved, as is the case in the trance dance of the bushmen. The phenomenon is well documented, but the physiology of trance still needs to be explored.[74] Dance, furthermore, allows man to act out situations and emotions through pantomime, but this is beyond the scope of this presentation. However, I would like to point out one aspect in this context, which is man's urge to express himself in his cultural nature, demonstrating his sovereignty over his biological nature to indicate his freedom of choice and action. Man is a cultural being by nature and exhibits a strong urge to control his behavior. Self-control in this context seems to be one of the universal virtues of man. Dance is often used to express man's triumph over nature, as exemplified by the Balinese Legong dance. Some of the movement patterns of this dance are so unnatural that they cannot be learned by imitation but must be taught by physical guidance (Fig. 22). Nevertheless, the dancer achieves perfect mastery of these new, unnatural movements and performs the dance smoothly and in perfect harmony with the grace of natural movements.

Poetry

Man's creative abilities in language can be said to be a characteristic which distinguishes him from all other animal species. Consequently, one would expect arts involving language to be the purest cultural expression of man, devoid of the limitations of phylogenetic adaptations, except for the very basic adaptations in the neuronal systems underlying man's capacity to acquire language and speak. Only recently have we become increasingly aware that matters are not that clear-cut. The metaphors we use, the way we speak, and how we express ourselves obey universal rules. I am not referring to the trivial fact that the basic themes – food, sex, fear, and offspring – occupy man's thinking in all cultures, but to the interesting fact that the subtleties of interaction seem to be governed by a system of rules which are universal.

This proposition occurred to me during our cross-cultural film documentation of unstaged social interactions, which I have pursued for over 10 years.

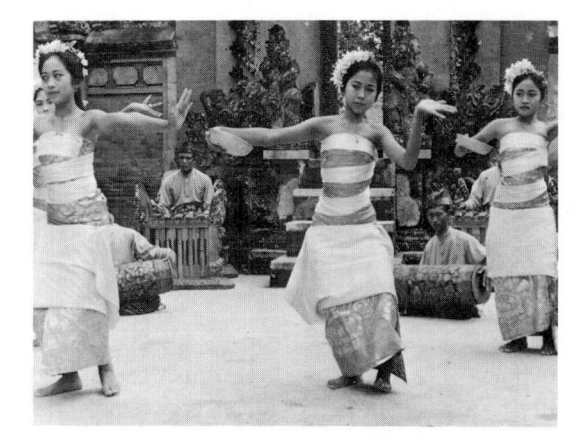

Fig. 22. In the Balinese Legong dance, man symbolically conquers nature. Elaborate and highly artificial movements are entrained to perfection.

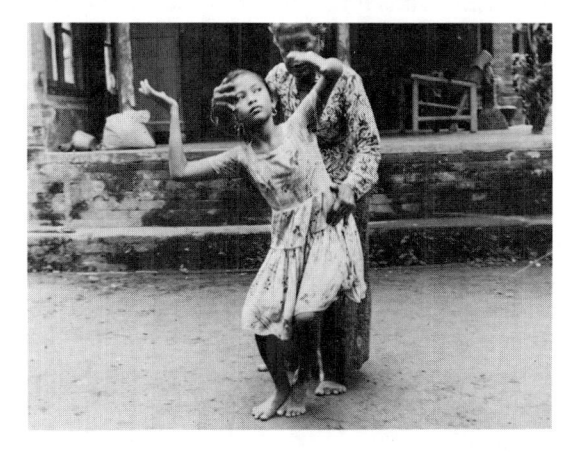

Some of the movements are so artificial they have to be entrained by physical guidance.
Photos: I. Eibl-Eibesfeldt

I found that there are only a limited number of strategies used by persons to achieve status, to ward off an aggressor, to comfort someone in distress, or to seek comfort. These strategies appear to follow the same principles in all cultures studied so far. Children act out these strategies similarly, regardless of specific cultural socialization, and adults verbalize them but also follow the same rules. They employ these basic strategies by verbal clichés rather than by actions as releasers, and they react verbally. Thus, verbal and nonverbal interactions alike conform to the same rules of etiquette. There exists, so to speak, a universal grammar of social interaction, structuring both verbal and nonverbal events alike.[75,76]

Let me give an example of how the symbolism of metaphor reflects these universal forms of perception and thought. In interviews carried out by Volker Heeschen and myself, we have found that the Eipo in New Guinea use the high-low symbolism in a similar way as we do to express high in contrast to low or negative esteem. In a similar way, right-left and bright-dark symbolism is used with right characterizing positive aspects. Handedness and the fact that we are a diurnal species seem to underlie these perceptions.[77,78] With words, phrases, and sentences triggering responses, it becomes possible for the artist to manipulate emotions at will, as he can in music.

Verbal communication is more differentiated than communication in music and the visual arts. Language permits communication of factual information, devoid of emotional overtones, as well as communication on an emotional level with varying intensity. The possibility of encoding messages by indirect reference and the use of metaphors constitutes one of the foundations of poetry. Metaphors are directly comparable to the allegorical presentation in painting, as in both we experience the pleasure of discovery of a hidden message. Words and phrases can evoke emotions directly by the use of verbal clichés, i.e., direct translation of social releasers. By language, we can also depict recurring themes in social relations, reinforcing and laying down the norms of altruistic behavior and loyalty towards family, clan, and those in need. With cultural evolution, conflict arises when the development of new cultural norms, such as making the killing of enemies a virtue, goes against our primary biological inhibition against killing a member of our species. With increasing social complexity, loyalty toward the group as represented by the king, for example, becomes the dominating loyalty overriding even the natural loyalty toward family and clan, a conflict commonly depicted in sagas. Poetry and song texts serve to indoctrinate these values, and art can become propaganda and an instrument of manipulation.

An examination of patriotic songs in our culture demonstrates this clearly. These songs take advantage of existing familial values but, at the same time, change them into group values. The text of the "Berlin-Garderegiment," a military song from the First World War, reads:

> "We wear the insignia of the guards on our jackets,
> and loyalty and honor in our hearts,
> faith in Germany and belief in God,
> and readiness to bear arms for our defence ..."

The family is not mentioned, since loyalty to wife and progeny does not need much reinforcement, but loyalty to the fatherland and to God must be constantly reinforced.

If kin terminology is used, then an effort is made to transfer the family ethos to the group by addressing nonkin group members, for example, as "brothers." In a similar way, attachment to one's native country is reinforced in songs, speech, and poetry, even among tribal people living as hunters and gatherers. Thus, the Nama-Hottentots, living as "strandlopers" from the products of the seashore and sea, glorify the sea in traditional songs of praise. Those living in the desert show attachment to their land in a special ritual described by Kuno Budack.[79] Upon returning to their land after a long absence, they take water in their mouths, sprinkle it onto the ground, and exclaim:

" /i //naoxan !hutse	"You, land of my forefathers,
!gaise !khoi !oa te re	Come and meet me well
eibe mutsi!"	Finally I see you."

The Eipo, in the songs translated by Heeschen,[77] praise their native mountains, the names of which they also call out during warfare to appeal to their ancestors, who came from there. Thus, the mechanisms which Western man applies to instill love for his nation or state seem to have ancient roots.

Other cultural values transmitted by language are those of heroism. This cultural adaptation is also found in tribal cultures. The Himba – a cattle-breeding Bantu people of the Kaokoland (Namibia) – praise the heroic deeds of their ancestors during social gatherings in ways similar to ours in songs and sagas. Social norm control is, furthermore, enforced in many cultures by speeches, songs of reproach, and the use of metaphors.

Speech allows detachment by indirect reference and can thereby serve to prevent disruptive emotional arousal. The art of speaking euphemistically allows, for example, a tactful approach in courtship. Through love songs, a partner may be addressed without any further obligations of consequence. If she or he refuses to accept the message, the existing social relationship need not suffer, since no direct refusal occurred. Some of the verbal appeals in love songs seem to be found in most cultures. In their love songs, the Medlpa refer to their lover as their "little bird," using the protective and nurturative appeal in a similar way that we do. In the contract songs of the Yanomami, the Himou, and the Wayamou, which were presented at one of our meetings by Kenneth Good (1980, Ritualized contract chants among the Yanomami, the Wayamou and Himou, unpublished work), the extensive use of metaphors and indirect reference is remarkable. In addition, verbal information is provided in short lines of three syllables, each line beginning with the last syllable of the prior one. This makes the text practically unintelligible for the uninitiated.

Such a culture-specific embellishment defines ingroup and outgroup, according to whether or not a person can grasp the meaning. A shared code creates a shared secret that bonds, a strategy often used by children who share secrets with close friends. Superstructure and metaphor obscure and demand reconstruction of the text by the listener to achieve understanding, which is aesthetically pleasing. The aesthetic criteria for poetry seem to be the skillful use of metaphors, rhythms, and regularity in structure while avoiding monotony, which allows the construction of supersigns to facilitate memorization and recognition (see chapter 3).

Discussion and Summary

In Keesing's excellent Anthropology[80], I recently read the statement: "It is the anthropoligist's special insight that these internal models we use to create a world of perceived things and events are largely cultural. What we see is what we, through cultural experience, have learnt to see."

This is only partly true. Our perception is initially biased by the existence of phylogenetic adaptations at different levels. These occur on the basic level of sensory physiology and on a level which we may call the ethological, because innate releasing mechanisms adapted for processing specific key stimuli and releasers are employed. Jung's idea of archetypes as an innate predisposition to think in categories of pictures and to symbolize accordingly comes close to this concept, although the concept that he used lacked the precision of the corresponding ethological concepts.

Art appeals in a variety of ways via our aesthetic perception by exploiting these mechanisms, depending in part on the particular role which the artistic creation is to play. Whereas aesthetic perception is an ability shared with higher animals, art is a creation of man alone and serves communicational functions specific to humans. Among these, the ideological reinforcement of shared norms and values is of prime importance as well as ideological indoctrination. It is this trait which sets man off from all other animals and which enhanced "cultural subspeciation."[81] Poetry and songs as well as visual arts are used in combination to serve this purpose. When discussing the indoctrinary power of song, it is clear that here we are not dealing with a very recent development but with a very ancient invention of man.

The rock paintings of Stone Age man in Europe and Africa and of the vanished South African Bushmen probably also served to indoctrinate the group with a sense of common identification. Rock paintings of the Australian Aborigines are found at sacred sites, which only men are allowed to visit and which are the symbolic centers of their territories. These paintings, which are restored during male initiations, depict the totemic animal of the local group (Fig. 23). The paintings symbolize identification, as do the sacred boards, which each initiated man owns, bearing similar insignia, including a highly symbolic narrative of the totemic ancestors' travels. During initiation at these sacred sites, the young men are instructed in the history of their group, and they pledge loyalty to it.

I often wondered why male initiation in particular plays such an impor-

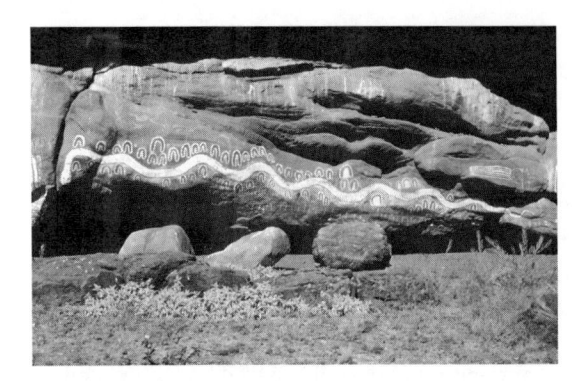

Fig. 23. A totemic site of the Walbiri (central Australia)
Photo: I. Eibl-Eibesfeldt

tant role in human societies. Now it occurs to me that by imprinting the symbols of the group, identification with symbols is achieved and, along with it, the readiness to attach prime importance to the welfare of the group as represented by the symbols. Group loyalty appears to be able to be indoctrinated in men to a stronger degree than loyalty to family and clan. This is particularly important for the men who are responsible for defending the group and must be ready to sacrifice their lives in case of emergency. To achieve this readiness, male initiation is characterized by hardship and humiliation. This creates a hierarchy between instructors and pupils and induces a readiness to obey and accept, thus facilitating learning. Up to our modern times, indoctrination takes advantage of these dispositions.

Art is one important instrument by which in- and outgroup are defined and by which groups are united by shared symbols, be it the Catholic church, a totem pole of the Kwakiutl, or a sacred site with paintings of totemic animals among the central Australian Aborigines. The symbols, whatever their origin, bind and enable man to identify with a larger group. Indoctrination can go so far that the group ethos reigns, a phenomenon which has important consequences for cultural evolution.[54]

Another feature that characterizes man and finds its realization in art is man's capacity to exploit his hedonistic mechanisms at will. Man as the "pleasure seeker"[48] creates art for art's sake, for the sheer enjoyment of the aesthetic experience of harmony and beauty, but also for the thrill of being terrified or saddened.

Perception can be rewarding in many ways: by providing sensory stimulation and excitement, by satisfying curiosity, by inducing awe and surprise, and by puzzling and satisfying our urge for discovery and a sense or order. Man strives to heighten his awareness to the extent of seeking altered states of consciousness. In addition to this, we have seen that art also serves many archaic functions, like status achievement and courtship. Music may be the purest form of art; in song, messages are encoded in the aesthetic experience, and art becomes a medium or vehicle for communication. Aesthetic perception attracts and holds attention and invites sensory exploration, which leads to the discovery of the encoded message – an experience which in itself is pleasurable. The discovered message is thereby reinforced. The presentation of exaggerated stimuli is another strategy of communication employed in art to convey a message.

Good, true, and beautiful are often attributes associated with art and science. We might contemplate this connection at the end of our biological excursion into aesthetics and art. In both science and art, man experiences discovery as an aesthetic experience. There is a special beauty in nature, which one has to learn to see and which one experiences when one discovers order and harmony. The enlightenment that accompanies scientific discovery is comparable to the discovery of supersigns, which we mentioned as creating an aesthetic experience in art. Gestalt perception is a most important source of scientific discovery.[82] It is awe-inspiring to experience the elegance with which problems are solved. Margulies'[83] investigation on the principles of beauty in chess, which were derived from the judgement of expert chess players, are worth mentioning in this context. Art and science both claim to aim at disclosing the truth. This is a preposterous claim when taken to mean the "final truth." Both attempt to present a current (valid) view of this world and to inspire new visions and ways to approach it. Here, science and art share one more common characteristic – their close relationship to ethics.

References and Notes

1. Tinbergen N (1963) The study of instinct. Oxford University Press, London
2. Gregory RL (1966) Eye and brain. Weidenfeld and Nicolson, London
3. Hochberg JE (1964) Perception. Prentice Hall, Englewood Cliffs, N.J.
4. Gombrich EH (1979) The sense of order. A study of the psychology of decorative art. Phaidon, Oxford
5. Schuster M, Beisl H (1978) Kunst-Psychologie "Wodurch Kunstwerke wirken". DuMont, Köln
6. Lawlor R (1982) Sacred geometry. Thames and Hudson, New York
7. Ertel S (1981) Wahrnehmung und Gesellschaft. Prägnanz in Wahrnehmung und Bewußtsein. Semiotik 3:107–141
8. Wertheimer M (1927) Gestaltpsychologie. In: Saupe E (ed) Einführung in die neuere Psychologie. AW Zickfeldt, Osterwieck am Harz
9. Sander F (1931) Gestaltpsychologie und Kunsttheorie. Ein Beitrag zur Psychologie der Architektur. Neue Psychol Studien 8:311–33
10. Frank H (1960) Über grundlegende Sätze der Informationsästhetik. Grundlagenstudien aus Kybernetik und Geisteswissenschaft 1:25–32
11. Metzger, W (1936) Gesetze des Sehens. Suhrkamp, Frankfurt/Main

12. Dörner D, Vehrs W (1975) Ästhetische Befriedigung und Unbestimmtheitsreduktion. Psychol Rev 37:321–334
13. Hospers J (1969) Introductory readings in aesthetics. The Free Press, New York
14. Forrest DW (1974) Francis Galton, the life and work of a Victorian genius. Paul Elek, London
15. Nguyen-Clausen A (1987) Ausdruck und Beeinflußbarkeit der kindlichen Bildnerei. In: von Hohenzollern J Prinz, Liedtke M (eds) Vom Kritzeln zur Kunst. Julius Klinkhardt, Bad Heilbrunn
16. Rensch B (1957) Ästhetische Faktoren bei Farb- und Formbevorzugungen von Affen. Z Tierpsychol 14:71–99
17. Rensch B (1958) Die Wirksamkeit ästhetischer Faktoren bei Wirbeltieren. Z Tierpsychol 15:447–461
18. Morris D (1962) The biology of art. Methuen, London
19. Ethology – objective research of human and animal behavior from a biological standpoint, especially considering species-specific adaption and the evolution of behavior.
20. Tinbergen N (1951) The study of instinct. Oxford University Press, London
21. Lorenz K (1943) Die angeborenen Formen möglicher Erfahrung. Z Tierpsychol 5:235–409
22. Simner ML (1971) Newborn's response to the cry of another infant. Developmental Psychology 5:136–150
23. Koenig O (1975) Urmotiv Auge. Neuentdeckte Grundzüge menschlichen Verhaltens. Piper, München
24. Eibl-Eibesfeldt I (1975) Ethology – The Biology of Behavior, 2nd edn. Holt, Rinehart and Winston, New York
25. Eibl-Eibesfeldt I (1975) Krieg und Frieden aus der Sicht der Verhaltensforschung. Piper, München
26. Eibl-Eibesfeldt I (1976) Menschenforschung auf neuen Wegen. Molden, Wien
27. Coss RG (1970) The perceptual aspects of eye-spot patterns and their relevance to gaze behavior. In: Hutt C, Hutt SJ (eds) Behavior studies in psychiatry. Pergamon Press, Oxford, 121–147
28. Bolk L (1926) Das Problem der Menschwerdung. Gustav Fischer, Jena
29. Schiefenhövel W (1984) Der Witz als transkulturelles ästhetisches Problem – Versuch einer biologischen Deutung. Mitteil d Anthrop Ges Wien (MAGW) 114:31–36
30. Rensch B (1963) Versuche über menschliche "Auslösermerkmale" beider Geschlechter. Z Morph Anthrop 53:139–164
31. Eibl-Eibesfeldt I (1970) Liebe und Haß. Zur Naturgeschichte elementarer Verhaltensweisen. Piper, München
32. Eibl-Eibesfeldt I (1984) Die Biologie des menschlichen Verhaltens. Piper, München
33. Cunningham MR (1986) Measuring the physical in physical attractiveness: Quasi-experiments on the sociogiology of female facial beauty. J of Personality and Social Psychology 50:925–935
34. Fauss R (1988) Zur Bedeutung des Gesichts für die Partnerwahl. Homo 37:188–201
35. Langlois JH, Roggman LA, Casey RJ, Ritter JM, Rieser-Danner LA, Jenkins VY (1987) Infant preferences for attractive faces: Rudiments of a stereotype? Developmental Psychology 23 (3):363–369
36. Eibl-Eibesfeldt I (1979) Ritual and ritualization from a biological perspective. In: Cranach M von, Foppa K, Lepenies W, Ploog D (eds) Human ethology: Claims and limits of a new discipline. Cambridge University Press, Cambridge

37. Ball W, Tronick E (1971) Infant responses to impending collision: Optical and real. Science 171:818–821
38. Ploog D, Blitz J, Ploog F (1963) Studies on social and sexual behavior of the squirrel monkey (Saimiri sciureus). Folia primat 1:29–66
39. Wickler W (1966) Ursprung und biologische Deutung des Genitalpräsentierens männlicher Primaten. Z Tierpsychol 23:422–437
40. Wickler W (1967) Socio-sexual signals and their intraspecific imitation among primates. In: Morris D (ed) Primate ethology. Weidenfeld and Nicolson, London, pp 69–147
41. Eibl-Eibesfeldt I (1970) Männliche und weibliche Schutzamulette im modernen Japan. Homo 21:178–188
42. Eibl-Eibesfeldt I, Wickler W (1968) Die ethologische Deutung einiger Wächterfiguren auf Bali. Z Tierpsychol 25:719–726
43. Basedow H (1906) Anthropological notes on the western coastal tribes of the northern territory of South Australia. Trans Roy Soc South Australia 31:1–62
44. Eibl-Eibesfeldt I, Sütterlin C (1985) Das Bartweisen als apotropäischer Gestus. Homo 36:241–250
45. Hansmann L, Kriss-Rettenbeck L (1966) Amulett und Talismann. Erscheinungsform und Geschichte. W. Callwey, München
46. Sütterlin C (1987) Mittelalterliche Kirchenskulptur als Beispiel universaler Abwehrsymbolik. In: Hohenzollern J Prinz v, Liedtke M (eds) Vom Kritzeln zur Kunst. Stammes- und individual-geschichtliche Komponenten der künstlerischen Fähigkeiten. J Klinkhardt, Bad Heilbrunn, pp 82–100
47. Fehling D (1974) Ethologische Überlegungen auf dem Gebiet der Altertumskunde. Monogr z Klass Altertumswissenschaft 61, CH Beck, München
48. Hass H (1968) Wir Menschen. Das Geheimnis unseres Verhaltens. Molden, Wien
49. Pawlik J (1973) Theorie der Farbe, 3rd edn. M DuMont Schauberg, Köln
50. Kreitler H, Kreitler S (1980) Psychologie der Kunst. W Kohlhammer, Stuttgart
51. Itten J (1961) Kunst der Farbe. Subjektives Erleben und objektives Erkennen der Wege zur Kunst. Maier, Ravensburg
52. Birren F (1950) Color psychology and therapy. McGraw-Hill, New York
53. Orians GH (1980) Habitat selection: General theory and applications to human behavior. In: Lockard JS (ed) The evolution of human social behavior. Elsevier, New York, pp 49–66
54. Eibl-Eibesfeldt I (1982) Warfare, man's indoctrinability and group selection. Zeitschrift f Tierpsychol 60:177–198
55. Wobst HM (1977) Stylistic behavior and information exchange. In: Cleland CE (ed) Papers for the director: Research essays in honor of James B. Griffin. Anthropology Papers. Museum of Anthropology, University of Michigan 61:317–342
56. Wiessner P (1983) Style and social information in Kalahari San projectile points. American Antiquity 48:253–276
57. Koenig O (1968) Biologie der Uniform. Naturwiss u Med (5) 22:3+19, 23:40–50, Boehringer, Mannheim
58. Koenig O (1970) Kultur und Verhaltensforschung. dtv, München
59. Biocca E (1970) Yanoama. The narrative of a white girl kidnapped by Amazonian Indians. E.P. Dutton, New York
60. Lommel A (1962) Motiv und Variation in der Kunst des zirkumpazifischen Raumes. Publikationen des Staatl Museums für Völkerkunde, München
61. Wickler W, Seibt U (1982) Alt-Ekuadorianische Spinnwirtel und ihre Bildmotive. Beiträge zur allgemeinen und vergleichenden Archäologie 4:315–419

62. Kneutgen J (1964) Beobachtungen über die Anpassung von Verhaltensweisen an gleichförmige akustische Reize. Z f Tierpsychol 21:763–779
63. Holst E von (1935) Über den Prozeß der zentralen Koordination. Pflüg Arch 236:149–158
64. Holst E (1936) Versuche zur Theorie der relativen Koordination. Pflüg Arch 237:93–121
65. Kneutgen J (1970) Eine Musikform und ihre biologische Funktion. Über die Wirkungsweise der Wiegenlieder. Zeitschr exp angew Psychologie 17:245–265
66. Bolinger D (1978) Intonation across languages. In: Greenberg JH, Ferguson CA, Maravcsik EA (eds) Universals of human language, 2, Phonology. Stanford University Press, Stanford, pp 471–524
67. Sedlácek K, Sychra A (1963) Die Melodie als Faktor des emotionellen Ausdrucks. Folia phoniatrica 15:89–98
68. Eggebrecht R (1983) Sprachmelodische und musikalische Forschungen im Kulturvergleich. Dissertation, University of Munich
69. Schröder M (1977) Untersuchungen zur Identifikation von Klageliedern aus verschiedenen Kulturen – Analyse der rhythmischen Struktur der Testlieder. Diplomarbeit Universität München
70. Eibl-Eibesfeldt I (1979) Human ethology: concepts and implications for the sciences of man. The behavioral and brain sciences 2:1–57
71. Pitcairn TR, Schleidt M (1976) Dance and decision: An analysis of a courtship dance of the Medlpa. New Guinea. Behavior 58:298–316
72. Eibl-Eibesfeldt I (1972) Die !Ko-Buschmanngesellschaft. Gruppenbindung und Aggressionskontrolle. Monographien zur Humanethologie 1. Piper, München
73. Sbrzesny H (1976) Die Spiele der !Ko-Buschleute unter besonderer Berücksichtigung ihrer sozialisierenden und gruppenbindenden Funktionen. Monographien zur Humanethologie 2. Piper, München
74. Eibl-Eibesfeldt I (1980) G/wi-Buschleute (Kalahari) – Krankenheilung und Trance. Homo 31:67–78
75. Eibl-Eibesfeldt I (1980) Strategies of social interaction. In: Plutschik R (ed) Emotion: Theory, research and experience. Theories of emotion, vol 1. Academic, New York, pp 57–80
76. Heeschen V, Schiefenhövel W, Eibl-Eibesfeldt I (1980) Requesting, giving, and taking: The relationship between verbal and nonverbal behavior in the speech community of the Eipo, Irian Jaya (West New Guinea). In: Key MR (ed) The relationship of verbal and nonverbal communication. Contributions to the sociology of language. Mouton, The Hague, pp 139–166
77. Heeschen V (1985) Probleme der rituellen Kommunikation. In: Rehbein J (ed) Interkulturelle Kommunikation. G Narr, Tübingen, pp 150–165
78. Eibl-Eibesfeldt I (1981) Ethologische Kommunikationsforschung: Ausdrucksbewegungen, Interaktionsstrategien und Rituale des Menschen aus biologischer Sicht. Medias res. Burda Verlag, Offenburg, pp 159–193
79. Budack KFR (1983) A harvesting people on the south Atlantic coast. South African J of Ethnology 6:1–7
80. Keesing RM (1981) Cultural anthropology. A contemporary perspective. Holt, Rinehart and Wilson, New York, p 82
81. Erikson EH (1966) Ontogeny of ritualization in man. Philos Trans Roy Soc London B 251:337–349
82. Lorenz K (1959) Die Gestaltwahrnehmung als Quelle wissenschaftlicher Erkenntis. Z angew u exp Psychol 6:118–165
83. Margulies S (1977) Principles of beauty. Psychological Reports 41:3–11

Part II
Three Enduring Pleasures

Metered Poetry, the Brain, and Time

Frederick Turner
School of Arts and Humanities, The University of Texas at Dallas, Box 830 688, Richardson, Texas 75083-0688, USA

Ernst Pöppel
Institute of Medical Psychology, University of Munich, Goethestr. 31, 8000 München 2, Federal Republic of Germany

This essay brings together an old subject, a new body of knowledge, and a scientific paradigm, which have not previously been associated with one another. The subject is poetic meter, a universal human activity, which, despite its universality and obvious importance in most human cultures, has received very little attention from humanists, except for the studies of a few literary prosodists, and virtually none at all from science. The new body of knowledge derives from the findings of the intense study of the human brain that has taken place within the last few decades. The new scientific paradigm has been developed by the International Society for the Study of Time. Its major postulates are that: 1. An understanding of time is fundamental to an understanding of the real world. 2. Time is not simple, but composite. 3. Time is a hierarchy of increasingly complex temporalities. 4. The more complex temporalities evolved as a part of the general evolution of the universe, and, in a sense, the evolution of time *constitutes* the evolution of the universe. 5. The hierarchical character of time as we know it reflects and embodies the various stages of its evolution.[1]

As a consequence of our assemblage of these three models, we have undertaken a cross-cultural study of poetic meter that reveals a universal temporal similarity in the verse of cultures as geographically and sociologically diverse as those of, for instance, classical Greece and Japan. This temporal commonality underlying poetic meter indicates a universal predilection for the creation and maintenance of meter as an ordering, creative mental process that possesses the capacity to establish a harmonious interaction among the various functional areas of the human brain. Because in this and in other ways, which shall be outlined, meter is so neatly attuned to the functionings of the brain itself, it can serve as a stimulant and reinforcer of those mental capacities that together contribute to and compose what we term understanding, in the fullest sense of the word. The first section of this essay presents an analysis of the primary characteristics of the human nervous system. We then summarize our findings concerning the meter and line of poetry as it is practiced in all cultures that we have analyzed. The third part of the essay is a description of human hearing and a discussion of its temporal organization. The conclusion of this essay will be devoted to the subjective experience of poetry as it is read or heard and an integration of the three preceding areas of study into a working description of the functional benefits of metered poetry in the brain and in the culture at large.

The radically interdisciplinary nature of this essay is not simply a consequence of the need to seek explanations across the boundaries of different fields. It also represents a commitment and a belief on the part of its authors. We are convinced not only that this type of study will cast light on its specific subject (poetic meter), but also that the scientific material will be reciprocally enhanced in value, taking its place within a framework which gives it a greater predictive power. We further believe that "understanding" itself consists of just such a union of knowledge with global significance.

At this point, it might be helpful to review the major characteristics of human cortical information processing as it has been determined by studies in perceptual psychology, brain chemistry, psychology, brain evolution, brain development, ethology, and cultural anthropology.[2] Individually, the characteristics of human brain activity listed below are commonplace and undisputed for the most part; collectively, they constitute a new and complex picture of the human mind.

Human information processing is, on the crude level of individual neurons, *procrustean*. That is, it reduces the information it derives from the outside world to its own categories and accepts reality's answers only if they directly address its own set of questions. In the macrocosm, human perception of electromagnetic radiation cuts out all but heat and the visible spectrum; in the microcosm, a given neuron in the visual cortex will fire only if certain characteristics – e.g., a moving vertical light contrast – fall upon the retina. The neuron will ignore all impertinent information. We possess, as it were, a certain domineering and arrogant quality in our dealings with sensory information, and our brain will "listen" only to replies to its own inquiries. In quantum physics, the familiar procrustean questions – Is light composed of rays or particles? Is this ray of light polarized north-south or east-west? – force reality into a certainty and definition which it did not originally possess, and this insistence on unambiguity is rooted in our neurons. Thus, we may say that human information processing is, secondly, *determinative*. With its insistence upon certainty, it overrules the probabalistic and indeterminate nature of the most primitive and archaic components of the universe.

Third, and in contrast to the "conservative" tendency we have described, the human nervous system seems designed to register differences; it is *habituative*. It tends to ignore repeated and expected stimuli and responds more eagerly to the new and unexpected. Although it frames the questions, it is more interested in odd answers than ordinary ones. Spatially, it sees contrasts and borderlines; temporally, it sees movements and hears changes. At this point in the essay, we are beginning to notice the seamless interfaces of poetic meter with the information-processing faculties of the brain; the variations within a given metrical system, which were used so often by Shakespeare and upon which Wordsworth elaborates in his preface to *Lyrical Ballads*, are tuned to the habituative capacity of the auditory nervous system.

Fourth, human nervous activitiy is fundamentally *synthetic* in its aim. It seeks form even when it is not there, and there is a serious ontological question as to whether definable form comes to exist when we postulate it.

It is (5) *active* rather than passive: the nervous system constructs scenarios to be tested by reality, vigorously seeks confirmation of them, and painfully reconstructs them if they are contradicted. The brain is at least as much an organ of action as it is an organ of knowledge.

It is thus (6) *predictive*: the patterns it extrapolates or invents are patterns that involve specific immediate expectations and, in the more distant future, expectations which await satisfaction and are tested by the senses. So dominant is human adaptation to predictive calculation that it might be said that the human senses exist to check our predictions rather than, as in most animals, triggers for appropriate behavior.

Human information processing is, moreover, (7) *hierarchical* in its organization. In the columns of neurons in the sensory cortex, a plausible reconstruction of the world is created by a hierarchy of the cells, the ones at the base responding to very simple stimuli and passing on their findings to cells programmed to respond to successively more complex stimuli. Likewise, motor decisions are passed down a long command-chain of simpler and simpler neural servomechanisms.

The coordination of these hierarchical systems, in which many kinds of disparate information must be integrated, requires a neural pulse within which all relevant information is brought together as a whole. For instance, in the visual system, many levels of detail – frequency, color, and depth – must be synchronized, or we would not be able to integrate the various features of a visual scene (I.Rentschler 1981, 1982, personal communications). Thus, brain processing is (8) essentially *rhythmic*. That these rhythms can be "driven" or reinforced by repeated photic or auditory stimuli to produce peculiar subjective states is already well known.

More controversial in detail but, in general, widely accepted is the proposition that the brain's activities are (9) *self-rewarding*. The brain possesses built-in sites for the reception of opioid peptides, such as enkephalin (the endorphins), as well as other pleasure-associated hormones. The brain controls the manufacture and release of these chemicals, and it has been shown that behavior can be reinforced by their use as a reward. The brain, therefore, is able to *reward itself* for certain activities which are, presumably, preferred for their adaptive utility. Clearly, if this system of self-reward is the major motivating agent of the brain, any external technique for calibrating and controlling it would result in an enormously enhanced mental efficiency. We would, by the utilization of such a technique, be able to harness all our intellectual and emotional resources to a given task. Indeed, as we will later argue, this is exactly what an aesthetic education, including an early introduction to metered verse, can do. It is, we believe, precisely this autonomous and reflexive reward system which underlies the whole realm of human values, ultimate purposes, and ideals, such as truth, beauty, and goodness.

Associated with the brain's capacity for self-reward is (10) that it is characteristically *reflexive*. It is, within broad limits, self-calibrating. Unlike a computer, it seems to have a capacity to convert software into hardware – short-term memory into long-term memory, for example, and vice versa. The brain can examine by introspection its own operations so that its hardware can become its input or even its program, if we extend this analogy. We might define consciousness, itself, as the continuous, irresolvable disparity between the brain as observer of itself and the brain as the object of observation.

The human nervous system cannot be separated from the human cultural system it was designed to serve, and it is for this reason that we say its operations are essentially (11) *social*. It is not only specific skills and communicative competences that are learned in a social context, but also the fundamental capacities of arousal, orientation, attention, and motivation. Clearly we possess genetic proclivities to learn speech, elementary mathematic calculation, and so on, but it is equally clear that we require a socio-cultural context to release that potential. Human society itself can be profoundly changed by the development of new ways of using the brain. Illustrative are the enormous socio-cultural consequences of the invention of the written word. In a sense, reading is a sort of new synthetic instinct, input that is reflexively transformed into a program, crystallized into neural hardware, and incorporated as a cultural loop into the human nervous circuit. This "new instinct" in turn profoundly changes the environment within which young human brains are programmed. In the early stages of human evolution, such new instincts (speech must have been one) had to wait for their full development while sexual selection established the necessary elaborate vocal circuitry in the cortex. Later on, we were able to use our technology, which required much less time to develop, as a sort of supplementary nervous system.

One of the most exciting propositions of the new brain science is that human information processing is (12) *hemispherically specialized*. While the jury is still out debating the consequences of these findings, we must caution against the popular view that the right hemisphere of the brain is emotional and the left hemisphere is rational and that artistic capacities, being emotional, are located in the right brain. More plausible is the position of Jerre Levy (chapter 9), who characterizes the relationship between right and left as a complementarity of cognitive capacities. In a brilliant aphorism, she has stated that the left brain maps spatial information into a temporal order, while the right brain maps temporal information into spatial order. In a sense, understanding largely *consists* of the translation of information to and fro between a temporal ordering and a spatial one – resulting in a sort of stereoscopic depth-cognition. In Levy's view, the two "brains" alternate in the treatment of information according to a rhythm determined by the general brain state and pass their accumulated findings on to each other. The fact that experienced musicians use their left brain just as much as their right in listening to music shows that their higher understanding of music is the result of the collaboration of both "brains," the music having been translated first from temporal sequence to spatial pattern and then "read," as it were, back into a temporal movement. The neurobiologist, Günter Baumgartner (chapter 7), suggests that the forebrain acts as the integrating agent between specialized left and right functions, and it is in this integrative process that we would locate the essentially creative capacities of the brain, whether artistic or scientific. The apparent superiority of the isolated right brain in emotional matters may well simply reflect the fact that emotions, like music, are temporal in nature, and their articulation requires the sort of temporal-on-spatial mapping that is the specialty of the right cerebral hemisphere.

Finally, human information processing can be described as (13) *kalogenetic* (Turner), a word coined from the Greek *kalos* (beauty, goodness, rightness) and *genesis* (begetting, productive cause, origin, source). The human nervous system has a strong drive to construct affirmative, plausible, coherent, consistent, concise, and predictively powerful models of the word, in which all events are explained by and take their place in a system that is at once rich in implications beyond its extant data and, at the same time, governed by as few principles or axioms as possible. The words that scientists use for such a system are "elegant," "powerful," and often "beautiful"; artists and philosophers use the same terms and also "appropriate," "fitting," "correct," and "right," all of which can be translations of the Greek *kalos*.

If this tendency is a true drive, then according to the theory of reinforcement, it is an activity for which the brain rewards itself. If these were techniques by which the endogenous reward system could be stimulated and sensitized, those techniques would enable us to greatly enhance the integrative powers of our minds.

Such a technique would have to meet certain qualifications. First, it would have to be culturally universal, since it would be based on neural and biochemical features common to all human beings.[3] Second, it would be very archaic, identifiable as an element of the most ancient and the most primitive cultures. Third, it would most probably be regarded by its indigenous practitioners as the locus of an almost magical inspiration and as a source of wisdom; it would have the reputation of having significantly contributed to the efficiency and adaptiveness of the societies in which it is practiced. Fourth, it would be associated with the social and cultural activities that demand the highest powers of original thought and complex calculation, such as education, the organization of large-scale projects, like war, cooperative agriculture, and the rituals that divert for social uses the dangerous and valuable energies implicit in sexuality, birth, death, sickness, and the like.

Metered poetry, the use of rule-governed rhythmic measures in the production of a heightened and intensified form of linguistic expression, nicely fulfills these requirements. In nearly all cultures, metered poetry is used in crucial religious, social, and economic rituals, and it has the reputation of containing mysterious wisdom; the learning of major poetic texts is central to the process of education in nearly all literate traditions. Much work – farming, herding, hunting, war, sailing and even mining – has its own body of poetry and song. Objective and universal traits can be identified across the whole range of poetic practice throughout the world and as far back into the past as we have records. From these universal characteristics, we can construct a general definition of metered poetry that applies to the ancient Greeks as well as to the Kwakiutl, Racine, and the Polynesians.

The fundamental unit of metered poetry is what we shall call the l i n e. This fundamental unit, while not designated by a written convention such as a line-break in all cultures, is recognizable metrically and nearly always takes from two to four seconds to recite, with a strong peak in distribution, according to the data we have collected, between 2.5 and 3.5 seconds.[4] The line is nearly always a rhythmic, semantic, and syntactical unit as well – a sentence, a colon, a clause, a phrase, or a completed group of these. Thus, other linguistic rhythms are accommodated to the basic acoustical rhythm, producing that pleasing sensation of appropriateness and inevitability, which is part of the delight of verse and an aid to the memory.

The second universal characteristic of human verse meter is that certain marked elements of the line or group of lines remain constant throughout the poem and thus indicate the repetition of a pattern. The 3-second cycle is not marked merely by a pause, but by distinct resemblances between the material in each cycle. Repetition is added to frequency to emphasize the rhythm. These constant elements may take many forms, the simplest of which is the number of syllables per line. Other poetic traditions arrange patterns of stress and cadence. Still other patterns are arranged around alliteration, consonance, assonance, and end rhyme. Often, many of these devices are used together, some prescribed by the conventions of a particular poetic form and others left to the discretion and inspiration of the individual poet. No verse convention dictates *all* the characteristics of a line, so every poem contains an interplay between prescribed elements and free variation.[5]

The third universal characteristic of metrical verse is *variation*. Variation is a temporary suspension of the metrical pattern at work in any given poem, a surprising, unexpected, and refreshing twist to that pattern. Here we must point out that variation can only be an effective or even a definable technique within the context of a prescribed metrical pattern, a pattern which cannot be abandoned. Meter is important in that it conveys meaning, much as a melody does in a song. Metrical patterns are elements of an analogical structure, which is comprehended by the right cerebral hemisphere, while poetry as language is presumably processed by the left temporal lobe. If this hypothesis is correct, meter is partially a method of introducing right brain processes into the left brain activity of understanding language. In other words, it is a way of connecting our much more culture-bound linguistic capacities with the relatively more primitive spatial pattern recognition faculties, which we share with the higher animals.

In the context of this hypothesis, we wish to introduce the major finding of this essay, which explains, we believe, the extraordinary prevalence of the 3-second line in human poetry. If we ask the question, "What does the ear hear?" the obvious answer is "sound". What is sound? It is mechanical waves in the air or another medium. This answer is not very enlightening. We can, for instance, perceive mechanical waves by the sense of touch: it would be as incorrect to say that a deaf man "heard" a vibrating handrail with his fingers as it would be to say a blind man "saw" a fire with the skin of his face. What characterizes hearing as such is not that it senses mechanical waves, just as what characterizes sight is not the perception of electromagnetic waves, but the perception of distinctions between electromagnetic waves.

For vision, those distinctions (except for color) are spatial distinctions, but for audition, they are mainly temporal. To put it directly: what the sense of hearing hears is essentially *time*. The recognition of differences in pitch involves a very pure and highly accurate comparative measurement of different frequencies into which time is divided. The perception of timbre, tone, sound texture, and so forth, consists of the recognition of combinations of frequencies. The recognition of rhythms necessitates the recognition of frequencies taking up longer periods of time.

Audition is not only a marvellously accurate instrument for detecting differences between temporal periods, but also an active organizer, arranging those different periods within a hierarchy as definite as that of the seconds, minutes, and hours of a clock. These different periods are also uniquely appraised. Pitch is an arrangement of that hierarchy into laws of harmony. New discoveries by Ernst Pöppel's group in Munich have begun to elucidate the role of the auditory hierarchy in the structure and function of the brain. This has led to a comprehensive understanding of the general hierarchical organization of the human sensory-motor system and a fresh approach to the production and understanding of language. We shall first briefly outline the auditory hierarchy.

Events separated by periods of time shorter than about three thousandths of a second (0.003 s) are classified by the auditory system as simultaneous. If a brief sound is presented to one ear and another sound is presented to the other ear less than 0.003 s later, the subject will perceive only one sound. If the sounds are a little more than approximately 0.003 s apart, the subject will experience two sounds. However, he will not be able to tell which of the two sounds came first until the interval between them is increased roughly ten times. Thus, the lowest category in the hierarchy of auditory time is *simultaneity*, and the second lowest is mere temporal *separation*, without a preferred order of time. The most primary temporal experience is timeless unity; next comes a space-like recognition – space-like because, unlike temporal positions, spatial positions can be exchanged. One can go from New York to Berlin or from Berlin to New York; but one can only go from 1980 to 1983, not from 1983 to 1980. Likewise, the realm of "separation" is a nondeterministic, acausal realm; events happen in it, perhaps in patterns or perhaps not, but they cannot be said to cause one another because we cannot say which came first.

When two sounds are about three hundredths of a second (0.03 s) apart, a subject can experience their *sequence*, accurately reporting which came first. This is the third category in the hierarchy of time, subsuming separations and simultaneities and organizing them rationally with respect to one another. At this stage, however, the organism is still a passive recipient of stimuli. We can hear a sequence of two sounds one-tenth of a second apart, but there is nothing we can do in response to the first sound before the second sound arrives.

We are helpless to alter what will befall us if the interval between the first signal and its sequel falls within this range. Events follow each other recognizably, but we cannot intervene.

If the temporal interval is longer than three-tenths of a second (0.3 s), however, we have entered a new temporal category – response. Three-tenths of a second is enough time for a human subject to respond to an acoustic stimulus. If we play two sounds to our subject one second apart, the subject could prepare to deal with the second sound in the time given him after hearing the first. The perceiver is no longer passive. For response to exist, there must be a temporal separation, and a further element, which might be characterized in a primitive sense as a purpose. The response to a given stimulus will differ according to the function of the responding organ and the purpose of the organism as a whole.

At several places in this analysis, it has been pointed out that a given familiar temporal relationship – chance, pattern, cause, purpose – only becomes possible when there is enough time given for it to occupy. The idea that an entity needs time to exist in has become commonplace recently. An electron, for instance, requires at least 10 to the negative twenty seconds (10^{-20}s, its spin period) in which to exist, just as surely as it requires 10 to the negative ten centimeters of space (10^{-10}cm, its Compton wavelength). The corollary to this observation is that entities that consist only of spatio-temporal relations are not necessarily less real than material objects, for spatio-temporal relations are a prerequisite for the existence of material objects, also. Although a given period of time may be sufficient for a given relation – chance, cause, function – to be recognized, it is not sufficient for the concept of the relation to be formulated. It takes much less time to recognize or speak a word once learned than it takes to learn the word in the first place. Many examples of the sequence or response relation between events must be compared before a causal or purposive order can be formulated and recognized in individual cases. However, comparisons require discrete parcels of experience between which the comparison can be made, and, since the entities being compared are themselves temporal in nature, these parcels of experience must exist in equal periods of time. The next lowest time division beyond the three-second response frequency must be sufficiently long to enable the completion and recognition of the temporal relations to be compared. The comparison of experience takes more time than experience itself; the recognition of a melody takes more time than the perception of the single notes.

This fundamental "parcel of experience" is about three seconds. The three-second interval, roughly speaking, is the length of the human present moment. (At least it is for the auditory system, which possesses the sharpest temporal acuity of all the senses. The eye, for instance, takes much longer than the ear to distinguish temporal separation from simultaneity.) The philosophical notion of the "specious present" – the present moment of a given organism – finds here its experimental embodiment.

A human speaker will pause for a few milliseconds every three seconds or so and, in that period, will decide on the precise syntax and lexicon of the next three seconds. A listener will absorb about three seconds of heard speech without pause or reflection and then stop listening in order to integrate and make sense of what he has heard. (Speaker and hearer are not necessarily "in phase" for this activity; this observation will be of importance later.)

To use a cybernetic metaphor, we possess an auditory information "buffer," whose capacity is three seconds' worth of information. At the end of three seconds, the "buffer" is full, and it passes the entire accumulated stock of information on to the higher information-processing centers. In theory, this stock should consist of about 1,000 simultaneities, 100 discrete temporal separations, and 10 consecutive responses to stimuli. In practice, however, the buffer has a smaller capacity – about 60 separations and 7 responses (the length of a local telephone number).

It appears likely that another mechanism is involved here, too. Different types of information take different amounts of time to be processed by the cortex. For instance, fine visual detail takes more time to be identified by the cortex than coarse detail. Some sort of pulse is necessary for all the various information to arrive at the higher processing centers as a bundle, correctly labelled as belonging together. At the same time, the sensory cortex "waits" for the "slowest" information to catch up with the "fastest" so that it all can be sent off at once. This three-second period constitutes such a pulse.

Beyond the two horizons of the present moment exist the two periods that together constitute *duration*, which is the highest or "longest frequency" integrative level of the human perception of time. Those two periods, the past and the future, memory and planning, constitute the widest arena of human thought.

It should be obvious from all of this that a remarkable and suggestive correlation exists between the temporal organization of poetic meter and the temporal functions of the human hearing mechanism. Of general linguistic significance is the fact that the length of a syllable, about 1/3 of a second, corresponds to the minimum period within which a response to an auditory stimulus can take place. To be efficient, speech must be as fast as possible, while, to be controllable, it must be slow enough for a hearer to react to a syllable before the next comes along.

Of more specific significance for our subject is the very exact correlation between the three-second line and the three-second "auditory present." The average number of syllables per line in human poetry seems to be about ten, so human poetic meter embodies the two lowest frequency rhythms in the human auditory system. The independence of poetic meter from the mechanism of breathing is explained by the fact that the master-rhythm of human meter is not pulmonary, but neural: we must seek the origins of poetry not among the lower regions of the human organism, but among the higher. An important series of questions present themselves to us at this point. How do we explain the cultural universality of meter? *Why* does verse embody the three-second neural "present"? What functions could be served by this artificial and external mimicry of an endogenous brain rhythm? Given the fact that poetry fulfills many of the superficial conditions of the brain's reward system, how might the three-second line serve that function? And what is the role of other components of meter – the rhythmic parallelism between the lines and the information-bearing variations upon that parallelism?

Here it might be useful to turn our attention to the subjective reports of poets and readers of poetry as an aid to our hypothesizing. These reports may help to confirm conclusions at which we have tentatively arrived.

Robert Graves speaks of the shiver and the coldness in the spine that accompany the experience of poetry, the hair rising on the head and body, as does Emily Dickinson. A profound muscular relaxation accompanied by an intense alertness and concentration has also been recorded. The heart feels squeezed and the stomach cramped. There is a tendency toward laughter, tears, or both, the taking of deep breaths, and a slightly intoxicated feeling. At the same time, there is an avalanche of vigorous thought in which new connections are made; Shakespeare's Prospero describes the sensation as a "beating mind." There is the sense of being on the edge of a precipice of insight – almost a vertigo – and the awareness of entirely new combinations of ideas assuming a concrete shape, together with feelings of strangeness and even terror. Some writers, Matthew Arnold for instance, speak of an inner light or flame. Outside stimuli are often blanked out, so strong is the concentration. The imagery of the poem can become so intense that it is almost like a real sensory experience. Personal memories, pleasant and unpleasant, are strongly evoked; there is often an emotional re-experience of close personal ties with family, friends, lovers, and the dead. There is an intense realization of the world and of human life, together with a strong sense of the reconciliation of opposites – joy and sorrow, life and death, good and evil, human and divine, reality and illusion, whole and part, comic and tragic, time and timelessness. The sensation is not a timeless one as such, but an experience of time so full of significance that stillness and sweeping motion are one entity. There is a sense of power combined with effortlessness. The poet or reader rises above the world, so to speak, on the "viewless wings of poetry," and sees it all in its fullness and completeness, but without loss of the clarity of its details. There is an awareness of one's own physical nature, of one's birth and death, and of a curious transcendence of both, and, often, a strong feeling of universal and particular love and communal solidarity. Of course, not all these subjective sensations necessarily occur together in the experience of poetry, nor do they usually take their most intense forms, but a poet or frequent reader of poetry will probably recognize most of them.

A further property of metered poetry, which goes beyond the immediate experience, is its memorability. Part of this property is undoubtedly a merely technical convenience: the knowledge of the number of syllables in a line and the rhyme, for instance, limits the number of words and phrases which are possible in a forgotten line and helps us logically to reconstruct it. But introspection will reveal a deeper quality to this memorability – somehow the rhythm of the words is remembered even when the words themselves are lost to us. The rhythm helps us to recover the mental state in which we first heard or read the poem, the gates of memory are opened, and the words return at once.

Equipped with the general contemporary conception of brain processing with which this essay began, with the temporal analysis of meter and its correlation to the hearing system, and with these last subjective reports of participants in the art, we may now begin to construct a plausible hypothesis of what goes on in the brain during the experience of poetry. Here we can draw upon a relatively new and speculative field of scientific inquiry, which has been variously termed "neurobiology," "biocybernetics," and "psychobiology." Barbara Lex's essay,"The Neurobiology of Ritual Trance,"[6] in which she summarizes much work in the field, provides many of the materials with which we may build an explanatory bridge between the observed characteristics of human verse and the new findings of the Munich group concerning audition. Although Lex is concerned with the whole spectrum of methods by which altered states of consciousness may be attained, and while her focus is on ritual rather than the art of poetry, her general argument coincides with our findings.

Essentially, her position is that various techniques of the alteration of mental states, generalized as "driving behaviors," are designed to add to the linear, analytic, and verbal resources of the left brain the more intuitive and holistic understanding of the right brain; to tune the central nervous system and alleviate accumulated stress; and to bring to the aid of social solidarity and cultural values the powerful somatic and emotional forces mediated by the sympathetic and parasympathetic nervous systems and the ergotropic and trophotropic responses they control.[7]

It has been known for many years that rhythmic visual and auditory stimulation can provoke epileptic symptoms in seizure-prone individuals and can produce powerful involuntary reactions even in normal persons. The rhythmic stimulus amplifies natural brain rhythms, especially if it is attuned to an important frequency, such as the ten-cycle-per-second alpha wave. It seems plausible that the three-second poetic line is similarly tuned to the three-second cycle of the auditory (and subjective temporal) present. The metrical and assonant devices of verses, like rhyme and stress, which create similarities between the lines, emphasize the repetition. The curious subjective effects of metered verse – relaxation, a holistic view of the world, and so on – are no doubt attributable to the very mild hypnotic state induced by the auditory driving effect – the stimulation by an external rhythmic sound of an endogenous brain rhythm.

Auditory driving is known to affect the right brain much more powerfully than the left. Thus, where ordinary, unmetered prose comes to us in a "mono" mode, predominantly affecting the left brain, metered language comes to us in a "stereo" mode, simultaneously calling upon the verbal resources of the left hemisphere as well as the rhythmic potentials of the right.

Furthermore, the accurate scansion (metrical analysis) of poetry involves a complex analysis of *grammatical* and lexical stress, which must be continually integrated with a nonverbal right brain understanding of metrical stress. The delightful way in which the rhythm of the sentence, as a semantic unit, counterpoints the rhythm of the meter in poetry is thus explained as the result of a cooperation between left and right brain functions. The "stereo" effect of verse is not merely one of simultaneous stimulation of different cerebral areas but is also the result of a necessary integrative collaboration and feedback between them. The linguistic capacities of the left hemisphere, which provide a temporal order for spatial information, are forced into an interaction with the rhythmic and musical capacities of the right hemisphere, which provides a spatial order for temporal information.

But the driving rhythm of the three-second line is not just any rhythm. It is tuned to the largest limited unit of auditory time – its specious present – within which causal sequences can be compared and free decisions made. A complete poem is a duration, a realm of values, systematically divided into presents, which are the realms of action. It, therefore, summarizes our most sophisticated and most uniquely human integrations of time.

There is, perhaps, still another effect at work at the cortical level. The various divinatory practices of humankind all involve a common element – a process of very complex calculation, which seems quite irrelevant to the kind of information sought by the diviner. A reader of the Tarot will analyze elaborate combinations of cards; an *I Ching* reader will arrive at his hexagram through a difficult process of mathematical figuring; a reader of the horoscope will resort to remarkable computations of astronomical positions and time. The work of scanning metered verse, especially when combined with the activity of recognizing allusions and symbolisms, and the combining of them into correct patterns seem analogous to these divinatory practices. The function of this demanding process of calculation may be to occupy the linear and rational faculties of the brain with a task that entirely distracts them from the matter to be decided – a diagnosis, a marriage, the future of an individual. Once the "loud voice" of reductive logical intelligence is stilled by distance, the quieter whispering of a holistic intuition, which can integrate much larger quantities of much poorer-quality information in more multifarious ways – although with less accuracy – can be heard. The technique is like that of the experienced stargazer, who can sometimes make out a very faint star by focussing a little to one side of it, thereby bringing its image to bear on an area of the retina which, though inferior in acuity, is more sensitive to light. The prophetic or divinatory powers traditionally attributed to poetry may be partly explained by the use of this technique. If the analogy is slightly unflattering to the work of some professional analytic critics of poetry, reducing their work as it does to the status of an elaborate decoy for the more logical capacities of the brain, there is the compensation that it is a very necessary activity, indispensible precisely because of its irrelevance.

On the cortical level, poetic meter serves a number of functions generally aimed at tuning up and enhancing the performance of the brain by bringing to bear other faculties than the linguistic. By ruling out certain rhythmic possibilities, meter satisfies the brain's procrustean demands for unambiguity and clear distinctions. By combining elements of repetition and temporal equivalence on the one hand with variation on the other, it fulfills the brain's habitual need for controlled novelty. By giving the brain a system of rhythmic organization as well as a circumscribed set of semantic and syntactic possibilities, it encourages the brain in its synthetic and predictive activity of hypothesis construction and raises expectations that are pleasingly satisfied at once. In its content, poetry has often had a strongly prophetic character – an obvious indication of its predictive function – and the mythic elements of poetry afford more subtle models of the future by providing guides of conduct. Poetry presents to the brain a system which is temporally, rhythmically, and linguistically hierarchical and, therefore, matched to the hierarchical organization of the brain itself. It does much of the work that the brain must usually do for itself by organizing information into rhythmic pulses, integrating different types of information – rhythmic, grammatical, lexical, and acoustic – into easily assimilable parcels and labelling their contents as belonging together. Like intravenous nourishment, the information enters our system instantly, without a lengthy process of digestion.

The pleasure of metered verse evidently derives from its ability to stimulate the brain's capacity for self-reward. The traditional concern of verse with the deepest human values – truth, goodness, and beauty – is clearly associated with its involvement with the brain's own motivational system. Poetry seems to be a device the brain can use in reflexively calibrating itself, turning its "hardware" into "software," and vice versa. Accordingly, poetry is traditionally concerned at its semantic level with consciousness and conscience. As a quintessentially cultural activity, poetry has been central to social learning and the synchronization of social activites (the sea-shanty or work-song is only the crudest and most obvious example). Poetry enforces cooperation between left brain temporal organization and right brain spatial organization and helps to bring about that integrated stereoscopic view that we call true understanding. Poetry is, *par excellence*, kalogenic – productive of beauty, of elegant, coherent, and predictively powerful models of the world.

A traditional charge against poetry is that, in doing all these things, poetry deceives us, presenting to us an experience which, because it is so perfectly designed for the human brain, provides a false impression of reality and separates us from the rough world in which we must survive. Much modern aesthetic theory is, in fact, devoted to reversing this situation and making poetry, and art in general, so disharmonious with our natural proclivities that it shocks us into awareness of stark realities. Clearly, poetry which is merely harmonious would be insipid, for it would disappoint the brain's habituative desire for novelty. However, mere random change and the continuous disappointment of expectations is itself insipid; we are as capable of becoming as habituated to meaningless flux as to mindless regularity.

Modernist esthetic theory may be ignoring the possibility that our species' special adaptation could, in fact, be to expect more order and meaning in the world than actually exists, and that such expectations may constitute, paradoxically, an excellent survival strategy. We are strongly motivated to restore the equilibrium between reality and our expectations by altering reality so as to validate our models of it – to "make the world a better place." The modernist attack on beauty in art would, therefore, constitute an attack on our very nature; and the modernist and post-modernist criticism of moral and philosphical idealisms likewise flies in the face of the apparent facts about human neural organization. What William James called "the will to believe" is written in our genes; teleology is the best policy and, paradoxically, it is utopian to attempt to resist our natural idealism. It is much more sensible to adjust reality to the ideal.

But our discussion of the effects of metered verse on the human brain has so far ignored the subcortical levels of brain activity. Let us substitute "metered verse" for "rituals" in the following summary by Barbara Lex:[6]

> "The *raison d'être* of rituals is the readjustment of dysphasic biological and social rhythms by manipulation of neurophysiological structures under controlled conditions. Rituals properly executed promote a feel-

ing of well-being and relief, not only because prolonged or intense stresses are alleviated, but also because the driving techniques employed in rituals are designed to sensitize and 'tune' the nervous system and thereby lessen inhibition of the right hemisphere and permit temporary right-hemispheric dominance, as well as mixed trophotropic-ergotrophic excitation, to achieve synchronization of cortical rhythms in both hemispheres and evoke trophotropic rebound."[8]

Lex maintains that the "driving" techniques of rhythmic dances, chants, and so on can produce a simultaneous stimulation of both the ergotropic and the trophotropic systems of the lower nervous system, producing subjective effects, which she characterizes as follows: trance; ecstasy; meditative and dreamlike states; possession; the "exhilaration accompanying risk taking;" a sense of community; sacredness; a "process of reviving the memory of a repressed, unpleasant experience and expressing in speech and actions the emotions related to it – thereby relieving the personality of its influence;" alternate laughing and crying; mystical experience and religious conversation; and experiences of unity, holism, and solidarity. Laughlin and d'Aquili[8] add to these effects a sense of union with a greater power and awareness that death is not to be feared, a feeling of harmony with the universe, and a mystical "conjunctio oppositorum" (unity of opposites). This list closely resembles our earlier enumeration of the experience of good metered verse as described by literary people.

If Lex is right, we can add to the more specifically cortical effects of metered verse the more generalized functions of a major ritual driving technique – the promotion of biophysiological stress reduction (peace) and social solidarity (love). Meter clearly synchronizes not only speaker with hearer but also hearers with each other so that each person's three-second "present" is in phase with the others, and a rhythmic community, which can become a performative community, is generated.

Laughlin and d'Aquili connect the mythical mode of narrative with the driving techniques of ritual, pointing out that mythical thought expresses the "cognitive imperative," as they call it, or the desire for an elegant and meaningful explanation of the world.[9] McManus argues that such practices are essential in the full development and education of children.[10]

The theory of the state boundedness of memory might also explain the remarkable memorability of poetry. If meter, with its unique variations, carries its own mood or brain-state signature, then it is not surprising that we can recall poetry so readily. The meter itself can evoke the brain state in which we first heard the poem and, therefore, make the verbal details immediately accessible to recall. Homer said that the muses were the daughters of memory, and this may be what he meant.

To sum up the general argument of this essay: metered poetry is a cultural universal, and its salient feature, the three-second line, is tuned to the three-second present moment of the auditory information-processing system. By means of metrical variation, the musical and pictorial powers of the right brain are enlisted to cooperate with the linguistic powers of the left. By auditory driving effects, the lower levels of the nervous system are stimulated in such a way as to reinforce the cognitive functions of the poem, to improve the memory, and to promote physiological and social harmony. Metered poetry may play an important part in developing our more subtle understandings of time and may thereby act as a technique to concentrate and reinforce our uniquely human tendency to make sense of the world in terms of values like truth, beauty, and goodness. Meter breaks the confinement of linguistic expression and appreciation within two small regions of the left temporal lobe and brings to bear the energies of the whole brain.

This new understanding of poetic meter endorses the classical concept of poetry as designed to "instruct by delighting," as Sir Philip Sidney put it in *The Defence of Poetry*.[11] It strongly suggests that "free verse," when uncoupled from any kind of metrical regularity, is likely to forgo the benefits of activating the whole brain. It also predicts that free verse could become associated with views of the world in which the tense structure has become very rudimentary, and the more complex values, being time-dependent, have disappeared. A bureaucratic social system, requiring specialists rather than generalists, might well find it in its interest to discourage reinforcement techniques like metered verse because such techniques put the whole brain to use and encourage world views that might transcend the limited values of the system. It might also encourage activities like free verse, which are highly specialized both neurologically and culturally. Prose, both because of its own syntactical rhythms and because of its traditional liberty of topic and vocabulary, is less highly specialized; but *bureaucratic* prose is often arhythmic and utilizes a specialized vocabulary. The effect of free verse is to break down the syntactical rhythms of prose without replacing them by meter, and free verse generally employs a narrow range of vocabulary, topic, and genre – mostly lyric descriptions of private and personal impressions.

The implications for education are very important. If we wish to develop the full powers of the minds of the young, early and continuous exposure to the best metered verse is essential, for the higher human values, the cognitive abilities of generalization and pattern recognition, the positive emotions, such as love and peacefulness and even a sophisticated sense of time and timing are all developed by poetry. Furthermore, our ethnocentric bias may be partly overcome by the study of poetry in other languages and the recognition of the underlying universals in poetic meter.

Φαίνεταί μοι κῆνος ἴσος θέοισιν
ἔμμεν' ὤνηρ, ὄττις ἐνάντιός τοι
ἰσδάνει καὶ πλάσιον ἆδυ φωνεί-
σας ὐπακούει

καὶ γελαίσας ἰμέροεν, τό μ' ἦ μὰν
καρδίαν ἐν στήθεσιν ἐπτόαισεν,
ὠς γὰρ ἔς σ' ἴδω βρόχε' ὤς με φώναι-
σ' οὐδ' ἒν ἔτ' εἴκει,

ἀλλ' ἄκαν μὲν γλῶσσα ἔαγε λέπτον
δ' αὔτικα χρῷ πῦρ ὐπαδεδρόμηκεν,
ὀππάτεσσι δ' οὐδ' ἒν ὄρημμ', ἐπιρρόμ-
βεισι δ' ἄκουαι,

ἔκαδε μ' ἴδρως ψῦχρος κακχέεται τρόμος δὲ
καῖσαν ἄγρει, χλωροτέρα δὲ ποίας
ἔμμι, τεθνάκην δ' ὀλίγω 'πιδεύης
φαίνομ' αι

ἀλλὰ πὰν τόλματον ἐπεὶ καὶ πένητα

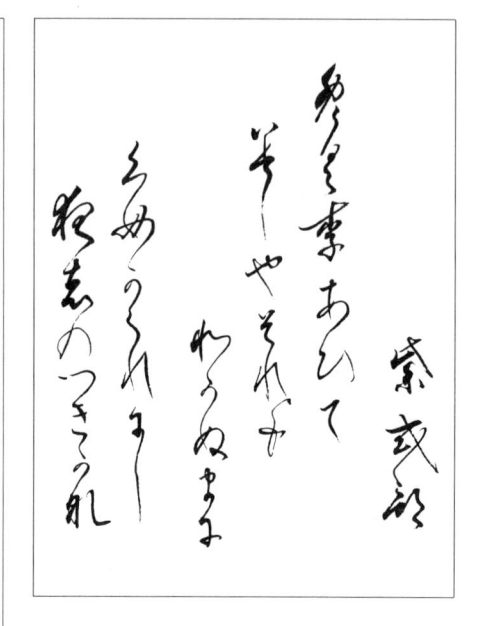

S'amor non è, che dunque è quel ch'io sento?
ma s'egli è amor, per Dio, che cosa e quale?
Se bona, ond'è l'effetto aspro mortale?
se ria, ond'è sí dolce ogni tormento?

S'a mia voglia ardo, ond'è 'l pianto e lamento?
s'a mal mio grado, il lamentar che vale?
O viva morte, o dilettoso male,
come puoi tanto in me, s'io nol consento?

E s'io 'l consento, a gran torto mi doglio.
Fra sí contrari venti in frale barca
mi trovo in alto mar senza governo:

sí lieve di saver, d'error sí carca,
ch'i' medesmo non so quel ch'io mi voglio,
e tremo a mezza state, ardendo il verno.

Fig. 1 Examples of metered poetry.

- Sappho, 6th century B.C., Greek *(Thalmayr A, Das Wasserzeichen der Poesie. Franz Greno, Nördlingen 1985).*
- Murasaki Shikibu, 11th century, Japanese *(Calligraphy. Maruyama Takao, Tokyo, 1988).*
- Hafez, 14th century, Persian *(Diwan-e-Hafez. Eqbal, Teheran).*
- Francesco Petrarca, 14th century Italian *(Thalmayr A, Das Wasserzeichen der Poesie. Franz Greno, Nördlingen 1985).*

Metered Poetry, the Brain, and Time

Amar el día, aborrecer el día,
   llamar la noche y despreciarla luego,
   temer el fuego y acercarse al fuego,
   tener a un tiempo pena y alegría.

Estar juntos valor y cobardía,
   el desprecio cruel y el blando ruego,
   tener valiente entendimiento ciego,
   atada la razón, libre osadía.

Buscar lugar en que aliviar los males
   y no querer del mal hacer mudanza,
   desear sin saber que se desea.

Tener el gusto y el disgusto iguales,
   y todo el bien librado en la esperanza,
   si aquesto no es amor, no sé qué sea.

شوق ہر رنگ رقیبِ سر و ساماں نکلا
قیسِ تصویر کے پردے میں بھی عریاں نکلا
زخم نے داد نہ دی تنگیِ دل کی، یا رب
تیر بھی سینۂ بسمل سے پَر افشاں نکلا
بُوئے گل، نالۂ دل، دودِ چراغِ محفل
جو تری بزم سے نکلا سو پریشاں نکلا
دلِ حسرت زدہ تھا مائدۂ لذّتِ درد
کام یاروں کا بقدرِ لب و دنداں نکلا
تھی نو آموزِ فنا ہمّتِ دشوار پسند
سخت مشکل ہے کہ یہ کام بھی آساں نکلا
دل میں پھر گریے نے اِک شور اٹھایا غالبؔ
آہ جو قطرہ نہ نکلا تھا، سو طوفاں نکلا

Ворон к ворону летит,
Ворон ворону кричит:
Ворон! где б нам отобедать?
Как бы нам о том проведать?

Ворон ворону в ответ:
Знаю, будет нам обед;
В чистом поле под ракитой
Богатырь лежит убитый.

Кем убит и от чего,
Знает сокол лишь его,
Да кобылка вороная,
Да хозяйка молодая.

Сокол в рощу улетел,
На кобылку недруг сел,
А хозяйка ждет милого
Не убитого, живого.

Mit gelben Birnen hänget
Und voll mit wilden Rosen
Das Land in den See,
Ihr holden Schwäne,
Und trunken von Küssen
Tunkt ihr das Haupt
Ins heilignüchterne Wasser.

Weh mir, wo nehm ich, wenn
Es Winter ist, die Blumen, und wo
Den Sonnenschein,
Und Schatten der Erde?
Die Mauern stehn
Sprachlos und kalt, im Winde
Klirren die Fahnen.

- Maria de Zayas y Sotomayor, 17th century, Spanish *(Thalmayr A, Das Wasserzeichen der Poesie. Franz Greno, Nördlingen 1985)*.
- Ghalib, 19th century, Urdu *(Diwan-e-Ghalib, No. 5. Taj Company Ltd., Lahore)*.
- Alexander Pushkin, 19th century, Russian *(Thalmayr A, Das Wasserzeichen der Poesie. Franz Greno, Nördlingen 1985)*.
- Friedrich Hölderlin, 19th century, German *(Hölderlin. Sämtliche Werke. Insel, Frankfurt a. M., 1965)*.

It may well be that the rise of utilitarian education for the working and middle classes, together with a loss of traditional folk poetry, had a good deal to do with the success of political and economic tyranny in our times. The masses, starved of the beautiful and complex rhythms of poetry, were only too susceptible to the brutal and simplistic rhythms of the totalitarian slogan or advertising jingle. An education in verse will tend to produce citizens capable of using their full brains coherently – able to unite rational thought and calculation with values and commitment.[11]

Acknowledgements

The authors would like to acknowledge the valuable editorial assistance of Arthur Redding and Barbara Herzberger.

References and Notes

1. Fraser JT (1975) Of time, passion, and knowledge. Braziller, New York Fraser JT, Lawrence N, Whitrow GJ (eds)(1972, 1975, 1978) The study of time, vols I-III. Springer, New York
2. Laughlin CD, d'Aquili EG (1974) Biogenetic structuralism. Columbia University Press, New York
   D'Aquili EG, Laughlin CD, McManus J (eds) (1979) The spectrum of ritual: A biogenetic structural analysis. Columbia University Press, New York
   Berlyne DE, Madsen KB (eds) (1973) Pleasure, reward, preference: Their nature, determinants, and role in behavior. Academic, San Diego
   Routtenberg A (ed) (1980) Biology of reinforcement: Facets of brain stimulation reward. Academic, San Diego
   Olds J (1977) Drives and reinforcements: Behavioral studies of hypothalamic functions. Raven, New York
3. Eibl-Eibesfeldt I (1970) Ethology. Holt Rinehart, New York
4. Turner F, Pöppel E (1983) The neural lyre: Poetic meter, the brain, and time. Poetry vol CXLII, 5: 211–309
5. Wimsatt WK (1972) Versification: Major language types. New York University Press, New York
6. op.cit. D'Aquili et al., pp 117–151
7. "Ergotrophic" refers to the whole pattern of connected behaviors and states that characterize the aroused state of the body, including an increased heart rate and blood flow to the skeletal muscles, wakefulness, alertness, and a hormone balance consistent with "fight or flight" acitivities. "Trophotropic" refers to the corresponding system of rest, body maintenance, and relaxation: decreased heart rate, a flow of blood to the internal organs, an increase in the activity of the digestive process, drowsiness, and a hormone balance consistent with sleep, inactivity, or trance.
8. op.cit. Laughlin and d'Aquili, p 144
9. op.cit. d'Aquili et al., pp 152–182
10. ibid d'Aquili et al., pp 183–215
11. Sidney P (1969) The defence of poetry. In : Kimbrough R (ed) Selected prose in poetry. Reinhart and Winston, New York, p 110

Tempo Relations in Music: A Universal?[1]

David Epstein
*Department of Music, Massachusetts Institute of Technology,
Boston, Mass., USA*

Performing musicians devote a good deal of their time to concerns about tempo. Small wonder, for tempo exerts one of the most powerful controls in music, affecting everything that will occur in the performance of a work. Curiously, for a musical factor so far-reaching in its scope, tempo is also a factor with the largest degree of variability in music. By contrast, for example, we can "bend" the pitches of a piece only minimally in the interests of intonation. The margin is small between "coloring" a note in this way and rendering it simply "out of tune." Likewise, we can bend the rhythms of a phrase only slightly for purposes of expressive nuance. Beyond a certain point, these changes distort the rhythmic shape inherent in the phrase. Again, the margin of variability is small.

Tempo, on the other hand, enjoys a much broader range of possibilities that we consider appropriate. Toscanini's Beethoven symphonies were on the fast side; Klemperer's were notably slow. Both made convincing performances of these works. Were the tempos of both men "right"? Where does the "truth" lie?

The question becomes all the more enigmatic when we consider tempo – that is, large-scale time durations – in contrast to rhythm, which involves durations on a smaller scale. The second movement of Beethoven's *Eroica* Symphony, for example, was marked by the composer as M.M. 80, a beat lasting 3/4 second, or 750 milliseconds (ms). Yet it is not uncommon to hear the movement played as slowly as M.M. 60, the beat thus a second long. Each tempo, as part of a strong musical concept, can be convincing.

Clearly our psychological sense of time, as it relates to musical character and affect, bears greatly upon these questions. Psychological perceptions of this kind are difficult to quantize, however, leaving us to seek some standard by which to convey a "right" sense of time and tempo to fellow musicians, especially via the printed medium of a score. Yet "right" tempo is a universal concern, for without it a performance is doomed. Tempo exerts a master control over the unfolding of all elements in a work – themes, phrases, harmonic progressions, sections, overarching relations, and proportions. Unfolded at the "right" pace, these fit together naturally. Our physiology, on whose coordination this performance depends, also functions naturally. In brief, we breathe, and so does the music.

The search for the right tempo involves a mixture of musical intuition and received information, communicated in a score by verbal description or metronome indications. Uncertainty seems to remain the product of it all. Intuitions vary. The vocabulary of tempo lacks a universal standard. (Allegro in Mozart, for example, suggests a faster tempo than allegro in Brahms.) Tempos conveyed by words often refer to musical character as much as they do to speed. (How do we convert "Allegro energico e passionato" – Brahms, Symphony No. IV, mvt.4 – into pace *per se* ?)

Nor are the precise, unambiguous markings of the metronome a solution. As all musicians know, this clocklike precision may or may not convey the complexities that inhere in a concept of tempo. Metronome markings become manditory at the peril of the music itself, for unspoken questions linger behind the comforting certainty of these numbers.

Did the composer, for example, sing just the opening bars of a movement to determine the marking? If so, how shall we deal with tempo fluctuations that inevitably occur later within the movement? Or did the composer take account of these fluctuations, arriving at an average tempo for his marking? Is the marking intended as an absolute or an approximation? Has the composer indicated this? (Rarely so, in nineteenth-century music.) Were these markings rechecked in mornings, afternoons, and evenings, when physical and psychological states may have varied, with a corresponding effect upon the perception of tempo? Were tempos checked against acoustics of differing halls? Do the tempos fit modern instruments? Was the composer's metronome itself accurate? Beethoven's, to cite one famous case, is believed not to have been – which casts light upon his often fast markings.

Another approach to questions of tempo offers solutions that embrace many of these concerns. This is the concept of proportional tempo, otherwise described as the theory of continuous pulse. Indeed, this inner pulse is the essence of music – and the quintessence of this study. The theory suggests that in works of different movements, or in single-movement works that contain different tempos (a classical overture, for example, with a slow introduction and subsequent allegro), all tempos are intrinsically related to one another. The relationships arise from the creator's conception of the work as a unified and coherent whole, in which all movements and ideas stem from underlying formative concepts of shape. Thematic contours and rhythmic form are aspects of this shape. So, too, is the inner pulse that gives rise to tempo.

These relationships of tempo can be expressed by whole number ratios (i.e. integral ratios). They are, moreover, ratios of a low order (1:1, 1:2, 2:3, 3:4, or the inverse). In this sense, the introduction to a classical overture might well be twice as slow as the subsequent allegro, thus related as 2:1.[2]

The mathematics of this is simple and serves as nothing more than a concise expression of a musical relationship. The musical notation of this relationship can often appear confusing, however (what note-value equals what other note-value); hence the value of depiction by ratio.

These relations suggest yet deeper aspects. For example, movements are bound together in their pacing by sub-pulses, which remain constant. In this manner, these inner sub-units of tempo serve to organize and to bind different parts of a work into a whole. They are felt as musical entities throughout. The theory further recognizes that there is not *one* feasible tempo alone for a given movement, or segment of a movement. A range of workable tempos exists (though it may be a limited range). In planning for a coherent performance, an artist must consider not only the possible tempos of individual movements but tempos that, through a continuous pulse, can further integrate all movements. On occasion, one movement in particular may demand a specific tempo. All else must be planned by working forwards and backwards from this point to interrelate the tempos of all other movements.

This is not a matter of music alone but of our biological system as well. This system has entrained[3] within it the beat or pulse that pervades the music. This beat remains a constant, embedded in the time clocks of our system. We organize these beats, or groups of beats or sub-beats, into collections that form the various tempos of a work.

There is a biological basis for pacing and tempo in the performance of music, which has psychological ramifications of the deepest sort. Pulse, and relationships of pulse, are a powerful unifying force in the organization of a work and in its presentation to an audience via performance. So powerful is this element of pulse that, if one violates it by distortion of tempo, one risks an unsuccessful performance. The performer seems to be violating not a "musical" factor alone, but a biological one as well, one which sets ground limits to our aesthetic perceptions. Thus the implications of this theory rapidly broaden to involve not just music but biology, as well as the understanding of our biological system and the feelings, pleasures, and experience of these sensations – in other words, aesthetics, communication, and so on.

Musicians have long been aware of this theory of temporal proportions, which has been the subject of a number of studies. It was developed at some length in sections of my book Beyond Orpheus[4], which was based on the instrumental music of the classic-romantic period (from Mozart and Haydn through Brahms and Mahler), the purview limited to the seminal German-Austrian (Viennese) tradition.

Clearly, however, this awareness of tempo relations is demonstrable on a broader plane. Much contemporary music is explicit about such relations of tempo, often depicting them in modern scores via quasi-mathematical formulations. Late medieval and Renaissance musicians were also concerned with this question, and many discussed it in their writings about music.[5] We are still not always certain what aspects of temporal change in Renaissance music are meant to be equal to other aspects. For example, do beats equal beats, or do metrical groupings equal different rhythmic figurations that follow them as this music goes from perfect (triple) to imperfect (duple) time? Nor is it clear whether these relationships signalled a universal practice in all European countries or in all eras. What *is* clear, however, is an awareness that some element of time, be it beat or another unit, serves as a constant in such transition, thus giving proportion and continuity to the music. It is just this fact that is our principle concern here.

In 1979 the ethologist, Irenäus Eibl-Eibesfeldt suggested that I might study the music of non-Western cultures to see whether these tempo relations, which I had found so constant in the music of Mozart, Brahms, etc. might be found in other musical traditions as well – whether, in fact, they might constitute a universal musical practice. Thus I studied, at the Max-Planck-Institut at Seewiesen, musical tapes from a number of non-Western cultures made during field work in these locations by members of the Institut staff.

To one steeped in the music of the Western tradition, especially its last three to four centuries, the initial suggestion came as something of a shock that the music of non-Western cultures, many of them of a way of life lacking the technological levels and intercultural contacts of the West, might have significant points in common with Western "classical" music. In brief, what could the music of Mozart have in common with, for example, an Eipo tribesman from the remote mountain highlands of New Guinea, whose contact with the world did not exceed relations with a neighboring tribe three kilometers away and whose physical life was not far removed from Stone-Age technology? Yet to Eibl-Eibesfeldt, whose career had been spent studying universal modes of behavior across varying cultures, such a suggestion seemed normal. He seems to have been proven right, as this study indicates, and I am greatly indebted to him for a suggestion that has opened many musical perspectives.

This report, then, deals with tempo in the music of seven non-Western cultures (or, more precisely, six cultures, one of them yielding musical examples from two sub-cultures in different geographical areas – the !ko and G/wi tribes of the bushmen in the Kalahari desert of Botswana, Africa). In all cases, the focus of inquiry was whether these musical traditions, as judged by the examples studied, show a practice similar to Western music in making tempo changes that can be characterized as proportional, the tempos lying in simple integral ratios to one another, integral ratios of a low order.

The theory behind this study involves several points, of which integral ratios are one. The theory itself can be simply stated:

1. Music is performed by means of a steady beat. The beat duration that is established and maintained is what we know as tempo.
2. This beat (tempo) is entrained within the "clock" mechanism(s) of our biological system.
3. If tempos change, either within a piece (i.e., a slow introduction and an allegro within one movement) or among many movements of differing tempos in a multimovement work, the various tempos will relate to each other by means of low order integral ratios, i.e., ratios of 1:2, 2:3, 3:4, or their inverse.

Point 3 assumes abrupt changes or juxtapositions of differing tempos. There are, however, other means of altering tempos. Paramount among them are: 1) rubato[6], 2) similar but less formalized modes of "playing" with tempo within a phrase, such as advancing the pulse or delaying the pulse in its arrival at some critical point, and 3) acceleration or slowing down from one tempo to another. We really know very little about these kinds of tempo changes, although they permeate our repertoire and are fundamental to our modes of performance and to the meaning and feeling of many musical works.

Rubati, for example, depart from the ground pulse of a work only to return to synchrony with this pulse, although the ways in which this is done need extensive study. *Accelerandi* or *ritardandi* between two tempos likewise embody the principle of proportion in unique fashion: The "departure" and "arrival" tempos framing these changes are very likely in simple integral proportion one to another. The mode of change, if done as high art, will involve a steady, small increment or decrement of pulse, beat by beat, until the new tempo is reached. The effect should thus be unobtrusive, natural, inevitable. This is a fascinating and complex process, for it involves several orders of tempo, all under the simultaneous control of our internal timing mechanisms. The beginning and the "goal" tempos, proportionally related, and the step-by-step decrement or increment of tempo toward the goal are really a measured calculus of change.

Often this process, in the *poco a poco ritard* (or *accelerando*) passages of Mahler or Tschaikovsky, may cover as much as a minute of real time. Complex as this phenomenon is, it takes place routinely in the making of music.

One of the signs of a truly gifted performer is his or her ability to make these changes with even increments or decrements of beat.

We can tolerate divergence from a master beat only at certain places in a work. Usually these are in the midst of phrases. Strict tempo relationships and strict fidelity to a governing beat must also be present at critical places. These are most common at the beginnings of phrases and at those points where tempos change abruptly. If we do not feel beat and ratio exactly at these moments, the music feels thrown out of proportion – out of temporal alignment. In this sense, it seems not to function, one of the parts does not fit properly. The result, in terms of feeling, or aesthetics, is a sense of impropriety or discomfort.

With these points as a theoretical framework, let us consider the investigation of music from seven different non-Western cultures viewed with respect to tempo.[7] Two preliminary considerations immediately arose in this study and had to be resolved. One was the problem of accurate time measurement itself. A second was finding criteria that could be used to judge whether two tempos were in *significant* relation to one another if their proportions deviated somewhat from the low-order integral ratios that are our concern here. In brief, *how much of a deviation is or is not significant*, and how is this to be determined?

Time Measurement

The problem of accurate time measurement turned out to be complex and difficult to solve. The first approach was to use a high-quality electronic stopwatch calibrated to hundredths of a second. It was not an ideal solution. Though the machine may have performed with great accuracy, the performer running the machine (myself) was prey to the usual well-known human failings involving accurate measurement. For if I snap the watch "on" and "off" to measure a beat, I must know if I snapped accurately right on the beat or not. There is no way to know, other than intuition, and there is no way to recheck the matter, for the moment has passed. Thus it became clear early in this study that timing data measured by stopwatch – in the absence of any other mode of measurement – might not be reliable.

The second approach developed was that of tape measurement. This technique, used in editing audio tape for phonograph recordings, turned out to be highly accurate. It involves listening for the point on an audio tape at which the note is articulated. The tape recorder is then stopped and the reels turned by hand, drawing the tape slowly over the playback head. Moving forward, one hears the abrupt starting-point of the note. Then, going in reverse, one hears a crescendo of sound leading to an abrupt cut-off at the attack point. By going back and forth continually, one can "zero in" on the attack point, mark it with a pencil, and then pass the pencilled point on the tape over the head to check whether the mark coincides with the attack. The mark can be endlessly rechecked and its accuracy refined. The same measurement is made for the next attack, and the distance between the two points is measured with a millimeter ruler. The distance is placed as the numerator of a fraction whose denominator is 190.5 mm (7.5 inches per second tape speed). The resulting number, carried out to three decimal places, gives the duration of the beat in milliseconds.

This mode of measurement seems accurate to within one millimeter, which, at a tape speed of 190.5 mm per second, means accuracy to within 5 ms. As will be seen in the following pages, this is well below what currently is regarded as the threshold of aural temporal perception. Thus these measurements seem highly reliable.

A fortuitous experience occurred while studying one of the pieces: Stopwatch measurements were made for eight successive beats. Subsequently, the tape measurement method was adopted, and these same eight beats were remeasured by that method. The highly accurate tape-measured durations were compared with stopwatch timings, and the latter were found to be 94.9% accurate. If this approximately 5% error is seen in relation to tape measurement timings, themselves accurate to within 1 mm (5 ms), then the stopwatch timing error is within 5% × 5 ms, or 0.00025 s (1/4 ms) – obviously a quantum of time of no consequence here.

There are other ways in which these measurements might be taken, for example, with an oscillograph. Intuitively we might expect that the rise point in a sound wave could easily be seen and determined as the attack point of a beat. Presumably this would be highly accurate and easily measurable. In reality, however, musical wave forms (the result of the amplitudes, various frequencies, overtones, and irregular envelopes) are exceedingly complex. Finding the attack point in these forms is extremely difficult; one cannot be sure of a correct reading. Thus, the oscillograph method turns out not to be viable.

Criteria Regarding Significant Deviations from Tempo Ratios

We come now to the question of deviation from a ratio, in terms of real time, and the further question of whether or not the quanta of time involved in this deviation are significant. We are dealing here with people, not machines. While human time systems are remarkably accurate, they are not like the cesium clock that sits in the Natural Bureau of Standards, functioning with an error of less than one second per year. How, then, are we to determine whether tempos are in significant relation to one another if, when measured to such great accuracy, they turn out to miss being in integral ratio by some (small) amount of time? How small (or large) can this amount of time be? And how are we to judge the importance or nonimportance of this deviation from an absolutely accurate ratio?

The question needs discussion: Let us suppose a performance, for example, where we find that the tempo (T_1) before a change is measured as 0.96 s per beat. The beat following the change of tempo turns out to be 0.49 s (T_2). Had it been 0.48 s, it would have been in an exact ratio of 2:1, with no deviation from this integral ratio. In reality, the second beat, 0.49 s, deviates from an integral ratio by a difference which can be expressed in two ways. One is by percentage; the 2:1 ratio is off by approximately 2% (1/48). The second mode of expression concerns the real time deviation of tempo T_2. This quantum of time can then be viewed and judged against the minimum amount of time we can truly perceive in temporal succession. Thus, we can say that this tempo deviates from a ratio of 2:1 by 10 ms. The significant question is: What does 10 ms represent? Is it a significant deviation from the absolute ratio or a nonsignificant deviation? What criteria can we use?

One criterion is the so-called "perception window" for temporal perception, which psychologists find to lie somewhere between 20 and 40 ms. This period may be the minimal level of perceptible time differences. Another criterion may be the "order threshold," that is, the minimum amount of time required for one to distinguish that one of two sounds comes either first or second, i.e., the *order* or *succession* of sounds.[8]

We also know from psychophysical studies that somewhere around 40 Hz – in other words, with a series of clicks given at a rate of about 40 per second – we begin to perceive these clicks not as separate sounds, but as pitch. At some point, time changes its face; our perception changes from one of duration to one of pitch. How critical is this? And if the critical frequency for this changed mode of perception lies around 40 clicks per second (cps), which would be 25 ms per click, then how should we regard temporal events separated by less than 25 ms? Are they perceptible *as* durational events?

It is essential to determine which of these various criteria we should choose in judging whether a discrepancy from an absolute ratio – for example, a discrepancy of 10 ms, constitutes a significant amount of time or an insignificant amount of time. The following observations seem pertinent: Some of the above data concerning time perception were derived from experiments made with timed clicks given in direct succession, in a laboratory environment where no context pertained other than the objective experimental condition. Judgements by the subjects in these experiments took place in a time frame of seconds.

By contrast, the musical examples discussed here are set in more complex frames of context. Furthermore, in the music in this study, the differences in elapsed time between contrasting tempos range anywhere from 30 s to 5 min. Time perception over such a durational framework is a totally different phenomenon from that of the laboratory tests referred to here. The signals used in these laboratory tests might well be called "dull time": Clicks are identified as longer or shorter, closer together or farther apart. In a certain sense, who cares? Time (and, of course, tempo) in music, however, involves time that is psychologically rich – time filled with experience. Our perception of that time and our psychological sense of that time is totally different from the bland time of an unchanging frequency given for a number of milliseconds.

We are continually forced here to think about time in its absolute, or mechanical, sense as well as time in its musical and psychological sense. These two different phenomena make even more difficult the question of where to place a lower limit on the time period that separates perceptible time quanta from those that are imperceptible – as well as the question of how this limit is to be determined. How high is this threshold of time perception? Moreover, what does it mean? Do we use criteria established from "absolute" time-empty time, a beat with no interest – as opposed to musically filled time? The criteria are indeed difficult to establish.

For the purpose of this study, I have set 20 ms as the criterion by which to make judgements. In other words, time quanta below 20 ms, such as a discrepancy in integral tempo proportions, were considered imperceptible. A deviation at or above 20 ms presumably is perceptible – hence the term perception threshold *(*PT*)* for the 20 ms quantum. However, it is important to note that this 20-ms barrier is relatively arbitrary, based upon laboratory studies far more than upon conditions and contexts that would seem to prevail in the performance of real music. Discrepancies in tempo ratios that meet these seemingly over-severe standards, however, must be insignificant by those less definable but more complex and flexible criteria that obtain with real music.

The Weber Fraction (WF), which has become a standard of measurement in experimental and behavioral psychology, may be a more relevant criterion in these studies than measurements of real-time differences. Both criteria are used here.

The nineteenth-century physicist, E.H. Weber, investigated how great the quantitative difference (or just noticeable difference) in stimuli must be in the various sensory systems for that difference to be perceived. How much more intense, for example, must a light be before the change in brightness can be recognized; how much heavier a weight before its difference is felt, etc.? Weber found that the various sensory systems have different thresholds and that the threshold for each system is not an absolute quantity, but a percentage of the stimulus itself. This percentage has become known as the Weber Fraction.

Weber's findings were elaborated by a younger colleague, G.T. Fechner, whose book *The Elements of Psychophysics* (1860)[9] was one of the major early works in the field. Weber's investigations were further pursued by the famous physicist, Ernst Mach, who was one of the first to test the Weber Fraction with respect to auditory time perception.[10] A recent test with respect to audition was made by David Getty, using mathematical techniques and electronic equipment for sound generation and for timing that were unavailable to Mach and other earlier scientists interested in Weber's findings.[11]

Weber found that, in the auditory perception of time, a stimulus would have to change by approximately 5% within a period of about 0.4 s – 2.0 s for the change to be perceived. The tests by Mach and Getty arrived at quite similar figures. Interestingly, the percentage is significantly higher for periods under 0.25 s and over 2 s. What we have earlier termed "deviation" is in fact an index that can be measured against the Weber Fraction to determine significant or insignificant deviation. A deviation less than the Weber Fraction would presumably be insignificant.

Like the 20-ms criterion, the Weber Fraction was arrived at through tests under laboratory conditions, not under circumstances of musical performance. Like the perception threshold, the Weber Fraction may impose stricter limits than found in the performance of music. Since the data in these studies largely satisfy these very strict criteria, the evidence is all the more convincing.[12]

Case Studies

Having established means of time measurement and criteria for determining significant deviations in tempo ratios, other questions arise. The first concerns universals: Anthropologists generally consider a sample of five cultures as minimal to determine a universal phenomenon, if the samples represent a good geographical distribution and a minimal-to-nil chance of intercultural influence exists. This study sampled seven cultures, with a geographical distribution of two from the Pacific, two from Asia, two from Africa, and one from South America. Furthermore, and very important, this is an unbiased set of samples. Available tapes were heard in random order.

The examples that follow come from the !ko and G/wi groups in the Kalahari desert of Africa, from a Tibetan monastery, from the Navari cast of Nepal, from the Yanomami Indians in the Orinoco River region of South American (Venezuela), from the Medlpa of the Papua coastal region of New Guinea, and from the Eipo of the mountainous central highlands of New Guinea (see also chapter 2).

!ko, Kalahari Desert, Botswana: Honey Badger Dance

The honey badger is a small, fierce animal of this region – so fierce that even lions and tigers avoid it. The honey badger dance seems to be a symbolic ritual of defiance towards this aggressive animal on the part of the dancers. They dance with great spirit and sense of fun, one person out of a group of 10 or 11 serving as the honey badger and making charge-like forays against his "foes." The others make passes, or sorties, at him, often leap-frogging over him.

The dance was seen on film and was already under way before filming had begun. The dancers, in a whispered sort of grunt, articulated a jazz-like rhythm (♩ ♩ ♫ ♩) whose tempo was consistently steady. After 59 s on the film, this episode of the dance ended, and the dancers rested for 1 min and 57s. They then began to dance again. In this way, the dance went on for about a half an hour, although only ten minutes of it were filmed.

Via the tape measurement technique described earlier, the duration of the first beat of the rhythmic motive was determined as chanted just before the rest period. The same beat in the motive was measured again as soon as the music began after the rest period. The duration of the beat, before and after the rest break, was 0.641 s – precisely the same tempo to within one ms. The tempos thus correlate 1:1, with no deviation.

It is also significant that, during the rest period of almost 2 min (1 min 57 s), the dancers showed no overt signs of continuing the beat – no foot-tapping, singing, etc. They lay on the ground to rest; they joked; the elder of the group, who was also a village elder, expressed annoyance because he felt the younger men were not performing the dance correctly; the others laughed at this and eventually resolved the argument; finally someone suggested they begin dancing again. The dance continued; clearly the pulse must have been internalized.

Tibet: Religious Ceremonial Music

The next example, Tibetan in origin, comes from the monastery in Dharamsala in the province of Himachal, Nepal, located just across the border from Tibet. Although this monastery is physically in Nepal, it is strictly Tibetan in its religious practice and is, in fact, the monastery where the Dalai Lama lives in exile. Annette Heunemann, of the research staff of the Max-Planck-Institut at Seewiesen, recorded this music during field work and made it available for these studies.

The music is a characteristic processional, recorded during a religious service. All celebrants were seated during the ceremony. This is important, for it suggests that there was little if any overt rhythmic entrainment – any kind of bodily motion – associated with the maintenance of tempo, a fact confirmed by Mrs. Heunemann. The music began with a group of men, in a baritone range, chanting in a manner that had no functional, felt, or in any way coordinated beat. After 29 s of this singing, a small orchestra of gongs and cymbals entered with music that was strongly rhythmic, whose beat duration could be clearly measured. This percussion stopped at 42 s of running time on the tape, and the singing began again as before, this time, however, with a chorus of children or young women – again with no perceptible rhythmic quality. Twenty seconds later the drums and cymbals entered once more.

The duration of the percussion beat heard the first time was 0.472 s. The duration of the percussion beat the second time was 0.231 s. These durations relate to each other as 0.489 (i.e., 0.472 : 0.231 = 0.489), which is a ratio of 2:1 (i.e. 0.472 : 0.236 = 0.5) with a deviation of 5 ms, or 2.1%. This amount of time is well below the threshold of perception, as defined earlier, and below the Weber Fraction, thus insignificant.

Nepal: Music from the Nevari Cast

This example, from Nepal, was from the religious music of the Nevari cast, played with percussion instruments and two flutes. Its tempo organization is quite fascinating: Within the total duration of 8 min and 8 s, the musicians, improvising on small motives, played passages at a steady tempo, and then began to accelerate. The points where these accelerations began were clear, as were their terminations, when a new tempo plateau was reached. Following a period in this new and stable tempo, another acceleration (or, at times, a ritard) followed, moving to yet another tempo level. There were also several points where a sudden tempo change was injected.

Twelve tempos were reached during this performance. Each tempo, as it followed the prior one, was in an integral, low-order ratio, with deviations in all instances that were below the level of perception. At the midpoint of the piece, a curious tempo "shift" occurred – almost a "hiccup" in tempo, which divided the piece in half. The tempo shifted via 4 : 3.5, or 8 : 7. The music at this point created the impression that the musicians were about to effect a change by a 4 : 3 ratio and somehow did not quite make it – they got only to the middle of the change, throwing the tempo out of phase by half a step.

Most fascinating of all, the ratio from the initial tempo to the final one is that of 3 : 2 (0.471 s : 0.325 s), with a discrepancy of -11 ms, or 3.5%, for the final tempo. Thus, although the piece was thrown out of phase in the middle, the tempo system functioned so precisely that from the beginning to the end, in over 6.5 min of time, the tempo ratio was exact, with a discrepancy below the level of perception as defined earlier by PT and WF.

Himou: Yanomami Indians, Orinoco River, Venezuela

The Yanomami Indians have a number of social customs that involve subtle and cautious "feeling out" procedures between individuals. One example is their custom for greeting strangers who come to the village. A respected village member will meet the stranger at the edge of the compound, speaking extensively with him until a point is reached where it is sensed that the newcomer has friendly intentions. Only then will he be welcomed.

The Himou is another such custom, studied extensively by the anthropologist Kenneth Good, a former member of the Seewiesen staff who has lived among the Yanomami. The Himou is a bargaining procedure, or, more precisely, it is the social intercourse of barter. It, too, involves extensive conversations before agreement is reached. It has more subtle psychological overtones as well, for during this ritual it is important that the "seller" not offend his fellow tribesman and potential "buyer" by asking so much for his property that he forces the other person to reveal that it is beyond his means, thus embarrassing him. By the same token, the buyer must not be driven to offend the seller – he must not be pushed to the point where he complains that the asking price is too great. There is thus much skirting around the central issue, as in all bargaining, although in this case, it follows the lines of ritualized decorum.

It is also a long-winded procedure. The Himou discussed here, recorded by Kenneth Good in 1979, lasted for over an hour, though Mr. Good's cassette tape ran out after 45 minutes. Almost 38 minutes of this tape was studied.

The Himou is a spoken affair, but it is a musical one as well, for its speech is chanted. It is in fact known as "bargain chant." The procedure is antiphonal, the seller stating a phrase that is echoed by the buyer, the alternation continuing at great length, always led by the seller. In this case, the seller's speech was exceptionally musical; it rhythmized and inflected very much like song. Moreover, it was organized in patterns, generally grouped in threes. Though his thoughts may have forced the seller's language to depart from this meter, he managed to return to it shortly. Thus, the entire ceremony had a musical cast – spoken in sung speech, indeed virtually directed by a truly virtuosic speaker, brilliant in his articulation and inflection.

As the seller proceeded along his discourse toward a point where a bargain seemed near, he became increasingly excited, with the result that the tempos of his speech fluctuated in speed. The first 18 min of this Himou were, in fact, a giant acceleration. In the virtually 38 min of the talk that were studied, 143 tempo timings were measured by stopwatch, each at a point where a tempo change was detected. These tempos and the points in the running time of the tape at which they occurred were then graphed, and the overall picture was studied by computer in various statistical modes to see what pattern provided the "best fit" for the data: that is, what pattern(s) most economically and pervasively characterized the varying tempos of the total performance.

The performance falls into four segments. Segments I and III are virtually exponential increases in tempo. Segment II is a positive linear regression, in other words, a continuous gradual slowing down. Segment IV is essentially a stable tempo.

A high degree of correlation, or pattern "fit," in all four segments is notable. Even more impressive are the tempo ratios within these patterns. The tempos in segment I not only accelerate "irrationally" or exponentially; they also reach temporary plateaus, or periods, when the beat oscillates at a rate that is almost steady, characterized by only minimal change. These plateaus fall into low-order integral ratios of 2:1 with minimal or, in one case, no deviation.

Segments II and III each move between tempo extremes in which the beat durations are 0.15 s – 0.30 s, that is, in an exact 1 : 2 ratio. The speed of 0.15 s at the end of segment III to that of 0.29 s at the start of segment IV, after a brief interruption, is also in a 1 : 2 relation, with a deviation of 10 ms, or 3.3% – a deviation below the PT and WF.

Two aspects of this performance and of this study may be of general significance. One is the rather remarkable fact that a performance lasting as long as 38 minutes, one influenced and even compelled by various emotions, moves through tempos that are tightly ordered by low-order integral ratios – so much so that discrepancies, or deviations from these ratios, are all below the level of perception. The second point of significance lies in the inherent exponential shapes of these tempo curves and their end points. They seem to confirm the intuition of many musicians that tempo changes, whether "irrational" or graduated by some calculus of change, take place within controlled or ordered limits. They function, that is, in relation to some governing pulse.

G/wi Group of the Bushmen People, Kalahari Desert, Botswana: The Dongo Player

The Bush people of the Kalahari Desert are a musical people. We have already seen one example of this in the honey badger dance of the !ko. The G/wi, like the !ko, are a subculture of the Bush people. The two peoples are of different and mutually unintelligible language groups, although they have limited intercultural contact.

The dongo is an African "finger piano." It consists of five or six strips of metal, each about 1/4 inch in width and of varying lengths, which lie parallel to one another, fastened to a wooden base at one end and passing over a low bridge with their other end free. The strips can be adjusted in length to give differing pitches, and the instrument is played by "plucking" the free end of the strips, or keys.

Some dongo players become quite virtuosic; the man whose music was studied here was rated by his fellow villagers as the second-best player in the village. By the standards of this Western observer, he was an impressive musician, very facile upon the instrument and possessing a keen rhythmic sense. The music itself abounds in jazz-like syncopations and asymmetrical meters of fives and sevens that interchange freely with more conventional duple and triple meters.

The music was continuously recorded over a period of 17 min 23 s. During the time of this performance, the musician played a piece and then stopped, retuned the dongo, improvised a few passages upon the retuned instrument, and continued with another piece. This went on for 11 pieces. In the course of each piece, the player either kept a steady tempo or altered tempos via accelerations and ritards to reach new tempos. Of all the tempos, 78% were in low-order ratios of 1 : 1, 2 : 3, or 3 : 4, most relating as 1 : 1.

Medlpa Group, Papua, New Guinea: Pig Exchange

The Medlpa live on the coastal region of Papua, New Guinea. The ceremony studied here involved a peace treaty with a neighboring group with whom the Medlpa had previously been at war. The war had been a bitter experience for both sides, so that this ceremony was a major event and an emotional experience in the lives of all concerned.

The ceremony consisted of a march by the former enemy into the settlement of the Medlpa. As part of this, the Medlpa were presented with some of the most choice possessions of the other group as peace offerings. Not surprisingly for a people living by agriculture, the proferred gifts were food, in this case pigs – some of the finest owned by the former enemy, thus constituting an offering of value and sacrifice.

As the visitors walked into the Medlpa community (from the sound of the proceedings caught on tape, it seemed like a large crowd of people walking in no particularly coordinated manner), they were accompanied by two distinct sets of drum beats. Within a time period of over 18 min 59 s, 16 different groups of slow beats were recorded.[13] The beats in each group were steady in tempo, and the average (mean) of these tempos was 1.11 s, with a standard deviation of 0.05 s (50 ms, or 4.5%). Of the beat durations (tempos) within this slow-beat group, 81.3% lay within ±1 standard deviation of the mean, and 9 of 16 cases (56.3%) lay below the threshold of perception.

The groups of fast beats on this tape occurred after periods of silence (no drums) that lasted from a minimum of 1 s to a maximum of 33 s. Six groups of fast beats were heard; the average duration of these beats was 0.36 s, with a standard deviation of 0.07 s (70 ms, or 19.4%). Here, too, a striking percentage of these beats (83.3%) lay within ±1 standard deviation of the mean (in a normal distribution, 68% of the cases would lie within ±1 standard deviation). Thus these figures correlated with the mean to a much higher degree than usual. Two cases (33%) of these fast beats lay below the threshold of perception. The percentage of variation from the mean was 68 ms, higher than most data in this study. Included in this mean, however, was one tempo duration of 0.497, which was a statistical exception ("outlier"). If this exception is disregarded, the mean and standard deviations fall within a much smaller range of tempo duration, and the variation from the mean turns out in real-time to be 11 ms.

The essential aspect of this data, as observed so far, is that within time periods that exceeded 19 min for the slow group of beats and more than 12 min for the fast tempo groups, 81%-83% of the beats varied from their average value by small amounts of time (within ±1 standard deviation), 9 cases varying by less than the threshold of perception. The fast beats, other than the exception, varied by 11 ms or 3.3%, well below PT and WF. The tempos of each group were constant (with the one exception) over these considerable time periods.

The two different tempo groups further correlate with each other. The fast beats in relation to the slow beats fall very close to a 3 : 1 ratio, deviating from this amount by 46 ms, or 12%. This amount of time is greater than deviations we have seen in other studies. Note, however, that the total duration of this recorded excerpt is over 12 min, during which the procession took place in a setting of much talking, general crowd noise, and the forward motion of large masses of people. To have deviated from an exact tempo ratio by 46 ms (12%) over this period of time and in these conditions hardly seems significant.

It is possible that 3 fast beats were conceived by the drummer as sitting within the time frame of 1 slower beat. This seems plausible, for in the sequence of beat groups as heard on the tape, the fast groups always follow the slow groups after a period of silence. It could be, therefore, that the drummer of the fast beats had as a reference the pacing of the slower beats just heard. It is striking that, if this were the case, 3 fast beats at an average speed of 0.36 s would fill a period of 1.08 s, only 0.03 s (or 30 ms, 2.7%) out of phase with the time frame of 1.11 s for the slower beat.

Eipo, New Guinea: Dance Festival

The Eipo are pygmies who live in the central highlands of New Guinea, a region surrounded by towering mountain peaks. The ethologists of the Max-Planck-Institut at Seewiesen have studied these people extensively, living among them for what at this writing amounts to a total of over 6 years.

The Eipo are a culturally distinct group from the Medlpa, studied earlier, although both groups live in New Guinea. They rarely travel more than 3 kilometers from their village, and this in large part to wage war with neighboring groups. Many hundreds of miles and 8000 feet in altitude lie between the Eipo village and the coast of New Guinea, the home of the Medlpa. The way is impeded by rugged mountains in all directions and dense jungle. It is thus unlikely that the music of the Eipo was culturally influenced by the Medlpa.

The music studied here took place during a festival that involved dancing and singing. Such festivals are common forms of celebration among the Eipo. They can last anywhere from 30 to 40 min to a whole evening. The entire village participates, performers numbering 40–50 people, primarily male. The festivities take place in the village center, where the performers dance for as much as 10–15 minutes, at the same time singing in a ritualized fashion. They then rest, while talking, laughing, etc., and again begin the same routine, alternating this way throughout the entire festival period.

These singing-dances were studied on audio tapes and on films. Two important points were clear from the films. First, when dancing, the performers as a group showed no distinctive rhythmic coordination. No unified dance pattern existed; dancers bobbed up and down in an unsynchronized fashion. Second, during the rest periods, no overt rhythmic activity could be discerned among the performers or among the others villagers present.

We will see shortly that the tempos of this festal singing and dancing were proportional. It seems from the two points observed above that these tempo relations must stem from some inner pulse and not from any explicit external act, such as a group-synchronized dance, song, clapping, etc.

The music for this dance festival consisted of three elements that followed a strict sequential order. They were, first, choral intonation, sounding something like a moan, which showed no beat or other rhythmic quality and was, thus, unmeasurable in terms of tempo; second, a kind of grunting, which was markedly rhythmic; third, a whistling made by inhaling through the nose.

Twenty-five minutes and 38 s of this music were studied from a festival that lasted throughout an evening. Tempos were measured from the grunting motive (16 samples) and from the whistling group (12 samples). The grunting motive, extending over a period of 13 min 18 s, showed an average tempo of

0.31 s, with a standard deviation of only 0.01 s (10 ms, 3.2%). Seventy-five percent of these beat durations lay within ±1 standard deviation of the mean tempo.

This is a rather remarkable phenomenon: in over 13 min, with all the distractions of dancing, pausing, talking, laughing, etc., these grunting motives, sung only intermittently, were all at virtually the same tempo, their tempo discrepancies (about 10 ms, 3.2%) lying well below PT/WF. The 12 samples of the whistling, extending over a time period of 11 min 46 s, show somewhat larger deviations from exact tempo ratios. The mean tempo of 0.641 s had a standard deviation of 0.077 s (77 ms, 12%); as with the grunting motive, 75% of the beats lay within one standard deviation of the mean. Of these 12 samples, however, only 4 had discrepancies from exact ratios that lay under the perception threshold. Finally, the two motives (grunting and whistling) were in precise temporal proportion, related by a ratio of 2 : 1, with a deviation of 11 ms (3.4%).

Summary and Conclusions

The data in these studies give the strong impression that tempos, when they changed in these various musics, changed by low-order integral ratios. This is seen in Table 1. Moreover, if the new tempo was not exactly in proportion, the deviation in the majority of cases was so small that it was below the threshold of perception. There is, however, no singular way in which this data can be analyzed, since the studies investigated a variety of musical settings in which tempos assumed various relationships and roles. The bases of the studies, therefore, were not uniform.

Only two tempos were studied in relationship, for example, in the !ko excerpt, whereas 143 tempo points comprise the Yanomami "Himou" case. The example from Nepal was of a straightforward linear nature, whereas the G/wi dongo player required a matrix of five different modes of analysis. The time periods in which all performaces took place vary from 1 min 30 s in the Tibetan example to some 4 hours in the overall duration of the Eipo festival.

Tables 1 and 2 represent two modes of data analysis. Table 1 uses as a criterion the 20 ms threshold of time perception (PT) for evaluating discrepancies from low-order integral tempo relations. Table 2 uses the Weber Fraction (WF) for the same purpose. Reading the tables horizontally provides a *per culture* summary in terms of PT (Table 1) and WF (Table 2). (For example, in the Yanomami Himou in Table 1, the 143 tempo points fall into six overall tempo ratios, 100% of which involve deviations less than PT.)

Table 1. Summary of deviations from low-order integral ratios in terms of a 20-ms threshold

Culture	No. cases (n)	Percentage of cases in which deviation (D) from ratio (in real time) was:			
		Below PT %	n	Above PT %	n
!ko	1	100	1		
Tibet	1	100	1		
Nepal	11	100	11		
Yanomami (Himou)	6**	100	6**		
G/wi	33***	94	30	6	3
Medlpa					
Slow beats	16	56	9	44	7
Fast beats	6	33	2	67	4
Ratios of beat groups	2	50	1	50*	1
Eipo					
Huh-huh	16	100	16		
Whistle	12	33	4	67	8
Ratios of huh-huh to whistle	1	100	1		
Total no. of cases	105		82		23

Notes for Table 1

1. * This figure includes an outlier.
   ** Total no. of time points = 143
   These fall into 6 proportional tempo relations characterized by integral ratios, as well as exponential curve- and straight-line regression-modes of acceleration and ritard.
   *** The data included here is a summary of four different modes which were used to analyze these 11 complex performances, whose pacing had various degrees of fluctuation. (The full data and analyses are found in the originally published article.) The modes were: a) the tempo difference from beginning to end of each piece, b) the tempo difference from beginning to beginning of successive pieces, c) the tempo difference from the end of one piece to the beginning of the next piece, and d) the overall tempo relationships from the beginning of Piece 1 to the end of Piece 11.
   In the data anlyzed here, 78% of the ratios lay in the category of the common low-order ratio of 1:1, 2:3, or 3:4, most of them relating as 1:1, as already recounted in the text. One case fell into a 4:5 ratio, and six cases (19%) were in ratios of 5:6 or 6:5. The ratios of 4:5 and 5:6/6:5 are somewhat anomalous, in the sense that they have appeared but rarely in the music of the other societies studied here and rarely in my earlier studies of tempo relationships in Western art music. Whether they are

true anomalies – "outliers" – that should not be considered as representing "valid" tempo proportions, or whether they are indeed valid but simply occur less frequently, is an open question. There is nothing intrinsically invalid about these proportions. They were, in fact, found quite often in music of the European Renaissance, and I discuss one such example in my study of Tschaikovsky's Fourth Symphony (publication forthcoming), to give but one sample from the "standard" repertory. In the present case, they seem the more likely in that many of the rhythms played by the dongo player fall into patterns of fives, alternating rapidly with patterns of twos and threes. These patterns could have provided a plausible set of heard and felt rhythmic proportions of 4:5 and 5:6, which in turn could have been the basis for these proportions as heard in the changes of tempo.
2. Total no. of cases $(n) = 105$
3. 78.1% of the total cases (82/105) include integral ratios with a deviation (D) below the threshold of perception (PT) of 20 ms
4. a) 21.9% (23/105) of the total cases include integral ratios with D above the 20 ms PT
   b) Of these 23 cases, 3 (from the G/wi) are D of 21–23 ms, just barely above what has been somewhat arbitrarily set for this study as the PT.
5. Of this data, therefore, 3 cases (in 4 b above) are marginal with respect to D<PT. These 3 marginal cases represent (3/105)=2.9% of n.
   Thus a more detailed spectrum with regard to D<PT would be:

$n=105$

D<PT	marginal D<PT	D>PT
78.1%	2.9%	19%

Reading the tables vertically provides a *cross-cultural* summary in terms of PT (Table 1) and WF (Table 2). In this case, all the data involved in the entire study are totalled, and the percentage deviations in tempo lying < PT and/or WF are determined. The notes to Table 1 suggest, particularly note 5, that 78.1% of the data are < PT, 2.9% are marginally at PT, and 19% lie above PT. As the notes to Table 2 indicate, 70.6% of the data are less than WF; 9.2% are marginally at WF. Thus, 79.2% are either less than or at WF.

The results are not significantly different by either mode of analysis. The striking correlation, however, is with tempos that relate so closely by these ratios that discrepancies from the ratios are imperceptible (variously, 78.1% or 79.8%). The study strongly supports the theory that tempos in musical performance change by low-order integral ratios.

There are many important aspects of this conclusion. For one, all the music studied was improvised in settings where conscious concern with specifics of tempo probably did not apply. Beyond the improvisational aspects of these instances, the distractions of ceremonies, dances, and social events would probably have precluded any thoughts the musicians might have about tempo *per se*, much less proportional relationships of tempos – if such arcane thoughts played a role in their music-making to begin with, which seems unlikely.

Tempo Relations in Music: A Universal?   111

Table 2. Summary of deviations from low-order integral ratios

Culture	No.cases (n)	Percentage of cases in which deviation (D) from ratio (in percentage) was:					
		Below WF		At WF margin		Above WF	
		%	n	%	n	%	n
!ko	1	100	1				
Tibet	1	100	1				
Nepal	11	100	11				
Yanomami (Himou)	6***	83	5	17	1		
G/wi	32	62.5	20	28.1	9	9.4	3
Medlpa							
Slow beats	16	100	16				
Fast beats	6	100**	5			16.6	1
Ratios of beat groups (See Table 1, item 4b)	2	100	1**			100	1*
Eipo							
Huh-huh	16	100	16				
Whistle	12					100	12
Ratio of huh-huh to whistle	1	100	1				
Total no.of cases	109		77		10		22

Notes for Table 2

1. * Including outlier
   ** Not including outlier
   *** Total no. of time points = 143. These fall into 6 proportional relations characterized by integral ratios, as well as exponential curve- and straight-line regression-modes of acceleration and ritard.

2. The discrepancy of n=33 (Table 1) and n=32 (Table 2) for the G/wi is explained by the fact that with one mode of comparison of the 11 pieces played by the dongo player (analysis mode D -see note *** in the notes for Table 1), discrepancies judged by Weber Fraction standards do not apply.

3. Total no.of cases (n) = 109. This includes calculations for Medlpa with and without outliers.

4. 70.6% of the total cases (77/109) include integral ratios with a deviation (D) < 5% (=D < WF).

5. 9.2% of the total cases (10/109) include integral ratios with a deviation (D) at 5%-7% (= D at WF margin).

6. 20.2% of the total cases (22/109) include integral ratios with a deviation (D) of +7% (= D > WF).

Secondly, the tempo-keeping phenomenon found in these studies – studies that cover six distinct cultures – agrees with the tempo proportions also found in Western classical music in studies carried out by myself and other theorists. Thus, we have virtually a worldwide geographical coverage with regard to this phenomenon – Africa, Asia, the Pacific, and South America (with multiple cases from the first three areas), to which can be added the art-music cultures of Europe and the practice of this European music in the New World. This data base and its geographical distribution more than fulfill the criteria usually demanded by anthropologists in determining whether a behavioral phenomenon may be universal. The evidence strongly supports the case for universality.

If in fact proportional tempo-keeping in music is universal, it seems inescapable that there must be a biological basis for this practice. The precision with which these proportions are rendered further supports the biological basis. It is hard to imagine even the most developed musical tradition effecting such precise proportions in tempo independent of some bodily system mechanically capable of this degree of exactitude.

The implications of this go further. There is an important psychological component allied with tempo and, therefore, with precise tempo correlations. We have seen earlier how a "right" tempo in performance seems to put "in place" so much else in the music. Associated with tempo are feeling, affect, and aesthetic perceptions and judgements, all of which relate to the tempo proportions discussed here. Tempo proportions, then, may in fact provide aesthetic constraints. Moreover, if a function of music is communication between performer and listener, then pulse (and thus tempo) may be a major component, if not *the* major component, in this communication. Pulse may well be the "carrier wave" upon which all else in music rides. If pulse and proportioned tempos are "wrong," imprecise, or unrelated, communication may be blocked or distorted.

It is notable in this study that proportional tempo is a constant – an unchanging factor – found in music of widely varying affect, emotional states, purposes, and settings: processionals, music for private entertainment (the G/wi dongo player), music of cermonies and large social gatherings (Medlpa, Eipo), of games (!ko), and even in the rhythms and tempi accompanying barter and bargain (Himou). This suggests a musical and an aesthetic *constant*, as well as the biological *constraint* mentioned above.

Last but hardly least, this study suggests an innate biological function as the foundation for a theory of tempo. Heretofore, tempo was exclusively musical in purview – i.e., a theory inferred from scores and their performance. Biology is a powerful foundation for this theory. We can always argue musical theories, which depend so much upon individual modes of perception. If there is a biological basis for such a theory, as this study suggests, the discussion moves to a higher plane of certainty, relevance, and significance.

Indeed, there may be a basis for telling a performer that if, for example, the tempos in a work of Mozart are not thought out and planned to relate proportionally, then the performance risks aesthetic failure. The playing may exceed fundamental parameters of perception intrinsic to our psychobiological make-up. Biological constraints may thus underlie musical performance and theories of performance. These constraints may further augment, as well as underlie, those other bases of authority, of tradition, and of intuition, which have heretofore been the sources of our musical training and musical thinking.

Another question arises from this discussion: Why, if proportional tempos are natural, does one hear some performances of Western art music where these relationships do not seem to apply?

A first response deals with what we might call "received tempos" – part of the "received knowledge" of our repertoire and its traditions. By the time most of us, as experienced musicians, come to prepare a work from this repertoire, we have heard it many times in concerts, rehearsals, and recordings. Its basic qualities are thus known to us, among them the "sound" of the music, how fundamentally it should "go," and what its general tempo ranges are. These basic properties of the score have been tried and tested by preceding generations. They form that unconscious (and often unquestioned) reference frame that often predetermines many of our initial thoughts and subsequent perceptions of the music. Tempo is no different in this respect than other aspects of the work, and we may well adopt without much concern the tempos that intuitively feel right. More often than not, these tempos *are* in the "right" range. Without a sense of the integral relationships and unifications that proportional tempos can provide, however, some tempos in the work may turn out more "right" than others. Again theory, if it is valid, can serve as a means to a more finely shaped and discerning concept of the music.

Second, the notion of competence and performance, as developed by Noam Chomsky[14] with regard to language, may be equally applicable to this area of music. Chomsky has determined that human beings everywhere possess an innate competence to understand grammar and syntax in language. It is this inborn ability that allows all of us to learn our native language as a part of our "natural" childhood development. Nevertheless, though virtually everyone learns his native tongue, individuals vary in the ability, complexity, and even elegance with which they speak ("perform") that language. Thus, performance varies within universal, innate competence.

This may also apply to music, specifically with tempo. We may well possess a universal competence to feel tempos in relation to a pulse and to relate that pulse itself in moments of changing tempos. The degree of precision (grace, elegance, fluency, etc.) with which we effect these tempo changes, however, may vary with our individual levels of performance. In brief, some of us are more gifted than others. Again, theory can serve as a guide for intuitions and perceptions, refining them and making them more precise, whatever one's initial gifts.

Obviously, much more must be learned about this subject, and the theory of proportional tempos itself needs greater elaboration than it has received here. This study suggests, however, that such a theory describes the inborn competence with which we feel tempo and tempo changes. It further suggests that this competence is universal and that our entrainment of tempo must lie within our biological system, with all the psychological, affective, and communicative consequences that this implies. It also seems that our aesthetic perceptions, as they affect our musical judgements and gestures, rest upon a physiological basis that exerts a precise and tightly regulated control upon our sense of tempo.

Acknowledgements

I am grateful to the Deutsche Forschungsgemeinschaft for a research grant during 1981-82, which made this study possible. I further wish to thank the Max-Planck-Institut für Verhaltensphysiologie in Seewiesen, West Germany, and Prof. Dr. Irenäus Eibl-Eibesfeldt, Director of its Forschungsstelle für Humanethologie, for the resources that provided the basis for this work and for Prof. Eibl-Eibesfeldt's initial suggestion that this subject be investigated. My thanks to Prof. Dr. Ernst Pöppel, Director of the Institut für Medizinische Psychologie of the University of Munich, and to Drs. Wolfgang Keeser, Wulf Schiefenhövel, and Polly Wiessner for their valuable help and suggestions.

References and Notes

1. A more extensive study on this subject has been published: Epstein D (1985) Tempo relations: A cross-cultural study. Music Theory Spectrum 7:34-71
2. Dealing with tempos related by proportion involves several steps. Step 1 consists of setting the two tempos (given in real-time durations of beat) in ratio to one another. The ratio should show the true progression through time of Tempo I leading to Tempo II, thus reading Tempo I : Tempo II. This is mathematically equivalent to Tempo I / Tempo II, and the two tempo values should be worked out by this formula, yielding a decimal that is, in effect, an index of the proportional relationship between the two tempos.
   When a musician makes such a transition in tempo, Tempo I, which is established at the outset of the piece, serves as a reference tempo. The subsequent tempo is

determined, that is, with reference to this initial tempo. Tempo II is the (new) goal tempo, which the player presumably achieves such that it is in meaningful proportion to Tempo I.

Obviously, any two tempos can be set in ratio to one another. What is significant in this study is that only low-number integers figure in these ratios. The ratios accepted here as workable are: 1:1, 1:2, 2:3, 3:4, and their inverse. The respective decimal equivalents are 1.0, 0.5, 0.67, and 0.75; the inverse being 1.0, 2.0, 1.5, and 1.33.

Having determined the proportion between two tempos, as described above, one next evaluates how close this proportion is to the accepted proportions just discussed. If it is close but not in 100-percent correspondence, it is of value to determine the extent of deviation.

Deviation has a special meaning in this study. It signifies the degree of discrepancy that the achieved Tempo II bears to the ideal Tempo II, the latter being in one of the proportions to Tempo I given above. This discrepancy (deviation, Δ) is given in percentage. In determining deviation, the difference between the ideal Tempo II and the actual Tempo II is found, and this difference is then set as the numerator of a fraction whose denominator is the ideal Tempo II.

This process is easily achieved by the following formula:

$$\Delta = \frac{t_2 - t'_2}{t_2}$$

where Δ = deviation; t_2 = ideal Tempo II; t'_2 = actual Tempo II

3. The term "entrainment" has only recently come into use in neurophysiological discourse. In this article, it refers to the process of perceiving a pulse and then, in effect, programming this pulse into our neuromuscular system. The simplest, most everyday example of this is the way we feel a pulse and then "beat time" with our foot.
4. Epstein D (1979) Beyond Orpheus: Studies in musical structure. MIT Press, Cambridge, Mass; Paperback edition (1987) Oxford University Press, Oxford
5. On this subject see:
   Apel W (1949) The notation of polyphonic music, from 900 – 1600. The Medieval Academy of America, Cambridge, Mass; Bank JA (1972) Tactus, tempo and notation in mensural music from the 13th to the 17th century. Annie Bank, Amsterdam; Dahlhaus C (1959) Über das Tempo in der Musik des späten 16. Jahrhunderts. Musica 13:767–769; Gullo S (1964) Das Tempo in der Musik des 13. und 14. Jahrhunderts. Haupt, Bern; Kümmel WF (1970) Zum Tempo in der italienischen Mensural-musik des 15. Jahrhunderts. Acta Musicologica 42 (3–4):150-163; Mertin J (1978) Alte Musik. Wege zur Aufführungspraxis. Lafite, Wien; Kümmel WF (1973) Tempoprobleme um den Tactus. Österreichische Musikzeitung 25:564–574; Planchart A (1981) The relative speed of tempora in the period of Dufay. Royal Music Association Research Chronicle 17:33 –51; Seay A (1981) The setting of tempos by proportions in the sixteenth century. The Consort 37:394–398
6. Rubato refers to fluctuations of speed within a musical phrase against a metrically steady background (beat).
7. More accurately, six cultures were studied, for as stated earlier, one of these cultures – the Bush people of the Kalahari Desert in Botswana, Africa – are represented by two sub-cultures: the !ko and the G/wi. These people are of different and mutually unintelligible language groups, although they do have limited intracultural contact.

It is questionable what effect this may have or have had over the centuries on the way either group keeps tempo in its music-making. These groups were selected for study, rather than a more broadly based selection, because tapes of their music were available, as was consultation with the anthropologists who had made these tapes during field trips.

8. Pöppel E (1978) Time perception. In: Held R, Leibowitz A-W, Teuber H-L (eds), Handbook of sensory physiology, vol. VIII, Perception. Springer, Berlin, pp 713–730
The article by Turner and Pöppel in this volume offers a number of figures concerning time perception which, at first glance, may appear contradictory to those offered here. They are in fact not contradictory in any significant way. The authors' figure of 0.003 s (3 ms) as the period by which a subject can discriminate two sounds as separate must be expanded by a factor of 10 to ca. 30 ms before the subject can further discriminate *order* – that is, which of the two sounds came first. Though this figure of 30 ms conflicts with my figure of 20 ms, used here as the minimum "perceptual window" for order discrimination, the difference is one of experimental design and subsequent observations.
The 20-ms figure was established by Hirsh and Sherrick (1961) as the "order threshold" below which one could not discriminate order, or succession, between two sounds. These researchers accepted a "confidence level" of 75% in their experiments, which means that 75% of the subjects tested confirmed this 20-ms interval. Pöppel and his associates in their experiments, which also involve order threshold, prefer a confidence level of 100%, which they find occurs at the time interval of ca. 30 ms. (See: Hirsh HJ, Sherrick CE jr (1961) Perceptive order in different sense modalities. Journal of Experimental Psychology 62:423–432.)

9. Fechner GT (1860) Elemente der Psychophysik. Breitkopf und Härtel, Leipzig; English translation (1966) Elements of psychophysics. Holt, Rinehart and Winston, New York
10. Mach E (1865) Untersuchungen über den Zeitsinn des Ohres. Sitzungsbericht der mathematisch-naturwissenschaftlichen Klasse der kaiserlichen Akademie der Wissenschaften 52, Abt. 2, Heft 1–5, pp 133–150
11. Getty DJ (1975) Discrimination of short temporal intervals: A comparison of two models. Perception and Psychophysics 18: 1–8
12. Engen T (1971) Psychophysics I. Discrimination and detection. In: Kling FW, Riggs LA (eds) Woodworth and Schlosberg's Experimental Psychology. Holt Rinehart and Winston, New York, pp 11–16
13. The tape recorder was turned off for periods ranging from 30 s to 4 min during this ceremony. Therefore, the time periods discussed here were in reality considerably longer.
14. Chomsky N (1965) Knowledge of language: its nature, origin and use. New York

Dance, the Fugitive Form of Art
Aesthetics as Behavior

Walter Siegfried
Lindwurmstrasse 74, 8000 München 2, Federal Republic of Germany

To analyze dance as an early form of aesthetics means to accept the idea that the aesthetic is not a quality of tangible objects alone. By stressing the fluent and fugitive side of art, dance emphasizes action and not a resulting object. The notion that artistic behavior does not always result in an object is often neglected, but here it is our main thesis. We shall focus on the dynamic character of art; aesthetics will be considered as behavior. Dance is most suited to visualize this dynamic side of aesthetics, which also can be objectified to demonstrate that something persisting has been created. The regularity of the generated rhythmic patterns or the stability of certain body orientations among the dancers provide prime examples. Dance, the fugitive art form, shows by such qualities as repetition, regularity, and constancy a tendency towards externalization. Since the beginning of this century, the value of isolated works of art has been questioned, and a reverse process can be observed. Interest is shifting from the graspable work of art towards the action of producing it. This first appeared in the expressionist school of art, and the result of the expression, the painting, remained an object of art. Since then, action has been increasingly stressed ("action painting"), but the result is still important. Finally, the action itself has become the aim (situationists [1], happenings, performances).

In emphasizing the behavioral aspect of the aesthetic, we shall focus on the specific qualities of dance movements and examine what separates them from ordinary motor activities. Such an analysis of dance movements is futile, however, without a concept for classifying the movements. Different classification systems have been proposed, most of the earlier ones in the context of choreography.

To get a clearer picture of the relationship between dance movement and ordinary movement, it is not enough to describe the isolated dance movements, which are often formally identical to everyday activities. Rather, we must look at the dancing group as a whole and ask what transforms those similar looking movements into something other than everyday activity. Two approaches, both holistic in their roots, have been chosen to determine the typical quality of dance movements: phenomenology and ethology.

Phenomenology, with its rich tradition in observing the human body in motion[2-4], presented a holistic approach. Only after a phenomenological description of dance movements had been undertaken[5,6], did it become clear in this investigation that it was not the movement itself but the context in which it occurred that necessitated further observation. In this investigation, "context" refers not to functions or cultural influences but to the movement context, i.e., what the dance movement is related to. What is the system within which the dance movements take place? The hypothesis of this study is that the system to which the dancers and their movements relate must be created by the dancers themselves and is the result of a group process. The reference points of the dance movements are elaborated by the dancers or, as Maxine Sheets[5] puts it: "A dance cuts into everyday time and space ... Consequently, one can speak of the specific temporal flow of a specific movement and the time of the dance as a whole as created temporality and created time ... Time and space are not containers in which dance occurs; they are intrinsic dimensions of the illusion, virtual force, and as such, they are immediately created with the creation of that force...." The measurable description of this spatio-temporal creation, as far as methodologically possible, is the essence of this study.

Regarding the ethological approach, it was precisely the analysis of movement patterns, especially of ritualized movements, with which ethology, a new branch of biology, contributed a new dimension to the theory of evolution.[7] As Lorenz showed in his article "On Dance-like Movements in Animals,"[8] ritualized animal movements resemble human dance. Because this study concentrates on human dance, the ethological perspective here focuses on the description of movement patterns, on the analysis of their coordination process, and on possible laws that govern this process rather than examining the whole richness of dance events. This approach, based on the most simple (and, probably, also the most original) forms of human aesthetic behavior, links dancing to the highly developed communicative behavior of animals and provides the best basis for the question of how behavior and aesthetics may work together in human dancing. In the domain of art, dance is the most suitable medium to demonstrate the cooperation between behavior and ideas, a cooperation that is also present – but less visible – in normal human movement. Aesthetic ideas, as conveyed through books, painting, sculpture, etc., are presented by the vehicle the human body in dance without the presence of an extraneous object. Therefore, the traditional analysis of aesthetic objects must be replaced in this study by the analysis of aesthetic behavior.

Investigating an Ephemeral Phenomenon

The working hypothesis of this study defines group dancing as a behavior in which dancers create, maintain, and vary a common space-time structure (S-TS), which, once created, is binding on the participants. This model of a specific S-TS links behavior and aesthetics by providing a *tertium comparationis* (the point in which two seemingly different phenomena are similar) between highly developed, ritualized animal movements and the early artistic expression of man in dance. Spatial as well as temporal structures established by the participants are crucial for both phenomena and provide a basis for comparison. In both cases, they provide a framework within which to behave.

What is meant by this "spatio-temporal framework" within which human dancing takes place? One of the most basic requirements of group dance is to be in the right place at the right moment, and this is essentially what is meant by the S-TS. But who determines the right place and the right moment? For ballroom dancing, this is obvious; the right moment is indicated by the rhythm of the music, and the right place results from learned dance movements, fixed by choreography. But if, for example, in children's play dances, there is no space-defining choreography and no time-keeping music, what then? We will show how the S-TS is established successively by the individuals dancing in the group. But first we must explain more clearly the meaning of the term space-time structure. We will initially analyze the space structure and then the time structure, since both processes are strongly interrelated.

The space structure is defined as the continuing spatial relationships among the dancers. Two methods will be used to show its development. First, drawings that were directly copied from film frames provide insight into the successive building up of the dance space. Second, a transcription method introduced by Kendon[9] and Deutsch[10] represents each body as a "transactional segment," thus defining the "shape of an individual's contribution to a joint interactional space" (Fig. 1).

Deutsch described the construction of the transactional segment as follows: "We can arrive at just what the shape of this space is by the following: Imagine a person standing erect with his hands at his sides. First we anchor this person in space and time by drawing a connecting line between the two points on the ground created by dropping a perpendicular line from the lateral extension of each shoulder. The length of this line (*line a* in Fig. 1) is approximately two feet for an average adult. We call this line the base of the transactional segment. From each of the two endpoints of this base we extend lines drawn at 45-degree angles to the straight ahead (*line b* in Fig.1). These lines were drawn at 45-degree angles because, as we saw, this angle is the maximum allowable discrepancy in the head-body orientation of an interactant.

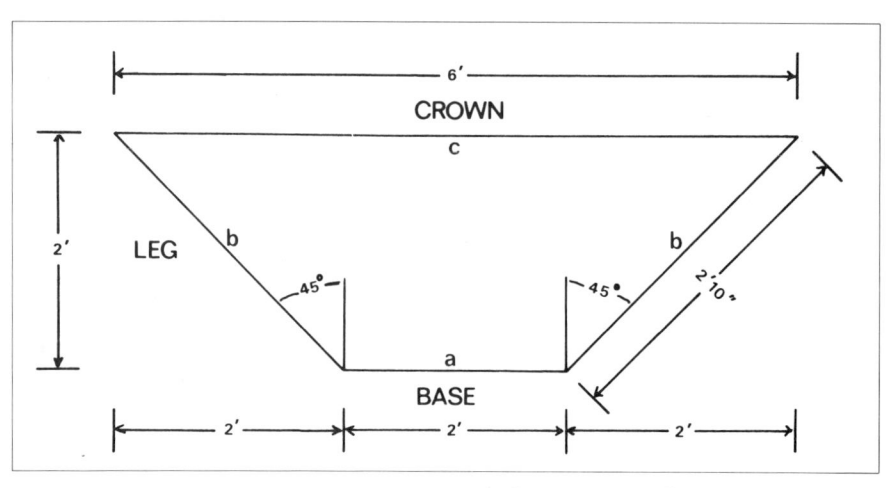

Fig. 1. Transactional segment according to A. Kendon[9] and R. Deutsch[10]

We call these lines the legs of the transactional segment. Finally, a line is drawn parallel to and two feet in front of the base (*line c* in Fig.1). This line is drawn thus because two feet is half the maximum distance (four feet) between two people interacting at Hall's "personal distance"; this line thus equally divides the space between the two interactants. We call this line the crown of the transactional segment. If we extend this crown in both directions until it intersects each leg, we create a bounded space with the legs being two feet ten inches long and the crown, six feet long. We hypothesize this transactional segment as an individual's contribution to the joint interactional space of a face-to-face interaction.

Just as face-to-face interactions may be viewed within this conceptualization of interactional space, so may dance groups. If one transcribes typical space configurations of simple dance forms by the interactional segment, the space structure and its characteristics are easily recognizable (Fig.2).

Such simple space configurations (floor patterns) as e.g.: a) the circle; b) and c) the line; d) and e) face-to-face differ fundamentally from one another vis-à-vis the relative positions of the bodies to each other. For instance, all participants are equal in the circle; in the line, there are a first, a last, and some middle positions; and in the face-to-face configurations, the pairs are emphasized.

In patterns A and B of Fig.3, the dancers always stand on the same spot in objective space and only change their orientations to each other slightly. But this slight spatial alteration provides a radical change in the meaning of the dance space; the members are embedded suddenly in a new spatial context. The changed context creates a new situation. For example, B1 is a

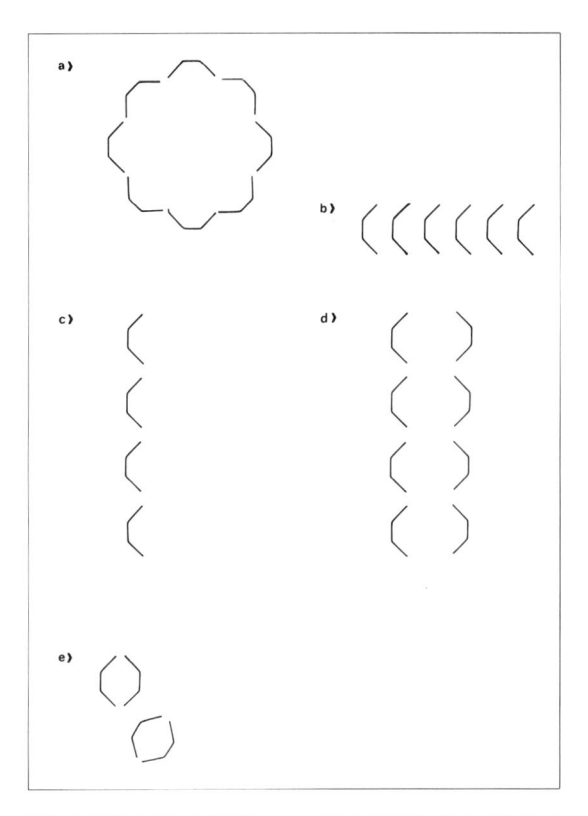

Fig. 2. The "transactional segment" in typical floor patterns of dances

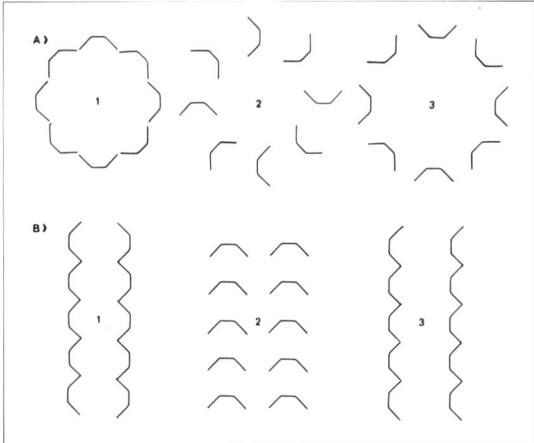

Fig. 3. A visualization of how slight changes in the spatial relationships of the dancers to one another alter the entire sense of the dance space

pronounced face-to-face situation, which could be characteristic of a courtship dance. B2 has a processional character, and B3, with its clear double front, can be found in war dances. Here are three versions in which each dancer remains on his spot in objective space but participates in very different dance spaces for very different purposes. The new spatial context in these examples is caused only by the changed relative positions of the dancers to each other and has nothing to do with the space surrounding the dancers.[11]

The inner coherence of the dance space has been neglected too long and requires further description. Such a description has caused and will cause methodological problems because no notation system exists, as far as I know, that allows description not only of the movements of the dancers but especially of their relationships to the whole, continually moving, dancing group. The only movement notation system that could be enlarged in the above-mentioned sense seems to be the one proposed in "A Choreography of Display" by Golani.[12] The aim here is not to develop such a notation system but to describe the specific space structure created by the dancers themselves, which separates them from surrounding space. In this context, it is important to remember that dancing often begins with the preparation of the dance site, with the cleaning of the floor, with different kinds of demarcations, with the fixing of a center (the most famous example being the maypole), and with the preparation of a specially delimited floor material – all acts that show how strongly the dance space is to be autonomous, separated from the surrounding space.

What is meant by the time structure is much easier to understand and, therefore, requires less explanation. It concerns the "tempo"[13] of a certain dance. The tempo of a dance could be defined by paraphrasing Epstein's definition of musical tempo as follows: It is the speed with which the dance goes through time.[14] The focus will be on the development of the specific speed within the dance group to answer the question of how the tempo is generated, maintained, and varied. We said that the basis of group dancing consists of being on the right spot at the right moment. The tempo defines the right moment, but who defines the tempo? If there is no accompanying music, the dancers themselves must establish a common tempo that synchronizes the individual rhythms.

Most dances are characterized by a series of strong underlying beats, which are referred to here as "pulse." This pulse must be established by the group, i.e., the members create their own time structure. The pulse can be formed by singing, stamping, clapping, etc. The method of analysis is chosen according to the method of production. We shall apply two types of analyses to determine pulse: whenever the pulse can be clearly seen, we use single-frame analysis, a method that is very effective for the optical segmentation of movements. If the pulse can be heard rather than seen, especially in large groups, the sound track provides the basis for analysis. Oscillogram transcriptions of the recorded pulse can be easily measured and compared. As the concrete definitions of the pulse beat vary with the dance forms, they will be introduced with the corresponding examples.

Given the concept of our research, it was clear that neither the analysis of stage dancing nor of ballroom dancing can be used to demonstrate the creation of space or time structures because, in those dances, the choreography or traditional positions dictate the space structure, and the given music dictates the time structure. We, therefore, looked for dance events that occurred without music. In such situations, the dancers are forced to create their common pulse themselves, and, during such opening phases, the relative positions among the dancers are not yet totally fixed so that the creation of the space structure can be observed. Children's dances and play dances meet these requirements.

Among the many documents in the Human Ethology Film Archives of the Max-Planck-Society, the film sequences of southern African dances provided the richest examples for our research. In this region, we find living dance traditions, and dancing children can often be observed.[15] However, only a few sequences of these films could be used for complete analysis.[16]

Other research material consists of documents of experimental dance groups, which consisted of medical students. The size of the groups varied from four to fifteen. In these dance groups, we played with spatial and temporal elements by grouping in different ways and producing different kinds of rhythms. Protocols, photographs, and tape recordings, partly transcribed by oscillograms, were the documentary tools used. As mentioned, this paper tries to emphasize dance not only as an aesthetic object but also as an act in which to participate. Therefore, our own experiences in dance groups were important.

The materials used in this study are obviously heterogeneous and are only examples to help illucidate the model proposed in the hypothesis. We do not intend to explain the meaning of the dances. To understand dancing fully, one must live within the dancing culture not only as an observer, but as a participant. Without such living participation, analysis intended to grasp the whole sense of dancing is open to all kinds of misunderstandings. Difficulties begin with the word "dance," whose corresponding terms in different cultures refer to different phenomena.[17] Because our study looks for very simple things, such as spatial orientation within a group or the temporal development of the pulse of a dance, the meaning of the analyzed dances can, at first, be neglected in our approach.

The Hypothesis

The core of this study's hypothesis is summarized in the term "common space-time structure." This structure is established at the very beginning of the group dance and is then binding on the participants by defining the spatial and temporal reference points for their movements. The development of the S-TS is the context of our endeavor.

Because dance is a fluent rather than a static, palpable art form, such as sculpture, the S-TS cannot be regarded as an object; it must be viewed as an ongoing process. Its aesthetic qualities must, therefore, be rooted in its dynamic creation and development. Focusing on the dynamic aspect of the dance, the S-TS must not only be created but also maintained and varied. Without active maintenance, the once established S-TS may break down very quickly; either the spatial coherence will become loose or the synchronized movements disintegrate into individual rhythms, causing a chaotic destabilization of the common tempo.

Maintaining the S-TS, i.e., continuing the same rhythm in the same spatial positions, soon becomes boring; there must be variation in the spatial configuration as well as in the temporal flow. It is especially these elements of playful variation that give dance the qualities that belong so fundamentally to aesthetic behavior and provide intrinsic reinforcement – thrill, pleasure, excitement, innovation, display of individuality, and so on. They need, of course, a background from which to evolve as variations. This background is not just space and time in general but the specific S-TS created and maintained by the participants.

Dance is not only the creation of a S-TS. As a dynamic process, it must constantly be regulated by the participants while it is being developed. This regulation may, at one time, consist of variation to avoid boredom. At another time, it may stress the basic S-TS to ensure continuity of the dance in a risky situation. Our description may be summarized in the following hypothesis: dancers create, maintain, and vary a common S-TS, which, once created, is binding on the participants. In the following sections, we shall present three aspects of the findings corresponding to the hypothesis:

Creation of the S-TS
Maintenance of the S-TS
Variations within the S-TS

In the last section, we shall discuss the consequences of this definition of dance for the concept of aesthetics. Special attention will be paid to the fact that dancers are the creators of the work of art, which they themselves represent and from which they personally benefit. This approach stresses perception as an active process. In dance, receptivity and activity do not exclude each other, but provide mutual reinforcement. This cooperation of perception and motion coincides perfectly with our concept of aesthetics, which stresses the unity of perception and behavior within a social context.

The Creation of the Space-Time Structure

Dance groups are defined by their specific space structures. If one decides to dance, one goes into the position required, but if dancing is happening without big decisions and defined beginnings, then finding the "right" position in space is a process. For example, the oryx-antelope dance or gemsbuck dance of the !ko-Bushmen (Kalahari Desert, Botswana) (Fig. 4) may be initiated by one man (A) stamping clearly the basic rhythm in the middle of a relaxed group (frame 0234).

A second man (C) stands up and begins to dance facing A, while B and D are still standing around in relaxed positions. A young member of the sitting group stands up (frame 0346) and enters the dance to challenge dancer A for a short period of the dance ; thus, an axis is created with A

Fig. 4. Sequence visualizing space creation in the opening phase of a gemsbuck dance (drawings from film documentation: !ko 1972, Eibl-Eibesfeldt)

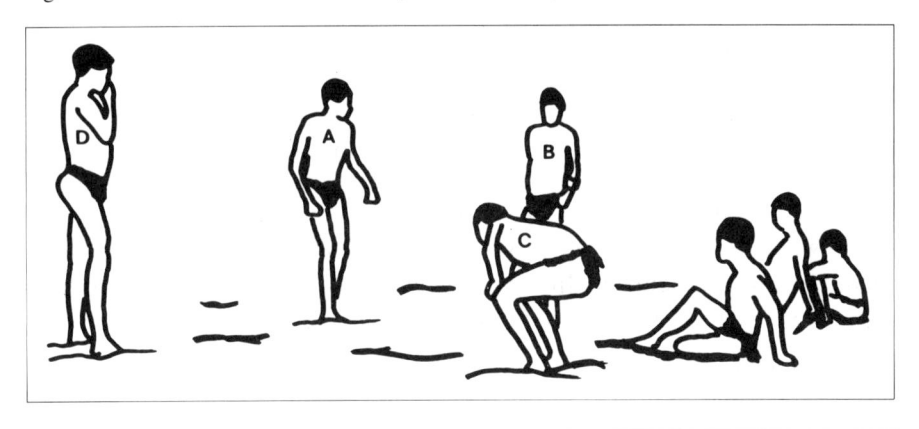

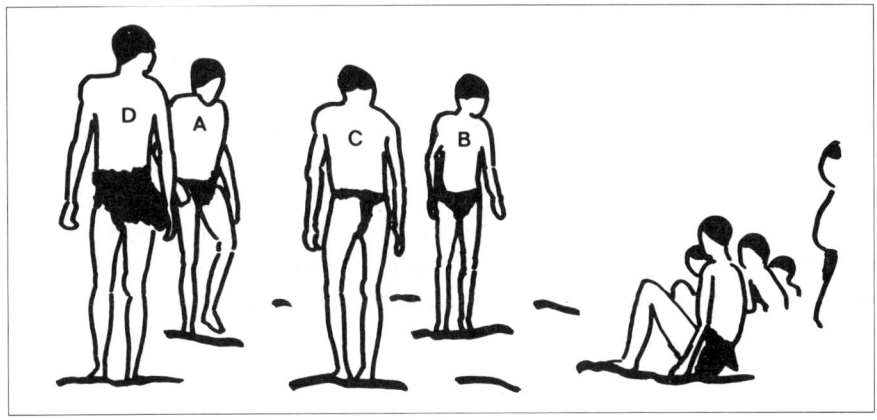

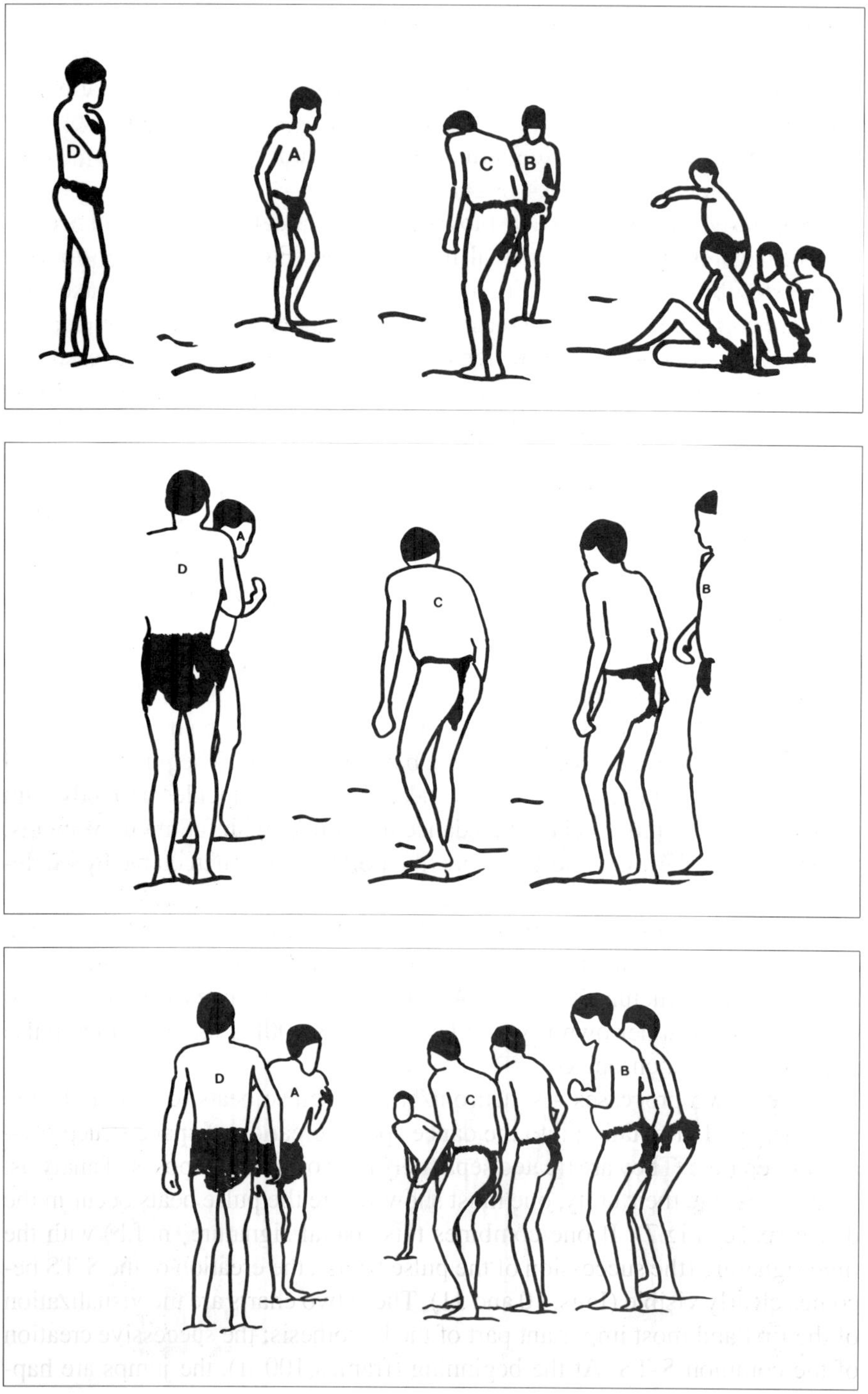
D
A
C
B
A
D
C
B
D
A
C
B

on one side and the boy and C on the other side. Now D moves closer to C, orienting his body axis towards A (frame 0652). All heads seem to be asking for participation of the sitting group . In frame 0924, a member of that group steps next to C, while B changes his orientation so that now, for the first time, the basic space structure is realized – the "antelope" in opposition to the group (frames 0924/1214).

Similarly, the girls, already moving in the typical pattern of a dance, do not yet have strong mutual spatial relationships (Fig.5). Only later do they create, step-by-step, a circle (Fig.6). At the beginning, neither body axes nor faces are correlated among the dancers, whereas later their mutual orientation creates the framework within which to behave. The time required to establish such a space structure varies from case to case and depends on many variables, such as mood, knowledge of the intended space structure, will of the participants to dance the same specific form, and so on.

Returning now to the group of girls that established a circle as a space structure, we ask how they created their time structure. In other words, how do they synchronize their individually generated movements? The girls dancing in this circle jump up and down, first in the middle position (m), later forward (f) and backward (b).

Figure 7 provides a schematic idea of this spatial development, which introduces the time factor by the jumping movements of the dancers. The rhythm, or pulse, of each individual can be defined as the succession of the jumps. Each jump is considered as one beat of the pulse. The jump is defined by the deepest point of flexion in the knees (Fig.8). It coincides perfectly with the feeling of the pulse beat in this dance that works with falling movements, with the force of gravity. Furthermore, the point is easily detectable by single-frame analysis.

If one uses this method to define the pulse beats for each individual in a dancing group and puts them together on a graph (Fig.9), the creation of the common time structure is visible. At the beginning (frames 100ff), each individual jumps in her own rhythm; later (frames 600ff), the individual pulse sequences are synchronized.

These two processes – synchronization of pulse beats (creation of time structure) and orientation into the dance space (creation of space structure) – are not separate. They are treated separately here only for purposes of analysis. To demonstrate their unity, one must show where the pulse beats occur in the dance space (Fig.7). If one combines this spatial signature (m,f,b) with the time signature (the succession of the pulse beats), the creation of the S-TS becomes clearly visible (Figs. 10 and 11). These two charts are the visualization of the first and most important part of the hypothesis: the successive creation of the common S-TS. At the beginning (frames 100 ff), the jumps are hap-

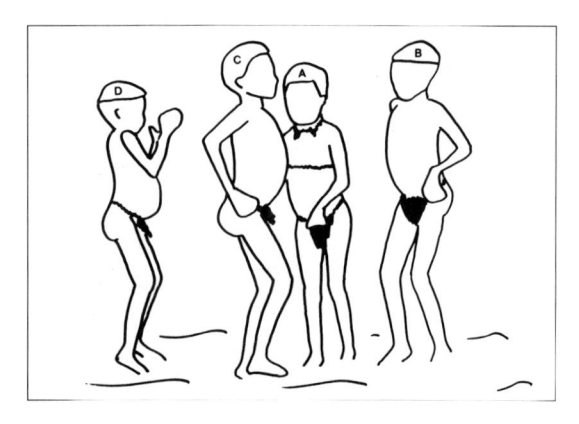

Fig. 5. Weak spatial relationship among the dancers (drawing from film !ko-Bushmen, Children Dancing, Part 1, Eibl-Eibesfeldt)

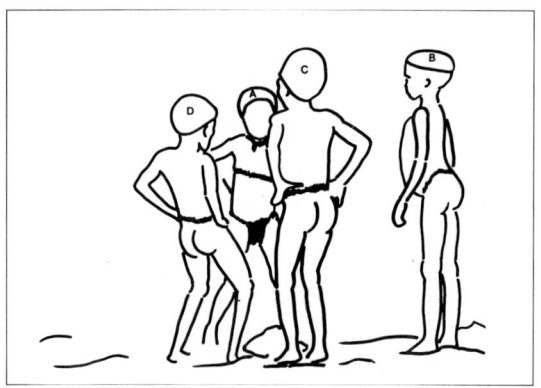

Fig. 6. Strong spatial relationship among the dancers (drawing from film !ko-Bushmen, Children Dancing, Part 1, Eibl-Eibesfeldt)

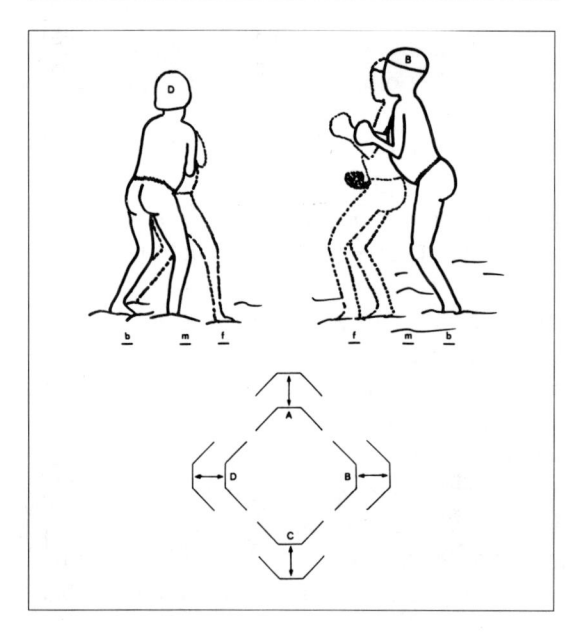

Fig. 7. Typical movements and space structure of a !ko-girls dance (drawing from film !ko-Bushmen, Children Dancing, Part 1, Eibl-Eibesfeldt)

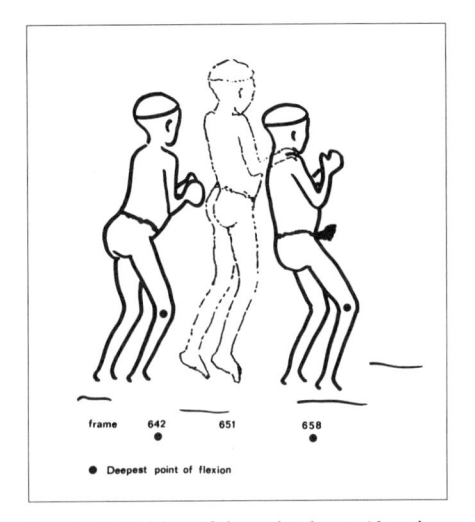

Dance, the Fugitive Form of Art: Aesthetics as Behavior 129

Fig. 8. Definition of the pulse-beats (drawing from film !ko-Bushmen, Children Dancing, Part 1, Eibl-Eibesfeldt)

Fig. 9. *(right)* Beginning and concluding phase of the synchronization process

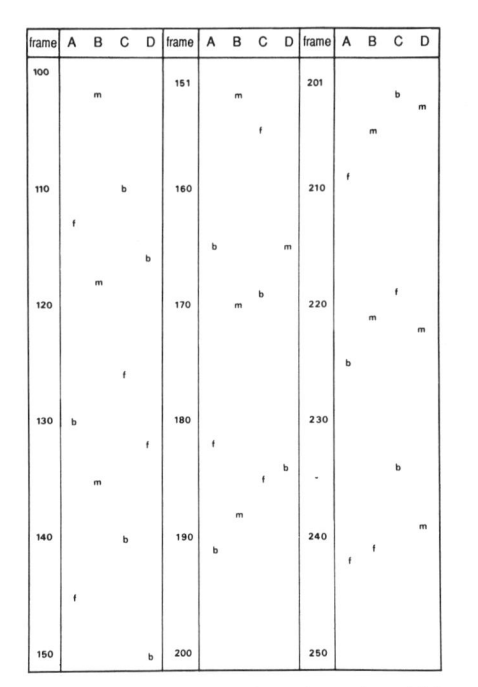

Fig. 10. Chaotic opening phase in which neither a space nor a time structure is established

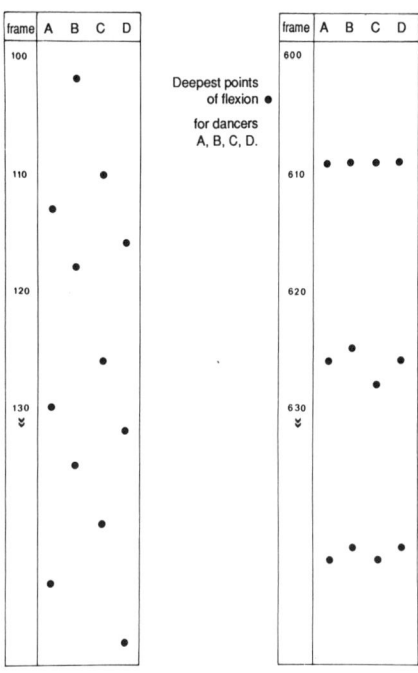

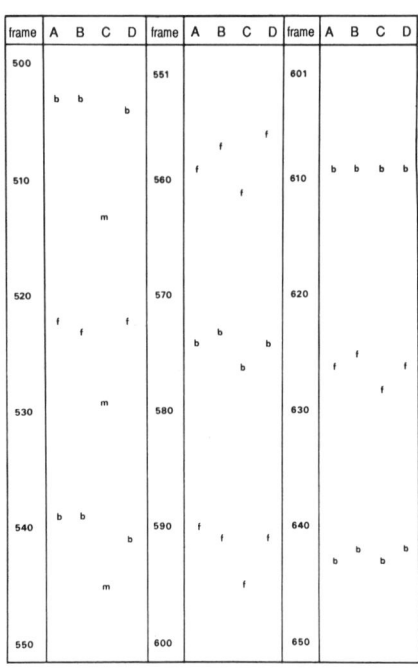

Fig. 11. Phase in which the common space-time structure is realized

hazard in space as well as in time, but the S-TS is clearly established around frame 560 – that is, after about 22 seconds.

The schematic transformation used here is a simple and rough version of what we were looking for in the methodological section. It shows how the framework, or the system of reference points, is created by the dancers themselves. The objective time represented in the succession of film frames is negligible, as it is not important whether something happens in frame 600 or 610. The importance for the dance is whether that something happens simultaneously among all four dancers or not. Similarly, it is not the coordinates in objective space that are of interest but the specific space structure of this dance form. This is the relative spatial relationship of the dancers to each other. Only when one understands the integrative form toward which the movements tend to be directed does the specific dance space become perceptible, allowing us to analyze, retrospectively, the creation process of the space structure by providing the reference points. These spatial and temporal reference points for the notation system can appear only step-by-step during the process of creating the S-TS. No external force integrates the dancers. The coherence of the group is not given, it must be realized while dancing, as the S-TS, which is then binding on the participants. The emphasis lies on the "realization," as it is clear that its structure cannot always be an absolutely new creation. More often it will be provided by tradition, but, unlike painting, it is not just "there"; it must be realized anew each time.

Maintenance of the Space-Time Structure

As we saw, the common S-TS must be created by the dancers. Once created, it must also be maintained. A created pulse can easily be destroyed or a circle broken if people lose interest.

To maintain the space structure means to control and continue the established spatial relationship of the dancers to each other. For instance, dancers in a line formation will control the distance between each other by taking shorter or longer steps. By such controlled distance, they guarantee continuity of the line formation. In some dances of the Trobriand Islanders (New Guinea), in which more then twenty participants dance behind one another, the control maneuver of one dancer influences all succeeding dancers in such a way that a correction can be seen as a wavelike movement going through the whole line of dancers.

An extreme example of the maintenance of a space structure has been observed during a courtship dance of the Himba people (South Africa). The women stand in a semicircle, which is opposed to the semicircle of the men. Two children behind the dancing women attract their attention. The women

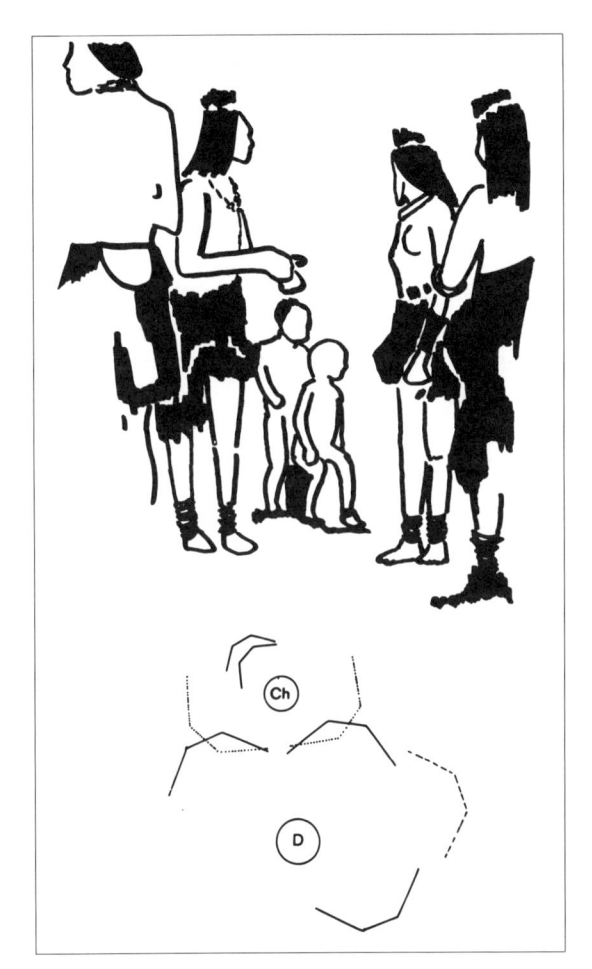

Fig. 12. Double orientation of two women over a period of about 16 seconds (drawing from film documentation Himba 1971, Eibl-Eibesfeldt)

turn toward them and stand, therefore, in a very uncomfortable position (Fig. 12). That this position is not a customary one is shown by Kendon, who reported to Deutsch "... that all interactants will not usually hold, for any sustained period of time, a discrepancy in their head-body orientation of more than 45 degrees. Rather, after momentarily adopting such a discrepant head-body orientation, a person will reorient himself so that his relative head-body orientation is less than 45 degrees. This position can and will be held for long periods of time in relative comfort...."[10] In our case, the unusual position is maintained over a period of about 16 seconds. I suggest that the women maintain it in order to make the dance space (D) continue to exist. With their body orientation (⌐⎯⌐), they maintain the dance space (D), while with their head orientation (⌐⎯⌐), they control the children space (Ch).

The maintenance of the time structure (the stabilization of a once-established tempo) can only be investigated if there is something like stability in the tempo behavior of dance groups. Some speak of such underlying stable structures as "meter."[17] For our purpose, "tempo" is more adequate, as it indicates the possibility of increasing, decreasing, or maintaining the speed. The term "meter" suggests that the stability is an extrinsic quality. This may be an effect of looking at music not as an experience but as a written text, with bars suggesting that musical time must occur within this outer framework. Music, however, does not have to fit within a metrical context; it creates its own context by establishing what we refer to as a maintained time structure. In dance, the maintenance of such created time is crucial to plan the movements of the body parts.

If one measures the pulse beats of the grasshopper dance (!ko) in the same manner as proposed in Figs. 8 and 9 with the method of deepest flexion of the knee, one sees that the created pulse is very stable (Fig.13). Two quarters correspond to x = 1150 milliseconds (ms) with a standard deviation of s = 60 ms. This is astonishing, if one sees the enormously complex movement patterns that are created in this stable pulse (Figs. 14-16).

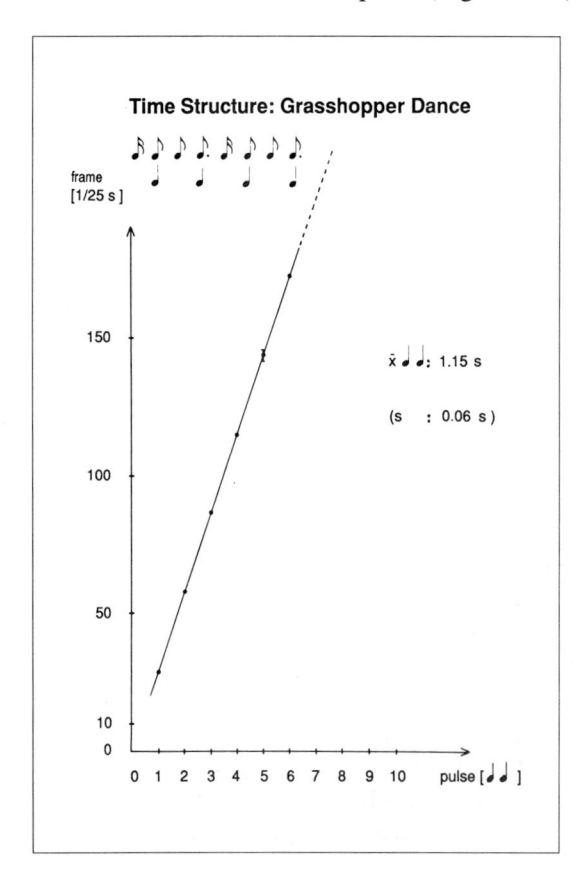

Fig. 13. The stability of a once-created time structure in the !ko-Bushmen grasshopper dance

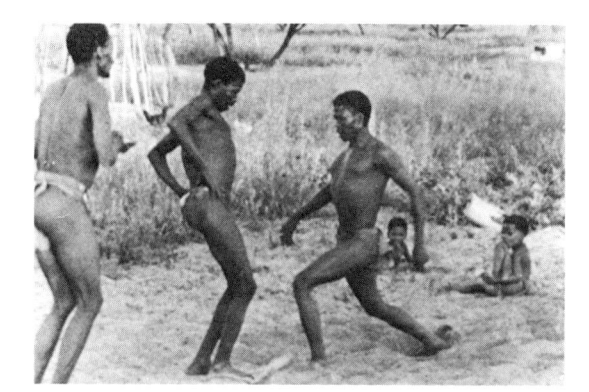

Dance, the Fugitive Form of Art: Aesthetics as Behavior   133

Figs. 14-16. Examples for the complexity of movement patterns in the grasshopper dance (frames from film !ko-Bushmen, grasshopper dance 1971, Eibl-Eibesfeldt)

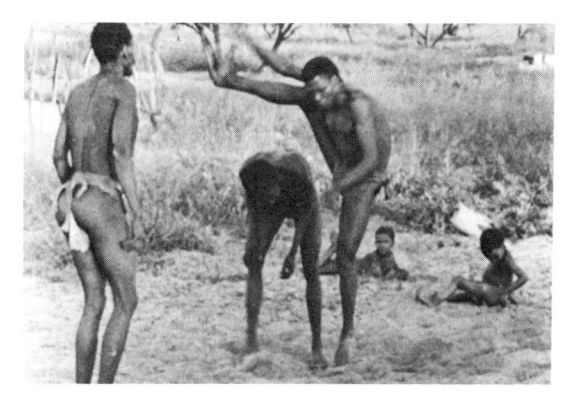

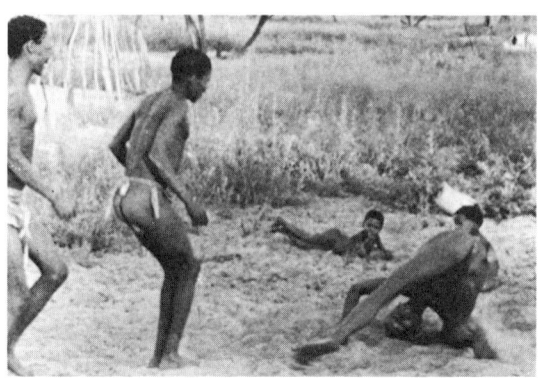

A similar stability of time structure was found in our experimental dance groups. This was not expected, since the members were not trained in dancing and did not have strong dance traditions. For instance, in a group of four dancing students, the oscillogram analysis showed a high stability of time structure and a standard deviation from the pulse similar to the one of the grasshopper dance (Fig. 17).

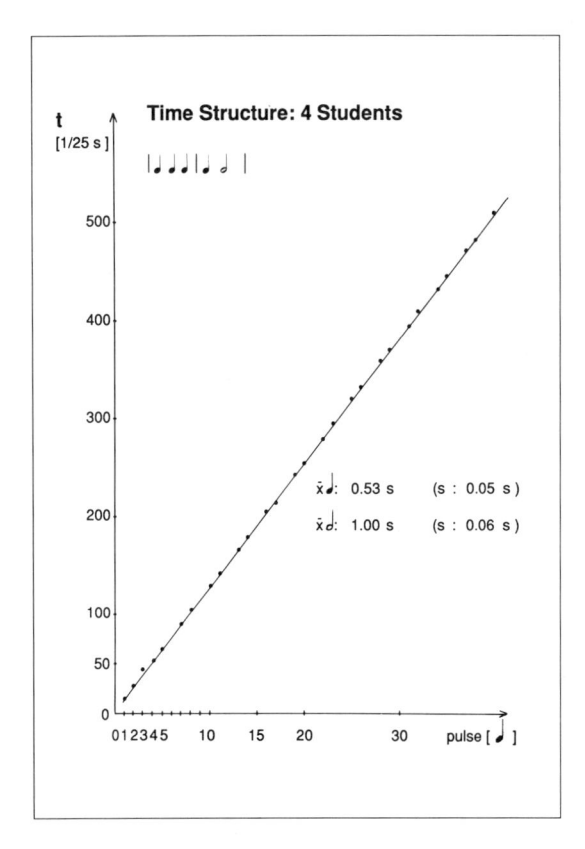

Fig. 17. The stability of a created time structure in a student group

It seems that stabilization of the dance tempo does not create large problems, particularly if it is compared with the difficulties in maintaining a certain tempo while singing in a chorus, for instance. The rhythmic movements that swing the body masses and stabilize the dance tempo are absent in singing. One could go further and suggest that the inertia of the moving bodies not only enhances the stability of a tempo but actually hinders tempo changes. This argument can be sustained by the following observation: in our dance groups, if the students were totally free in their tempo choices, an established tempo would normally be maintained. If the students changed their tempo, it was not through a commonly controlled increase or decrease of speed but rather through a short period of chaotic destabilization, from which a new stable tempo emerged. It is as if each individual accelerates or decelerates the first tempo in his own manner, thereby causing the general acoustic mass (Fig. 18a) out of which a synchronization at a new tempo level occurs (Fig. 18b). One could speak of a trend toward stabilization of tempo levels. There are traditional dances in which sudden changes in tempo levels have become fixed rules, as in the previously discussed Himba courtship dance. After a period of

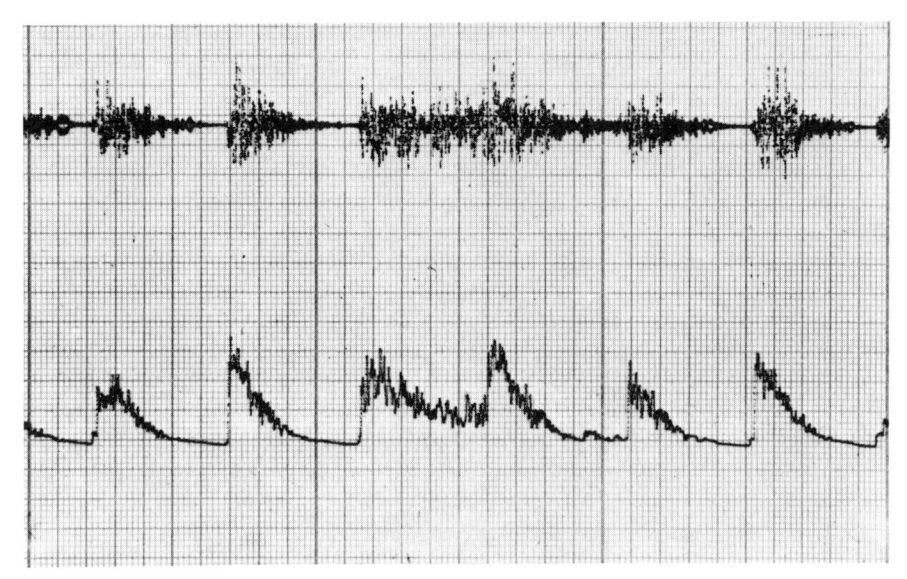

Fig. 18a. Oscillogram during a destabilized phase between two stable tempi

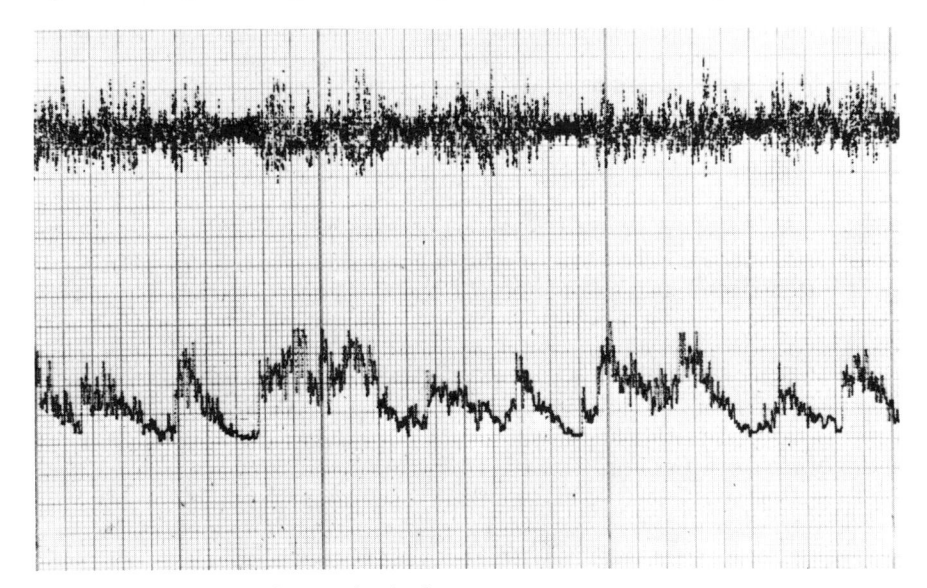

Fig. 18b. Oscillogram during a maintained tempo

allegro (about 480 ms), the speed is almost doubled as soon as a soloist leaves the common circle, which initiates a prestissimo of the dance (about 270 ms). After a variably long pause, the group begins again with the allegro tempo, which is always between 460 and 500 ms.

This rather long description of the phenomenon of tempo levels does not suggest that this process is the only possible way to change tempi. Further experiments with the students showed that we are able to produce constant accelerandi or ritardandi while dancing, and many elaborate dance forms (e.g., a wallaby dance of the Australian Aborigines from the Wik tribes) work in fascinating ways with just this possibility of constant accelerando or ritardando. The point here is that in simple dance events there is a tendency to maintain tempo levels. If tempo changes, it often occurs in such a way that an established tempo (A) breaks down in a chaotic phase out of which a new stable tempo (B) emerges.

Does the relationship between two or more tempi such as this follow certain rules? Do these tempi correspond to the time proportions of low integer ratios, e.g., 1:2, 2:3, 3:4, that have been found in examples of Western classic music[14,18] and later in examples of non-Western music?[19] We found such time proportions of low integer ratios in some experiments with our student dance groups (Fig.21). The students accelerated in such a way that, after a short phase of destabilization, a second tempo was established in the proportion 3:2 com-

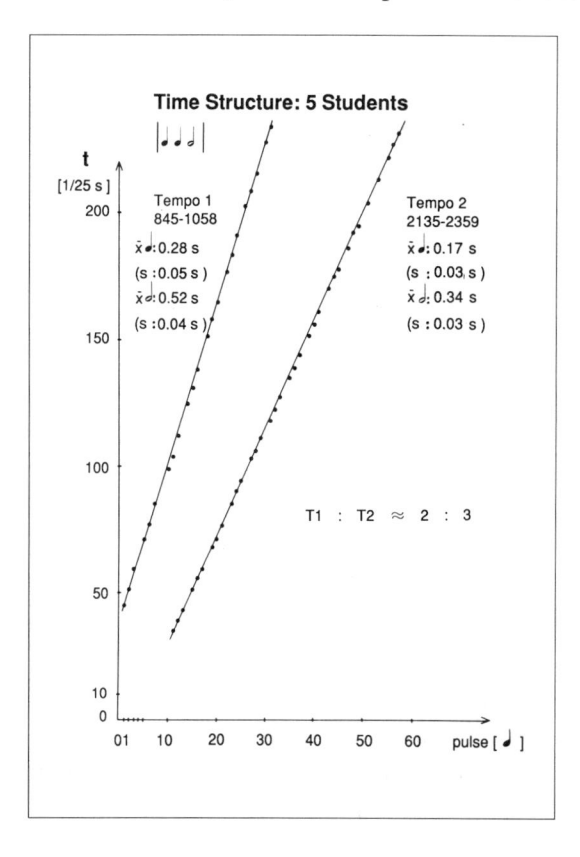

Fig. 19. Two tempo levels in student groups

pared to the first tempo. We need, of course, many more examples of such tempo shifts to be able to decide whether the observed proportions indicate parallels to Epstein's findings (see chapter 4) on the temporal relationships in music.

The maintenance of the S-TS guarantees the continuity of the basic dance structure by controlling the spatial relations of the dancing bodies to each other and the temporal framework within which the movements take place. The S-TS must be maintained because of the fluent character of the dance. It is the only stable element in the dynamic process of dancing. The maintenance of the S-TS establishes invariance during all transformations. It continues the created gestalt within the dynamic process, thus providing the contextual frame that dictates when the dancers or parts of their bodies must be where.

Variations within the Space-Time Structure

As we demonstrated, maintenance of the S-TS guarantees the continuity of an invariant pattern that organizes the movements of the dancers. To attain this common pattern is fascinating; to maintain it by repeating the movements strengthens the feeling of community and can be exciting, too, especially in trance dances, for example. But one of the most thrilling experiences while dancing is the variation of the S-TS or even allowing it to desintegrate to create a new one.

Variations of movements represent such alterations within the S-TS. Instead of a space used to go directly from point A to point B in the simplest dance movement pattern, the way from A to B becomes a zone of more elaborate and richer movement possibilities. The framework of invariant points in space and time remain the same, while the empty zones between the fixed points are open to all kinds of inventions.

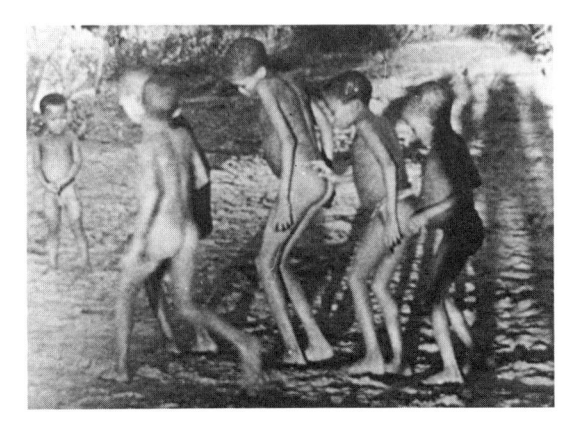

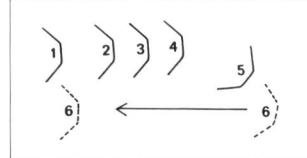

Fig. 20. Spatial variation within a line formation: A boy breaks out of the space formation (frame from film documentation G/wi 1973, Eibl-Eibesfeldt)

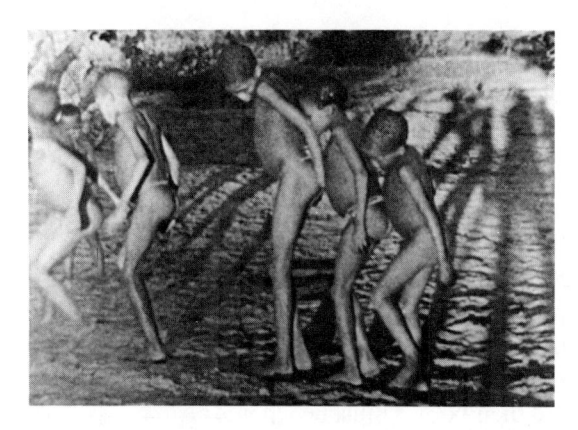

Fig. 21. Spatial variation within a line formation: The boy reintegrates in a new position of the old line formation (frame from film documentation G/wi 1973 Eibl-Eibesfeldt)

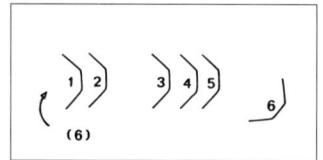

To illustrate a variation within a given space structure, we shall describe a simple dance of G/wi children (South Africa): One girl crosses the children's playground with typical dance movements and is followed by other girls and boys. They create a line formation and synchronize their movements, thus establishing and maintaining a S-TS. They then begin to move more freely; one boy does not seem happy with his sixth position in the line formation, breaks out, and runs alongside the line (Fig.20). He then jumps in front of the first dancer. The former leading dancer then becomes the second, and the boy who moved in front becomes the new leader (Fig.21). The line formation is maintained, but, with the changed position of this one dancer, all participants are in a new situation. The framework here is the line formation, which represents an absolute schema that can be varied; it provides organized positions without indicating who has to take which position. The variation within the space struc-

Fig. 22. Temporal variation within a stable pulse in the grasshopper dance

ture takes place during the time between leaving the old position and reentering the line formation in the new position.

Our example for the variation within the time structure is more complex. It is based on observations of the already discussed grasshopper dance of the !ko-Bushmen. As we have seen, its pulse is very stable (Fig.13). But within this pulse, a highly developed division of time takes place (Fig.22). While the group maintains the rather simple pulse, the individual dancers in the center of the group perform complex variations. They break up the time between two pulse beats in different manners (variations 1-3). Sometimes this changing division of time can go so far that a pulse beat may be left out (variations 4-6). The different structuring of time between two or three pulse beats may be experienced as a subjective elongation or contraction of the same objective span of time. For the active dancer, such possibilities to play with time create the feeling of moving back and forth between the common pulse, breaking away from it and then falling back again into the common time structure.

The grasshopper dance example also demonstrates a possibility (frequently used in Himba and !ko-Bushmen dancing) to divide the functions of maintainance and variation among the participants. A group of dancers maintains the S-TS and invites one or two participants, either by fixed rules or by stimulation, to perform rich individual variations. After a certain time, the soloists return to the core of the group maintaining the S-TS to allow others to invent variations. The solo phase stresses the possibilities for competition and individual display; the group phase puts emphasis on the community, the binding character of dance. This ambiguity and tension between competition and community is an important topic in Andrew Strathern's conception of aesthetics discussed in chapter 12 of this volume.

The variations need the unchanging background provided by the maintained S-TS. If there is no such continuity, the variations would not be possible. In our example of G/wi children, when a child left the line formation, the dance would end if all participants did the same at the same time, and no one maintained the line. We have observed that the variations get richer as soon as the common S-TS reaches a certain stability. If the variations begin before this stability has been reached, they risk disintegration of the S-TS, as the points to relate to become vague. In such phases of impending disequilibration, we have observed regression to the most simple movement patterns, which are then performed with formal exaggerations similar to those during the opening phases of dances.

In other words, the elements of maintenance and variation are not independent. The labile equilibrium opens manifold possibilities of relationships between two extreme poles. If maintenance is too strong, dancing becomes rigid and boring (except, of course, in those situations in which maintenance has a specific sense, as in trance dancing). If the variations are overemphasized, the movements become totally individualized. Although the latter may be very expressive, the sense of community, which is essential for group dancing, is lost. Other possible relationships between stabilization and variation within a group could be analyzed.[20]

Research on this relationship between maintenance and variation within the body of just one individual dancer could reveal interesting phenomena. It may be possible that some body parts maintain simple movement patterns, allowing others to perform rich variations. The temporal development could be similar to the one in group dancing. Variations are only possible on the foundation of a strong invariance. The typical movement patterns of Black African dances are summarized by Dauer[21] as: relaxation, isolation, polycentricity, and multiplication. Based on our analysis, one should now ask how these processes develop temporally within the body of one dancer. We suggest that isolations of movements are only possible after the creation of a strong basic movement to which the isolations are related.

Variation normally takes place within a given S-TS. Sometimes, however, a new structure can be heard or seen within the variations of the old structure. If these emerging new rhythms or space formations are emphasized by some of the participants, a struggle between the two structures begins. In this labile phase, the old S-TS may break down totally, so that the new structure is heard and seen clearly and may then be maintained by all the participants, who provide the basis for new variations.

Dance as Aesthetic Behavior

We have analyzed simple dance forms from the perspective of our approach – aesthetics as behavior. Dance has been viewed as a fluent art form that is regulated by the dancers while it is being developed. An important question remains: does this perspective provide some insight for understanding aesthetics?

This view of aesthetics stresses other factors than those elaborated through the analysis of literature, painting, sulpture, etc. We will discuss here the two most important ones: the dynamics of aesthetics and the social aspect of aesthetics.

Theodor Adorno[22] said that "there is no question that art does not begin with works"; he then went on to speak of "aesthetic behavior." This term is ideal to characterize what happens in dance: perception (aisthesis) and behavior – often thought of as being the opposite – are strongly linked in dance. The S-TS must be created by the dancers, and this creation can only take place if already created elements (spatial configurations as well as temporal structures) are perceived. This unity of perception and movement was described by Viktor von Weizsäcker as early as 1940[23], and Rudolf zur Lippe [24] expanded on this matter in his "anthropological aesthetic."

Aesthetic behavior in dance means perception of the ongoing movements and modification of one's own movements while perceiving those of others. It seems that we share this behavior with animals, as some birds modify their movements while "dancing" in relation to the mate's movements. One of the most beautiful examples is the mating dance among the male birds of paradise, in which they coordinate their movements on the pairing tree. But this behavior does not comprise the creation of a S-TS because there is no continuity that indicates intentionality. A S-TS can only be established if the projection of temporal and spatial structures is possible: the dancer must know in advance exactly when he wants to be where. It is not enough to react to a partner; this will always be too late.

Intentionality is, therefore, crucial. It enables the dancers to plan their movements to be in the right place at the right moment. It is astonishing how often children, energetically perceiving and moving, try to get into such a S-TS (Figs.20 and 21), and it is wonderful to see their happiness when they are "in phase" with the group. After a certain time, the maintained S-TS may become boring, so that variations within the structure may begin. Sometimes these variations lead to the end of the dance; sometimes they are the beginning of a transformation phase from which a new S-TS evolves.

The creation of common norms, their maintainance, their variation, and their desintegration are not only stages of dance events, they also correspond to important phases in problem solving[25] and creative processes.[26] The stages can be detected in both the individual process of creation, as in the development of Picasso's "Guernica"[27] and in phenomena of art history, such as the construction, variation, and destruction of linear perspective.[28,29] As dance leaves no traces or constructions, there is nothing left to be destroyed. In dance, something is or is not. To dance means to transform.[30] Destruction is linked to construction – to material objectification that can be destroyed. The density of such objectification on our planet demands "objectless" art, through which we can relearn transformation instead of destruction.[31]

The first essential change caused by the "dance model" was to abandon the common supposition that aesthetics predominantly deals with ideas fixed in works of art (objectifications). The triangle – creator, work of art, and receptor – is replaced by the moving subject that is at once creator, vehicle of the message, and receptor. The comprehensive term for this changed attitude is aesthetic behavior. The specificity of this behavior lies in the fact that it is not a simple action or reaction but a permanent play with the self-created rules.

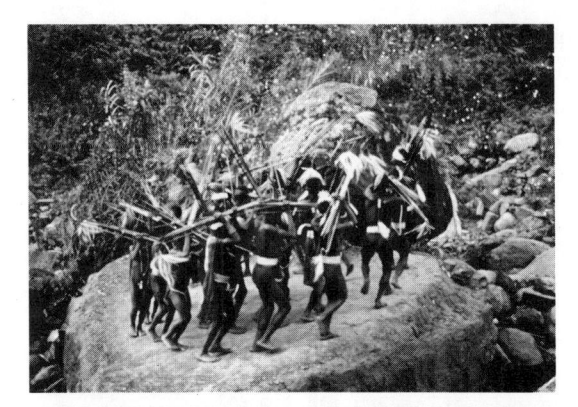

Figs. 23 and 24. Embodiment of the space-time structure. Eipo tribesmen, Papua-New Guinea, W.Schiefenhövel (1978)

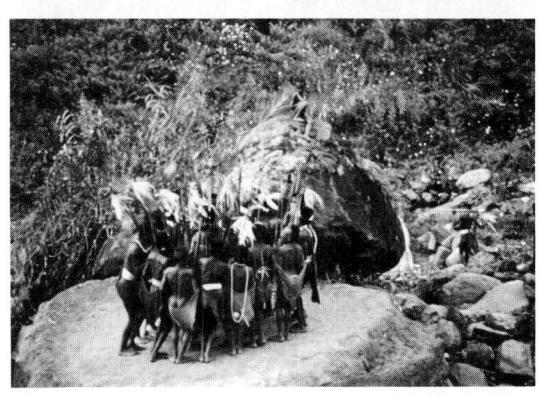

The rules provide a framework within which the dancer can cause shivers by trying new exciting movement combinations. The power lies in his hands. The pure shock does not provoke the aesthetic thrill but the fear that there is no more possibility to handle it. Therefore, the playful character of aesthetic behavior is important. It permits regulation of thrill, stimulation, and the degree of novelty, which make art experiences so wonderful.

Another common supposition concerning the relationship between aesthetic events and the social context has been amended. The belief still prevails that creation occurs in solitude. From our perspective of group dancing, creation cannot be an act of just one individual – only the consent of the participants leads to a group dance (Figs. 23 and 24). The consent is expressed in the S-TS, which can be considered a unifying norm. The "group-binding function" of dance, described by Eibl-Eibesfeldt[32], may have one of its roots in this common S-TS. Strong and weak individuals must integrate if they do not want to be excluded from the dance event. The norm binding the participants does not mean that individual display is suppressed. It is this very common S-TS that allows and even demands individual variation.[33] This is especially true for small groups. The rhythms of very big groups dominate the individual movements without being influenced by their specific dynamics. The rules become laws and lose their playful character. The dance has changed into a military march. Instead of encouraging variation, it dictates uniformity.

Human movement – a very simple form of creation – needs the answering movement of other human beings. Only if these movements are authentic expressions of personalities and not the jerking movements of marionettes, can real communication occur. Only in small groups will individuals be able to learn to trust their own rhythms, dynamics, and movements. Sometimes, society delegates the creation of aesthetic norms and their maintenance to a few specialists. Then the aesthetic domain loses not only wide ranges of individual variations, it also risks being increasingly secluded from everyday life. The public may be confronted with works of art whose meaning is no longer comprehensible to them. The works of art denote a foreign world.

The masses, who are condemned to passive spectatorship or are forced to perform in a preconceived manner, lose interest in experimenting with their individual possibilities. Instead of revealing their personalities to others and having fun, they become narcissistic, or worse, just boring.

Acknowledgements

This research project was made possible by the Swiss National Foundation. I am especially obliged to Prof. Irenäus Eibl-Eibesfeldt – Research Unit for Human Ethology in the Max-Planck-Society in Seewiesen, BRD – who generously allowed me to use his film documents and to Prof. David Epstein who, as a guest of the Institute of Medical Psychology at the University of Munich, encouraged me to go on with my work. He contributed as well as Joyce Nevil-Olesen and Barbara Herzberger to the editing. Furthermore, I thank Prof. Edwin Wilmsen for his help during the translation, Renate Krell for her photographic collaboration, Dr. Wulf Schiefenhövel and Dieter Heunemann for their information about the social background of the southern African dancers, Peter Heinecke for his technical help during the experimental dance groups and for the oscillogram production, and Daniel McKee for his computer instructions. Last but not least, I thank the medical students from Munich and the city dancers for their active dancing in our groups!

References and Notes

1. Nautilus (ed) (1976) Situationistische Internationale. MaD, Hamburg
2. Buytendjik F (1956) Allgemeine Theorie der menschlichen Haltung und Bewegung. Springer, Berlin

3. Plessner H (1970) Philosophische Anthropologie. S.Fischer, Frankfurt
4. Sartre JP (1943) L'être et le néant. Gallimard, Paris
5. Sheets M (1966) The phenomenology of dance. University of Wisconsin Press, Madison
6. Siegfried W (1977) Mensch – Bewegung – Raum. Thesis, University of Zürich
7. Lorenz K (1975) Die Rückseite des Spiegels. Piper, München
8. Lorenz K (1952) Über tanzähnliche Bewegungsweisen bei Tieren. Studium Generale 1:1-11
9. Kendon A (1975) Organization of behavior in face-to-face interaction. Mouton, The Hague
10. Deutsch R (1977) Spatial structurings in everyday face-to-face behavior. Asmer, Orangeburg
11. There are also situations in which the surrounding space influences the dance space. In cosmic dances, the orientations and the movements of the dancers are guided by qualities of cosmic space (e.g., the sun or the moon). In processional dances, a spatial configuration created by the dancers moves through a surrounding space (i.e. the village).
12. Golani I (1952) Auf der Suche nach Invarianten in der Motorik. In: Immelmann K (ed) Das Bielefeld-Projekt. Paul Parey, Berlin
13. If we speak of tempi in metrical terms, it will be expressed throughout as the duration in milliseconds between two beats of the pulse.
14. Epstein D (1983) Das Erlebnis der Zeit in der Musik. Die Zeit, vol 6. Schriften der Carl Friedrich von Siemens Stiftung, München
15. Sbrzesny H (1976) Die Spiele der !ko Buschleute. Piper, München
16. Selection was limited by the multitude of criteria that had to be met for the planned investigation and by the fact that the films had originally been made to fulfill other purposes. To mention some problems: the films began at the moment when the dance group had already been constituted; people danced out of the frame; dancers stood in front of one another so that individual movements could not be analyzed; etc.
17. Hanna JL (1979) Movements toward understanding humans through the anthropological study of dance. Current Anthropology 20:313-339
18. Epstein D (1979) Beyond Orpheus: Studies in musical structure. MIT Press, Cambridge
19. Epstein D (1985) Tempo relations: A cross-cultural study. Music Theory Spectrum 7:34-71
20. It would be interesting to know whether the general principle that a strong background S-TS allows richer variation within this S-TS can also be delegated to one element of the S-TS. Does a strong space structure allow the movements more temporal variation? Does a strong time structure free them from spatial limitations?
21. Dauer AM (1969) Zum Bewegungsverhalten afrikanischer Tänzer. Research Film. 6(6):517-526
22. Adorno TW (1984) Aesthetic theory. Routledge and Kegan Paul, New York
23. Weizsäcker V von (1940) Der Gestaltkreis. Thieme, Leipzig
24. Lippe R zur (1987) Sinnenbewußtsein. Rowohlt, Hamburg
25. Rohr AR (1975) Kreative Prozesse und Methoden der Problemlösung. Belz, Weinheim
26. Kubie LS (1965) Neurotische Deformation des schöpferischen Prozesses. Rowohlt, Hamburg
27. Arnheim R (1962) Picasso's "Guernica". University of California Press, Berkely
28. Francastel P (1951) Peinture et Société. Audin, Lyon
29. Novotny F (1938) Cézanne und das Ende der wissenschaftlichen Perspektive. A. Schroll, Wien

30. Siegfried W (1987) Danse, Dessin, Destruction. Cahiers du Centre de Recherche Imaginaire et Création. Université de Chambéry 3:122-141
31. Siegfried W (1988) Stadttanz, Übungen zur Ganzheit. Poiesis 4:92-97
32. Eibl-Eibesfeldt I (1972) Die !ko-Buschmanngesellschaft. Piper, München
33. This relationship between the group and the individual seems to be a fertile field for research. Polly Wiessner (1984) investigates this subject in her study: Reconsidering the behavioral basis for style: A case study among the Kalahari-San. Journal of Anthropological Archeology 3:190-234

Part III
The Eye of the Beholder

Biological Aspects of Color Naming

Heinrich Zollinger
Technisch-Chemisches Laboratorium, Eidgenössische Technische Hochschule (ETH), 8092 Zürich, Switzerland

Introduction: Characteristics of Sensation and Perception in Color Vision

When we speak of colors, we generally specify the color of objects, i.e., "the apple is red," and "the leaves are green." Certain things are given an obviously incorrect name ("white wine") or attributed a constant color, even if it often varies greatly (the "blue sea").

In this way, we give the impression that color is a property that these things possess, that it represents fact. We do not realize that colors are sensed and experienced and are not an objective property of the environment. This must be one of the most important causes of the difficulties in their total comprehension. We experience them through an extremely complex path of physical, chemical, neurological, and mental processes.

Isaac Newton laid the foundations of modern color science. In 1672, he published his observations concerning the refractive separation of sunlight by a prism into the various parts of the visible spectrum[1]. In addition, he demonstrated that a recombination of the spectral colors gave the sensation of colorless ("white") light to the human eye.

A hundred years later, Johann Wolfgang von Goethe strongly contradicted Newton's theory. Goethe's book, *Farbenlehre* (Theory of Color), is the most voluminous work he ever published.[2] According to Goethe, it is inconceivable for white to be a combination of all spectral colors. Even today, most people would probably agree intuitively with Goethe – without, however, questioning the validity of Newton's observations.

In the next 160 years, many people investigated the correlations between the scientific (physical and neurobiological) and the psychological (including aesthetic) aspects of color. By psychological aspects, we refer to the conscious and unconscious adaptive activity of a person when he/she experiences color sensations.

Color vision deals with one of the major sensory receptors, the eye, and its primary stimulus, light. In animals, the evolutionary development of the five senses proceeded in a fairly orderly manner[3], indicating that they have definite functions for survival. For example, touch, smell, taste, vision, and hearing are important for nutrition. In that context, color is related to the capability of differentiating the suitability and ripeness of fruit or vegetables. The good color differentiation demonstrated by insects and birds and the relative insignificance of color perception among nocturnal beasts of prey are typical examples. A bee not only differentiates flowers and the location of honey in a flower by color vision, it also easily learns to locate the appropriate entrance in a beehouse. Cats, on the other hand, pay little attention to differences in color; training cats to respond to color has had little success.

Color vision in man is highly developed. That innate capacity has diminished in importance, however, in our technological civilization. It has been subordinated by man's cultural development and his industrial activities. Color vision is less important for survival today than it was earlier. Examples for the cultural and technological influence on the conversion of color sensations in the eye into cognitive concepts will be provided later in this chapter.

As discussed in chapters 7–10, the transformation of visual sensations in the brain into perception is complex, but it is scientifically accessible. Much more difficult to investigate and to understand are the gaps between perception and cognitive experience.

Today the view of the Gestalt psychologists that visual perception is creative or constructive rather than being an analytical process has gained increasing acceptance. It is also clear that previous experience plays an important role for the interpretation of the sensory input to the brain. A significant amount of knowledge has been accumulated in recent decades on the major areas of the brain that are active in the perception of visual sensations. However, we still know very little about the nature of perception as the basis of cognition, particularly because the interplay between the perceptual and the cognitive system is complicated by experience and emotions.

The relative size and complex organization of the human brain is significantly greater than that of animals. Aside from the development of sight, *language* has contributed to the dominance of the human brain.[4,5] The fact that only man has language is, biologically, still a mystery. Many animals can signal observations to other animals, but only man has the ability to represent the steps of an argument with an ordered sequence of verbal signals. The biological basis of man's language capacity appears to be confirmed by the observations that: (a) all children acquire language at nearly the same age, although various languages have very different degrees of complexity in lexicon and grammar, and the children may be raised under quite different circumstances; and (b) that the degree of similarity between the first and the second language acquired is quite irrelevant to the ease of learning the second language when it is learned during the biologically optimal period, namely, during childhood.[6]

In the following sections, we shall discuss linguistic studies that are related to color perception, i.e., naming of color samples and the development of color naming in various languages. Such psycholinguistic investigations demonstrate the "psychological response function" of the biological processing of light stimuli in the brain.

Neurobiology of Color Vision

Thomas Young[7] assumed early in the nineteenth century that *all* conceivable colors can be obtained by mixing three appropriate principal colors. His hypothesis was later verified and is called the tristimulus (or trichromatic) theory today. It is important in technology: color printing, color photography, and color television are based on it.

The tristimulus theory is also supported by physiological, biochemical, and biophysical studies. The eyes of fish, mammals, and man contain two types of photoreceptive cells in the retina – rods and cones. Rods are sensitive to dim light or at night and to light and dark only. Cones are responsible for color sensation under daylight conditions. There are three types of cones, as discovered in 1964 by Marks et al.[8] for primates, and by Brown and Wald[9] for man. The three types of cones have peak sensitivities in different parts of the visible spectrum. These cells have often been called blue-, green-, and red-sensitive cones, respectively.

In the classical tristimulus theory, it was assumed that each cone is associated with its own specific nerve fiber, which is correlated with one of the three fundamental color sensations, namely blue, green, and red. Yellow was assumed to arise from combined red and green excitations, white from excitation of all types, and black from no excitation (Fig. 1).

As the tristimulus theory explained much of the data on color vision fairly well, another theory, namely Hering's opponent color theory, was almost forgotten in the mid-nineteen-fifties. In 1874, Ewald Hering, a German physiologist, proposed that there are three pairs of opponent physiological processes for vision, the members of each pair being antagonistic. The three pairs were thought to correspond to black/white, red/green, and blue/yellow sensations (Fig. 2).[10] Hering's postulate of positive and negative responses (called "assimilation" and "dissimilation") of the same nerve cell was not accepted by physiologists for a long time because negative excitations of a nerve cell were not conceivable. Later, however, physiologists

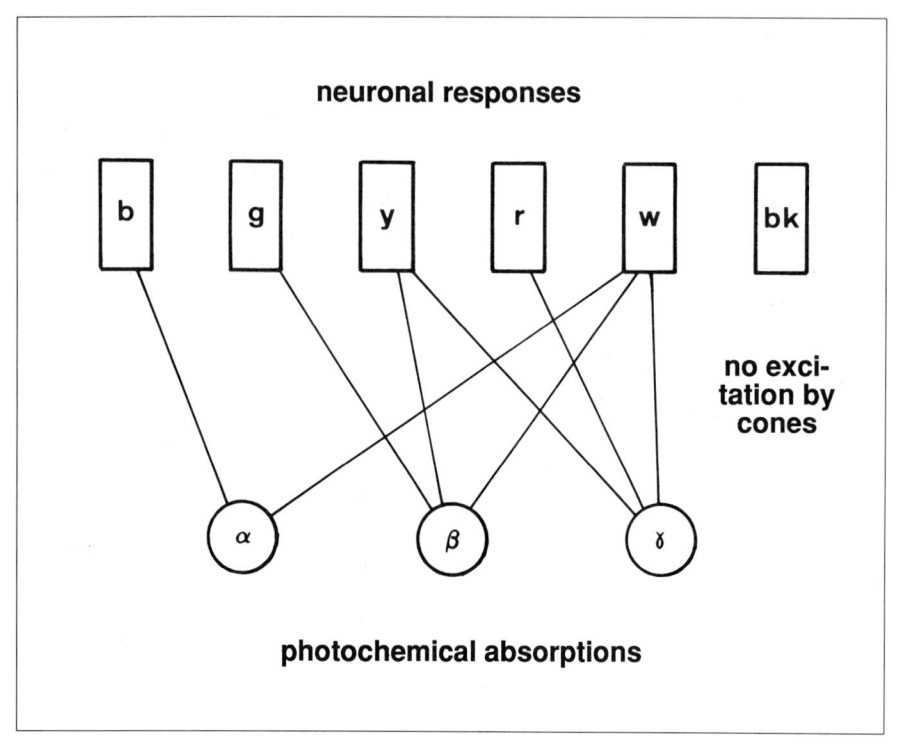

Fig. 1. Schematic representation of the tristimulus theory of color vision
(b: blue; g: green; y: yellow; r: red; w: white; bk: black)

experimentally discovered antagonisms in neural processes, and this led to a renaissance of Hering's theory.

Direct experimental support was found by Svaetichin[11] and by De Valois et al.[12] in the late fifties. They found several types of nerve cells in the retinas of fish (Svaetichin) and in the lateral geniculate body of the monkey

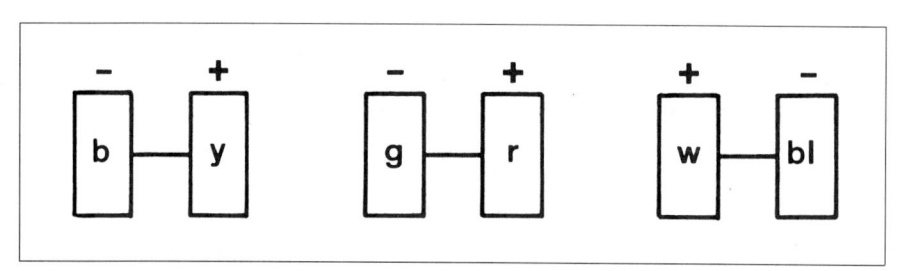

Fig. 2. Original representation of Hering's opponent color theory
(b: blue; y: yellow; g: green; r: red; w: white; bk: black)

(De Valois), the relay station between the retina and the cerebral cortex. Such cells were excited by retinal stimuli of one group of wavelengths and were inhibited by stimuli of the complementary band of wavelengths, both for red/green and for yellow/blue light. In addition, cells were found whose excitation correspond to the overall sensitivity of the eye, i.e., for achromatic ("white") light.

At the time they were proposed, Hering's concepts were far ahead of the knowledge of neurophysiology. This situation changed with Svaetichin's and De Valois' pioneering studies, but subsequent research revealed that the visual system is even more complex. Beginning with the retina, each photoreceptor is connected to several bipolar cells, making synapses with many secondary neurons and vice versa. These bipolar cells are connected in a similarly complex manner with the retinal ganglion cells.

The first two biological stages in the processing of color vision can be found in the retina and in the lateral geniculate body of the thalamus. The function of the three types of cone cells in the retina corresponds to the principle of trichromatic color discrimination. The subsequent stage – the bipolar and ganglion cells in the retina as well as the cells in the lateral geniculate body of the thalamus – is color opponent, as predicted by Hering.

The third, basically different stage, was discovered simultaneously by Daw[13] and by Hubel and Wiesel[14] in the primary visual cortex. It consists of double opponent cells. Their receptive fields have a center with opponent response characteristics to two different bands of wavelength and a surround

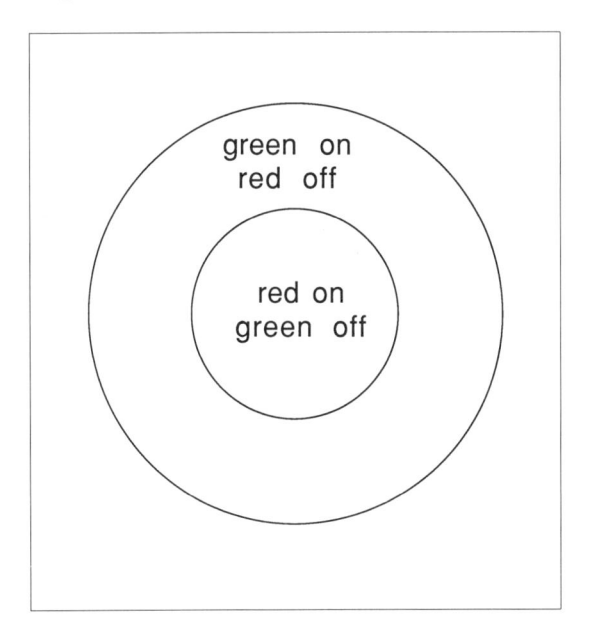

Fig. 3. Schematic representation of a double opponent receptive field

with the same type of spectral sensitivity but opposite sign of response (Fig. 3).

Fibers from the primary visual cortex project to a number of additional areas, including an area called V2. V2, in turn, projects to area V4, where a high percentage of color-coded cells was found by Daw[15], Zeki[16], and others.

In summary, we see that the trichromatic scheme operates only in the very first stage, i.e., in the cone cells. Afterwards, simple and more complex opponent color schemes are found. They are based on three pairs of main color categories, namely black/white, red/green, and yellow/blue. Perception of white is not a simple addition of all chromatic colors as in optical color mixing, but a different type of perception as compared to the perception of chromatic colors. All this is basically related to Hering's proposal, as shown schematically in Fig. 4.

On the basis of Hering's opponent color scheme, Goethe's view[2] that white is not an additive mixture of chromatic colors becomes understandable. Indeed, achromatic stimuli are treated trichromatically only on the photorecep-

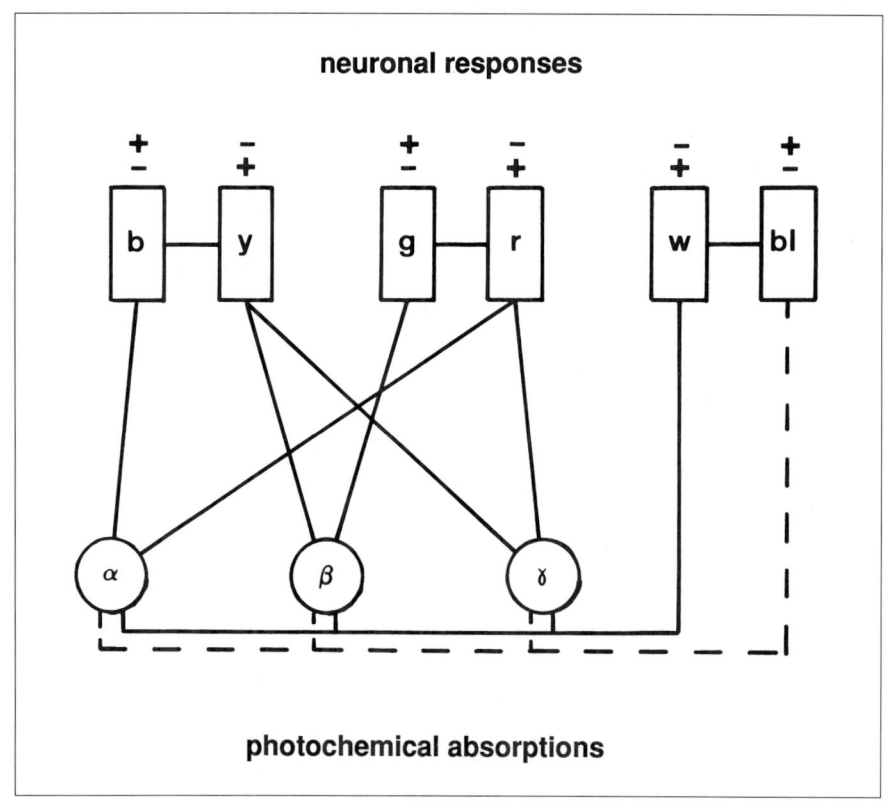

Fig. 4. Hurvich's[18] representation of Hering's opponent color theory

tor level of the retina. In the ganglion cells of the retina and in subsequent processing stages, achromatic information is treated separately from chromatic information.

Psycholinguistics of Color Naming

If Hering's opponent color scheme is reflected in man's brain, psychophysical investigations should demonstrate a dominant role for black, white, red, green, yellow, and blue and, in psycholinguistics, terms for these colors should be of primary importance. With respect to psychophysical investigations, this conclusion was first reached by Jameson and Hurvich[17] in 1955. They carried out color-mixture experiments by matching chromatically colored lights in proper proportions. The results clearly demonstrated a correlation in the occurrence of the two opponent chromatic pairs red/green and yellow/blue.

We can even go a step further, i.e., from a psychophysical experiment to an evaluation of color term usage and to color sample naming in various languages. In the 1970s, we developed a color test and administered it to German, French, English, Hebrew, and Japanese science students.[19,20,21] It was later repeated with German and Hebrew art students[22], and in a slightly different form, with illiterate, monolingual Indians in Central America (Misquito and Quechi).[23] First, the subjects were asked to write down color terms considered to be absolutely necessary for a minimum color lexicon; next, they were shown and asked to name a set of 117 Munsell color samples. In the Munsell system of colors, the samples are perceptionally equidistant from one to the next sample in the three basic dimensions of color space, i.e., hue, brightness ("value" in Munsell's nomenclature), and saturation (chroma; Fig. 5). Each sample had to be named within 20 seconds.

Evaluation of the first part of the test showed that in all languages the terms for red, green, yellow, and blue were listed as absolutely necessary. Added to these were black and white in Japanese, and there is an obvious explanation for this. In German and in English, color can be used as an antonym for the achromatic "colors" black, white, and grey. In this sense of "color," black and white photographs are not "colored." In contrast to German and English, the words for color cannot be used as an antonym for the achromatic colors in Japanese. Black and white are considered genuine colors by native speakers of Japanese. When color photography was introduced in Japan, it was, therefore, not called "color photography" because black-and-white photography is, for a Japanese, a "two-color photography." Hence, "color photography" was called "natural photography."

The second part of the test involved the frequency of occurrence of color terms and the certainty of determination, a figure derived from the ratio of the

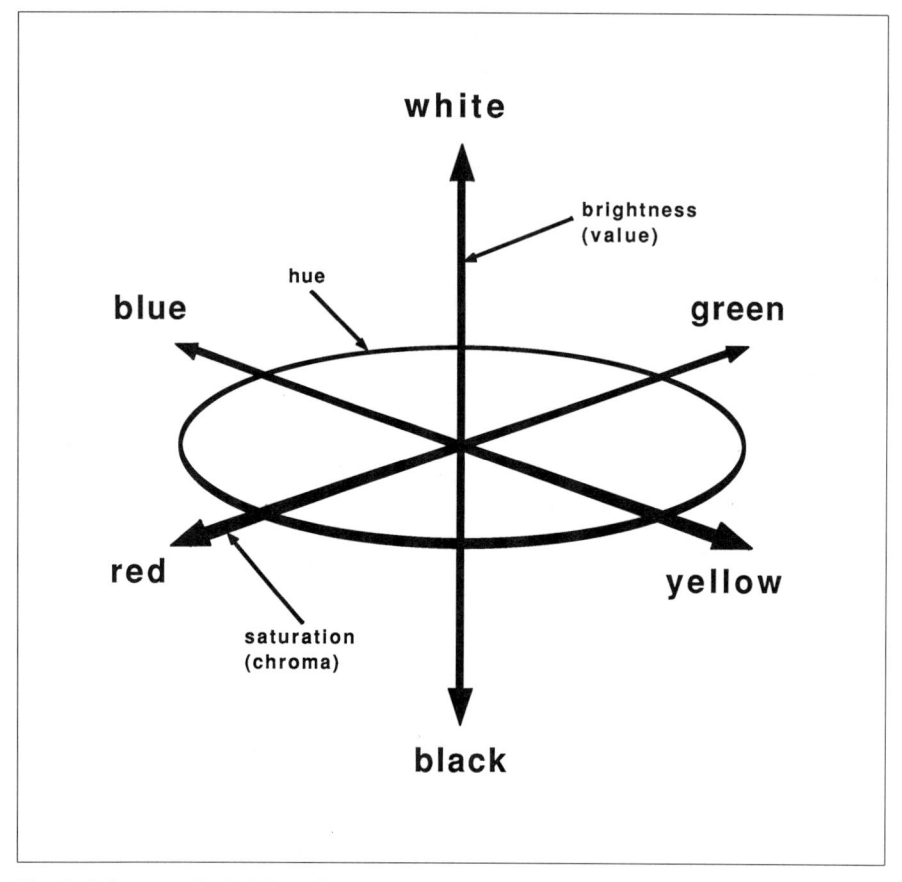

Fig. 5. Color space in the Munsell system of colors

sum of all names given to a sample to the total number of subjects. The certainty of determination demonstrated that, for samples of high saturation ("pure hues"), a correlation with the principal hues red, green, yellow, and blue exists (no achromatic samples were included in this part of the test). Figure 6 shows the frequency of occurrence and the certainty of determination of the highest level of saturation for German-speaking science students. The positions of psychologically pure green, yellow, and blue are indicated with an arrow (not given for red because psychologically pure red is a mixture of the blue and red end of the physical spectrum).[24]

This relatively good correlation disappears, however, as soon as we compare hues on a lower level of saturation. Obviously, the higher relative content of polychromatic ("white") light of these samples interferes with the simple relation between opponent color perception and color naming.

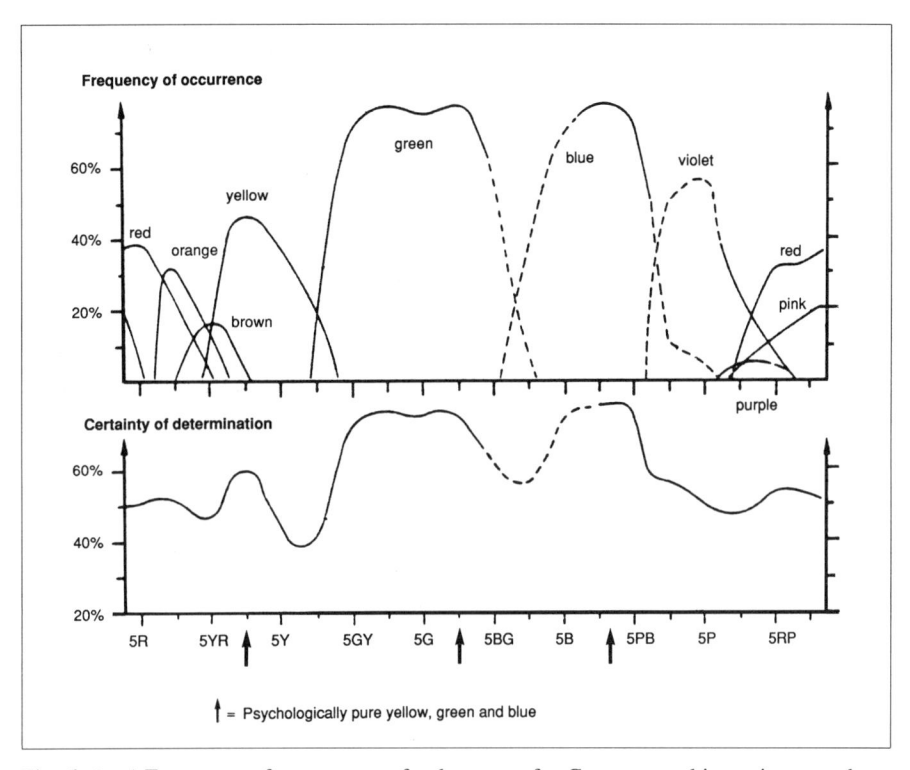

Fig. 6. *(top)* Frequency of occurrence of color terms for German-speaking science students (color samples with relatively pure hues) and location of psychologically pure yellow, green and blue[17]
(bottom) Certainty of determination: percentage of subjects who named respective color samples within 20 s with *any* color term

Color naming is also influenced by cultural differences. The most striking examples of cultural components in color naming in our tests were found for the Japanese[21] and the Quechi[23] languages and in comparing color naming of science students with that of art students in German and in Hebrew.[22] For the certainty of determination of color samples, the following sequence was found:

Quechi Indians > science students > science > art students
                 (German, Hebrew,   students   (German,
                 French, English)   (Japanese) Hebrew)

In our opinion, this sequence of *decreasing* certainty of determination reflects a series of *increasing* "concern" with the phenomenon of color perception. The more the color naming is influenced by personal concern, the less evident the physiological basis of perception becomes. Hence, the physiological basis can best be detected with subjects who do not show any concern at all in color naming.

The reasons for a lesser or greater concern with color are many. The Quechi Indian has a very restricted color lexicon; it is easy for him to make a choice between the five color terms that he has in his language. We speculate that monolingual speakers of this and other languages with a limited color vocabulary do not use their language in such an elaborate way as we do. For them, color is a phenomenon that is always related to some material, like food, but color itself is not an isolated phenomenon with an independent (absolute) value. Quechi Indians are, however, as capable of differentiating hues as we are. This is shown clearly from our color grouping tests.[23] These Indians put green and blue color samples clearly into two categories in spite of the fact that they use the same word to name blue and green samples.

Science students generally have no personal relationship to color; they are not particularly concerned with color names. Art students, in contrast, attempt to describe color impressions, not only the perception of a physical sensation. Within 20 seconds, it is impossible to achieve this perfectly. The color vocabulary of art students is much more elaborate than that of science students; therefore their speed in color naming is slower.

For Japanese science students, the task is also more difficult than for their Western counterparts. The relationship to the person to whom one speaks is much more important (and difficult) in all situations for a Japanese than for Europeans; this also applies to color naming. It takes a Japanese longer to name a color sample. In our test, when a subject waited more than 20 seconds to decide how to name a specific sample, he or she received the rating "not determined" for that sample.

There is a hypothesis in the linguistics of color naming that human races with different skin pigmentation see and, therefore, name colors differently, as pigmentation may also be different in the eye.[25] Although there is, in our opinion, no good experimental biological evidence for this hypothesis, one might argue that biological differences may be the cause for the different importance that Japanese and Europeans, respectively, attribute to the achromatic colors, white, grey, and black. None of our data support the conclusion that any of the differences which we observed in linguistic tests with Japanese relative to Europeans depend on a different underlying physiology.[26] This conclusion was verified recently by Uchikawa and Boynton[27] in a careful comparative study of color sample naming in English and in Japanese.

Positive evidence for our claim that the physiology of color vision is the same for Japanese and for Europeans and that the linguistic differences are influenced by culture derives from an investigation in which we examined[28] whether Western influence changes color vocabulary and color naming characteristics of native speakers of Japanese. For this purpose, we performed our tests with three groups of Japanese children of the same age (12-15) at the following locations: (1) Yonezawa (Yamagata Prefecture), a town of about 100,000 inhabitants; (2) Suginami-ku, Tokyo; and (3) the International Japanese School in Düsseldorf (Federal Republic of Germany), where Japanese children live with their families in a European environment. It can be assumed that the Western influence increases in the sequence of locations given above.

The results demonstrated, first of all, that such an influence was not detectable in the color vocabulary test with respect to the six color terms of the Hering scheme. Changes, however, are observed for terms of colors that are not primary in the sense of the Hering scheme: For the term "cha-iro" (brown, literally "tea color"), a remarkable increase in frequency from only 18% in Yonezawa to 45% in Tokyo and 62% in Düsseldorf was obtained. The frequency of 62% in Düsseldorf corresponds closely with the frequencies of "braun" (57%) and "brown" (62%) observed with German and English science students. It seems plausible to conclude that the Japanese participants in Düsseldorf have adopted for the term "cha-iro," emphasizing the greater importance of the corresponding terms in English (first foreign language at the Japanese school in Düsseldorf) and German (language of their environment).

Interesting cases are the terms orange (or "orange-iro") and pink, borrowed from English. Each of these terms is mentioned with about the same frequency in Japan (Y: 22%, 20%, T: 40%, 42%), but with significantly different frequencies in Düsseldorf (58% orange, 34% pink). In the order Yonezawa, Tokyo, Düsseldorf, the frequencies of orange increase, but pink is listed in Düsseldorf less frequently than in Tokyo.

This asymmetry has an obvious explanation. The English term orange but not the term pink has a German counterpart. Many Germans, even those who speak English, do not know what pink means, while the French word orange is frequently used in German. We conclude that the use of orange but not of pink was reinforced in the German-speaking environment of the Japanese children in Düsseldorf. Again, as in the case of "cha-iro," the frequency of orange corresponds to that found among German science students.

The original Japanese color terms "daidai" (orange) and "momo-iro" (pink) are listed less frequently. "Momo-iro" is listed in Yonezawa (6%), but does not occur at all in Tokyo and Düsseldorf. For "daidai," a frequency decrease is observed (Y: 26%, T: 6%, D: 4%). It is opposite to the increase found for orange (Y: 22%, T: 40%, D:58%). It appears that, from Yonezawa via Tokyo to Düsseldorf, a partial switch of labels for the same basic color category occurs.

New color terms may be formed for technological reasons. This is the case for the increased importance of turquoise in English and analogous terms in other languages in industrialized countries during the last decades. It can be shown[29] that, today, turquoise is an often-used term. This is probably due to the development of synthetic dyes and their use in dyeing textile fibers, plastics, and other material. Dyeing of turquoise shades which do not fade has been possible only for about 45 years, since the invention of the synthetic dyestuff phthalocyanine and its introduction in the dyeing industry.

Previously, it was difficult to dye textiles turquoise. A word for that color was used rarely; it existed in some Italian dialects ("turchino") because expensive textiles dyed turquoise were imported from Eastern Mediterrean countries, like Turkey.[30]

Another interesting linguistic basis for color words relating to turquoise can be found in Bolton and Crisp's study[31] of color terms in folk tales from 40 cultures. In these cultures (including eight European ones), a term for turquoise never occurs except in the Tiwa language of Hopi Indians in Taos (New Mexico). The Taos collection of folk tales contains eight references to turquoise because turquoise stones are the most important gems in that culture. These stones are found frequently in that part of America. It is likely that such color terms are also present in the folk tales of other Indian tribes, e.g., Navajos in that part of the Rocky Mountains. Such languages were, however, not included in Bolton and Crisp's study.

Finally, we will refer to the most extensive and most general study on color-term linguistics, namely Berlin and Kay's book on basic color terms.[32] It was a landmark for understanding the universality, evolution, and categorization of color vocabularies in almost 100 languages. From naming tests carried out with subjects in 20 languages and with the help of a color chart containing 329 color samples and additional evaluations of linguistic publications on color terms in 78 other languages, Berlin and Kay concluded that the most simple color lexicon contains words for black and white (or dark and light). If the color lexicon contains three words, a word for red is added to black and white; the fourth word is an expression for green or yellow or "grue" (blue and green). Languages with five color terms have words for black, white, red, green (including blue), and yellow. Those with six words include a term for blue; next an expression for brown is added; and, finally, in an irregular sequence, expressions follow for pink, violet, orange, grey, etc.

Although slight modifications had to be made to that evolutionary scheme later by Kay and McDaniel[33] and by Sun[34], it is consistent with the biological scheme of opponent colors in as much as the six opponent colors are also primary colors linguistically.

In summary, it is clear that the six basic colors of the Hering opponent scheme are recognizable by a purely psychological response function, namely in linguistic studies on color lexica and color naming in a large number of languages. As shown in this section of our chapter, that scheme, however, is very often masked by psychological, social, cultural, and technological influences.

Mutual Influences of the Senses: Linguistic Relations

Very often, color perception of certain objects seen by a person is influenced by one or more of the other senses. This is particularily important for the evaluation and acceptance of food, in which at least four of the five senses are involved. Watson[35] demonstrated that, if water is colored orange by artificial coloring and, at the same time, made to taste like pineapple by means of artificial taste additives, subjects tend to reply that it tastes like oranges. Obviously, the visual sense is dominant in this test. For the case of vision, the shape is less important than the color for the acceptability of a food, e.g., potatoes are eaten in forms of very different types, but the color has to be between white and medium brown.

These and other examples of synesthesias (correlated sensations of two or more senses) fit into a linguistic scheme of the senses which was studied by Williams.[36] He investigated the metaphorical use of adjectives which are related to the five senses. He found that adjectives belonging to a certain human sense are transferred metaphorically to the area of another sense almost without exception only in those directions indicated in Fig. 7.

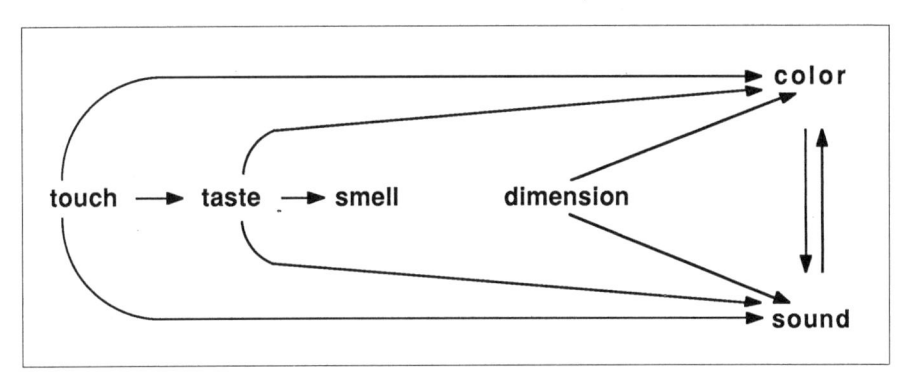

Fig. 7. Metaphorical transfers of sensory adjectives to other senses, according to Williams.[36] The visual sense is referred to in two areas, color and dimension (spatial perception).

As the senses are arranged in this illustration, metaphorical shifts take place in general only from left to right. Examples which are interesting in the context of color vision are:

"warm brown" (touch – color)
"full red" (dimension – color)
"acrid violet" (taste or sound – color)
"C major is a bright key" (sound – color)
"a loud color" (sound – color)

Yet statements like "the taste of this tomato is red" are not understandable. Williams demonstrated that Fig. 7 applies not only to English, but also to Japanese.

There is strong evidence that the directions of transfer shown in Fig. 7 parallel the biological evolution of the senses, i.e., their phylogenetic development in animals and man. The hindbrain of early vertebrates processes touch, taste, and balance. The midbrain of higher vertebrates is specialized in processing olfactory and visual stimuli. The acoustic sense probably developed parallel to the visual sense. This leads to a sequence of sense development from touch to taste, smell, and finally, to hearing and sight (or vice versa). The fact that the visual and the acoustic senses cannot be put in a distinct sequence parallels their position in William's scheme of metaphorical transfers.

The Evolution of Color Vision in Man

Relations between food color and the perception of various colors are interesting. The daylight sensitivity of the human eye begins with light of wavelengths around 400 nanometers; it passes through a maximum at 555 nm and ends at 700 nm. The highest sensitivity is found in the perception of yellow to green objects (500–600 nm). It may well be that this maximum in sensitivity is related in human evolution to the capability of differentiating the ripeness of fruits and vegetables.

The evolution of color terms as discovered by Berlin and Kay[32], i.e., the sequence white/black – red – yellow/green – blue – brown, etc., may be related also in part to food: white and black are important as the basis of light in general, e.g., day and night. Red relates to life (blood), yellow and green to food. The sixth color category in the neurobiological opponent color scheme (blue), however, has no relation to the basic needs of life. In nature, it exists almost only in objects which cannot be physically grasped, such as the sky, or which lose their color when caught hold of (i.e. water).

In concluding this chapter, we hope to have demonstrated two major points:

1. The physiological mechanisms used by the eye and the brain to analyze light stimuli and synthesize color perception can be recognized in a purely psychological response function, namely in the color lexicon of various languages and in color naming tests.
2. The results of such linguistic tests are not unchanged reproductions of those physiological mechanisms.

Psychological, social, cultural, and technological influences are superimposed on the innate physiological reactions. Brain research during the last two or three decades has shown clearly that cortical mechanisms are not completely preprogrammed genetically. The nervous system is influenced by the surrounding world after birth. This process of learning is based on the plasticity of the brain. It is, therefore, not astonishing that this plasticity is also reflected in psycholinguistic studies on color vision.

References and Notes

1. Newton I (1672) Trans Roy Soc London 80:3075–3087
2. Goethe JW (1810) Zur Farbenlehre. Cotta, Tübingen
3. Sarnat H, Netsky MG (1974) Evolution of the nervous system. Oxford University Press, London
4. Lenneberg EH (1967) Biological foundations of language. John Wiley, New York
5. Lieberman P (1984) The biology and evolution of language. Harvard University Press, Cambridge
6. Kucera H (1981) The abduction algorithm: A computer model of language acquisition. Perceptives in Computing 1:28–35; see also Lieberman[5], chaps 2 and 9
7. Young T (1802) On the theory of light and colours. Phil Trans Roy Soc London, 12–48
8. Marks WB, Dobelle WH, MacNichol EF (1964) Visual pigments of single primate cones. Science 143:1181–1183
9. Brown PK, Wald G (1964) Visual pigments in single rods and cones of the human retina. Science 144:45–52
10. Hering E (1874) Grundrisse einer Theorie des Farbensinnes. Sber Akad Wiss Wien, math-nat Kl III 70:169–204; Hering E (1876, 1920) Zur Lehre vom Lichtsinne. Carl Gerold's Sohn, Wien (1876), reprinted by Springer, Berlin (1920)
11. Svaetichin G (1952) The cone action potential. Acta physiol scand 29, suppl 106:565–600; ibid. 39, suppl 134:17–46
12. De Valois RL, Smith CJ, Karoly AJ, Kitai ST (1958) Electrical responses of primate visual system. J comp physiol Psychol 51:662–678
13. Daw NW (1967) Goldfish retina: Organization for simultaneous color contrast. Science 158:942–944
14. Hubel DH, Wiesel TN (1968) Receptive fields and functional architecture of monkey striate cortex. J Physiol 195:215–243
15. Daw NW (1984) The psychology and physiology of colour vision. Trends in Neurosciences 7:330–335

16. Zeki S (1985) Colour pathways and hierarchies in the cerebral cortex. In: Ottoson D, Zeki S (ed) Central and peripheral mechanisms of color vision. MacMillan, Basingstoke, pp 19–44
17. Jameson D, Hurvich LM (1955) Some quantitative aspects of an opponent-colors theory. J opt Soc Am 45:546–552, 602–616
18. Hurvich LM (1981) Color vision. Sinauer, Sunderland
19. Zollinger H (1973) Zusammenhänge zwischen Farbbenennung und Biologie des Farbensehens beim Menschen. Vjschr Naturf Ges Zürich 118:227–255
20. Zollinger H (1976) A linguistic approach to the cognition of colour vision in man. Folia linguist IX–1–4:265–293
21. Wattenwyl von A, Zollinger H (1979) Color term salience and neurophysiology of color vision. Am Anthropologist 81:279–288
22. Wattenwyl von A, Zollinger H (1981) Color naming by art students and science students. A comparative study. Semiotica 35:303–315
23. Wattenwyl von A, Zollinger H (1978) The color lexica of two American Indian languages. Quechi and Misquito. Int J Am Linguistics 44: 56–68
24. Psychologically pure colors are those which do not possess a tinge of neighboring colors, e.g., psychologically pure green is neither yellowish nor bluish.
25. Bornstein MH (1973) Color vision and color naming: A psychophysiological hypothesis of cultural differences. Psychol Bull 80:257–285
26. Iijima T, Zollinger H (1980) Colour naming in Japanese – some remarks on cultural factors (in Japanese). Nippon Shikisaigaku Kaishi (J Color Sci Ass Japan) 4 (4): 2–7
27. Uchikawa K, Boynton RM (1987) Categorical color perception of Japanese observers: Comparison with that of Americans. Vision Res 27:1825–1833
28. Iijima T, Wenning W, Zollinger H (1982) Cultural factors of color naming in Japanese: Naming tests with Japanese children in Japan and Europe. Anthropol Linguistics 24:245–262
29. Zollinger H (1984) Why just turquoise? Remarks on the evolution of color terms. Psychol Res 46:403–409
30. Kristol AM (1980) Color systems in southern Italy: A case of regression. Language 56:137–145
31. Bolton R, Crisp D (1979) Color terms in folk tales. A cross-cultural study. Behavior Sci Res 14:231–253
32. Berlin B, Kay P (1969) Basic color terms. Their universality and evolution. University of California Press, Berkeley Los Angeles
33. Kay P, McDaniel CK (1978) The linguistic significance of the meanings of basic color terms. Language 54:610–646
34. Sun RK (1983) Perceptual distances and the basic color term encoding sequence. Am Anthropologist 85:387–391
35. Watson RHJ (1980) Colour and acceptance of food. In: Counsell TN (ed) Natural colours for food and other uses. Applied Science, London 27–38
36. Williams JM (1976) Synaesthetic adjectives: A possible law of semantic change. Language 52:461–472

Physiological Constraints on the Visual Aesthetic Response

Günter Baumgartner
Department of Neurology, University Hospital, 8091 Zürich, Switzerland

Most biologists agree that living organisms have evolved over millions of years, and it seems possible to trace evolutionary processes back to the prebiological molecular level.[1] One of the most important steps of evolution was the development of the central nervous system and of the cortex of the cerebral hemispheres in mammals. This part of the brain is most directly related to the growing differentiation of behavior and, consequently, reaches its climax in man. One could say that, in the human brain, the first principle of evolution, learning, has become the main function. Most noteworthy is the fact that the brain may adapt to environmental changes within seconds, whereas learning by evolution is a slow process requiring thousands and more years. This enormous acceleration of learning by the brain has consequences of utmost importance. It enabled mankind to develop and hand down its cultural achievements independently of the slow pace of evolutionary processes. It also implies that there is little chance that evolution will be able to correct what went wrong during this development.

Despite the fact that it is the capacity of the brain that allowed the human race to initiate "cultural evolution," we may find it difficult to accept that our perceptive and cognitive abilities are the direct consequence of the functional organization of our brains and, especially, of our cerebral cortices. Part of the reason for this may be that the wonders of our mental world seem unlimited, whereas the brain is a finite structure. Yet both physiological research and clinical experience suggest that what we perceive is not the reality of the physical world but a model thereof, which has been constructed by using relatively few sensory signals. The mystery of the relationship between the discontinuous neuronal activities within the brain and our apparently continuous mental experience is deepened by the fact that the brain's model of the world never manifests itself as such but is inevitably interpreted as the world per se.

This brain-mind paradox has received so much attention by the most brilliant scholars and yet may remain unexplained forever.

It is important to note, however, that within the last three decades there has been both an acceleration and a convergence in the developments of objective and subjective research in sensory physiology. As a consequence of the possibility to record the activity of individual nerve cells in the brain, neurophysiologists began investigating the behavior of neurons within a given sensory system (e.g., vision, audition, or somatosensation) under well-defined conditions of stimulation. The results of such studies could then be related to psychophysical observations, that is, to responses obtained from conscious subjects under identical conditions of stimulation, or, in behavioral experiments, from animals trained to react differently to various signals. It turned out that the activity of certain cells in the cerebral cortex is necessarily and directly correlated with the perception of, say, red, or of a well-defined sound. It became also clear that the constraints on perception are directly reflected by the response properties (e.g., resolution, spectral sensitivity) of such cells. This conclusion is supported by the clinical observation that the ability to perceive a quality of sensation disappears when the cells related to it are destroyed. These findings do not provide an answer to the question of why the activation of the nerve cells under investigation is associated with such a wealth of sensory impressions like the gradation of color or tone quality, etc. Yet it is inevitable to conclude that mental experience can be split and is as limited as the brain, itself.

The study of correlations between neuronal activities and perception has been applied successfully to the investigation of man's cognitive competence. Thus, it seems legitimate to extend this type of research to the possible relationships between aesthetic experience and activities within the neuronal networks of the brain and also the rules that define the interaction among neurons. Even if one considers the aesthetic as "inimical to quasi-scientific treatment,"[2] its prerequisites are accessible. However, it is neither desirable nor probable that aesthetic responses will become predictable as a consequence of such an approach. By virtue of the extreme complexity of possible neuronal networks and their ongoing modification by learning, they will almost certainly remain unpredictable, and this must continuously lead to new kinds of aesthetic evaluation. Physiological constraints on the aesthetic experience should, therefore, not be understood as an attempt to explain the aesthetic per se. Yet if we were able to demonstrate their existence, this would explain why theories concerning aesthetics have been and will remain unsatisfactory.

To better understand the relationship between aesthetics and perception, we ought to note that without perception there cannot be be any aesthetic experience. Hence, the nature of perception must influence the evaluation of the aesthetic. It is, therefore, of interest to pose the question of how external stimulation modifies the activity of sensory systems. As previous experience influences aesthetic judgements, we shall also discuss the role that learning plays in the modification of sensory processes. There are no straightforward answers to these questions since the relationships between brain function, perception, and cognitive experience are far from being understood. We shall not attempt to answer the question of how and why the organized activity of brain cells is associated with mental activity. We shall, instead, concentrate on elucidating the conditions under which a certain perception occurs and, if known, its neuronal correlate. From such a narrowed perspective, some physiological constraints on aesthetic exerience can be demonstrated.

What is known about vision derives from many disciplines. Neuroanatomy investigates the connections within and between the neuronal networks subserving perception and cognition. Its results constitute the basis for any discussion about sensory systems. In the present context, however, it is sufficient to say that the visual system is widely distributed within the cerebral cortex and also deeper brain structures. It is also important to note that the different visual areas of the cortex are not only connected in series but also parallel.

The quantitative relationships between sensory stimuli and the resulting perceptions have been extensively studied by psychophysicists.[3-5] Aspects of sensory quality – the essence of aesthetic experience – received much less attention. Here it suffices to mention the work of the physiologist Ewald Hering[6] and artists like Leonardo da Vinci[7] and members of the later schools of impressionism and neoimpressionism. Their studies concentrated on the effects of the distribution of brightness and color in more qualitative terms.[8] The main concern of the Gestalt psychologists was form as the primitive unit of perception.[9-12] They assumed an isomorphic mapping of the perceived form onto the patterns of neuronal activity.

A topology of higher brain function has been established in neuropsychology, the discipline investigating the neuronal correlates of disorders in perception, language, and action.[13-15] Its results have been confirmed by recent studies of local cerebral blood flow and metabolism[16-18] and electrophysiological brain mapping.[19] During such investigations, human subjects receive some form of sensory stimulation and/or have to do something while the ongoing activity in their brains is monitored by means of a detector system. The latter is connected to a computer that analyzes the responses with respect to the characteristics of the stimulus and/or task. Probably the most significant result of neuropsychological research is that specific functions of perception and cognition depend on the hemispheric site of the activation, and the same is true for defective perception and cognition in the presence of circumscribed brain damage. These findings have been corroborated by the observation that both metabolic energy consumption and the generation of electrical activity vary in different regions of the brain, depending on the task being performed by the subject.

A related clinical observation is the functional loss of a visual hemifield (to the left or the right of the vertical meridian) as a result of the destruction of the central visual areas in the contralateral cerebral hemisphere (e.g., the left hemisphere if the right hemifield is lost). The reason for this is the convergence in one hemisphere of the nerve fibers of both retinae carrying information from the contralateral hemifield (see diagram p. 246, chap. 10). In much the same way, visual stimulation of one hemifield increases metabolism in the contralateral visual areas in the cerebral cortex.

The visual loss as a consequence of a lesion of the visual cortex can be predicted according to the location of the lesion. What cannot be predicted, however, is that the loss may go unnoticed by the patient. Even complete blindness following a lesion of both visual areas may be negated. Hence, it appears that the destruction of the visual areas in the brain also implies a loss of visual memory, and this unexpected finding demonstrates that we do not really understand the process of sight. There are also locations in the brain where circumscribed lesions can abolish the recognition of objects, colors, or faces, etc., a clinical condition previously called *seelenblindheit* (blindness of the mind). Furthermore, such lesions can also lead to a neglect of one visual hemifield or a part of the body.

The dependence of the consequences of a cortical lesion on the hemispheric localization can be demonstrated by means of the work of artists who suffered such visual defects. Figure 1 shows a sequence of self-portraits by the German painter, Anton Räderscheidt, who suffered a stroke in the parietal lobe of the right cerebral hemisphere.[20] In the first picture he painted two months after the stroke, the artist completely neglected the space to the left of the midline. This side is predominantly related to the sensory and motor systems of the damaged right cerebral hemisphere. Three and a half months after the event, the artist tried to represent a whole face in the still accessible right half of space. Half a year later, there are a few and distorted image elements beyond the midline. Even after a recovery period of nine months, the representation of the left hemispace is still distorted. This artist did not suffer a deterioration of speech, but the infarction in the right cerebral hemisphere affected his style of pictorial representation and his perception of space.

Completely different was the condition of the French artist and caricaturist, Sabadel, who suffered a stroke in the left cerebral hemisphere.[21] He immediately lost the capacity of speech, and the right side of his body became paralyzed. Although under the impression that he would never be able

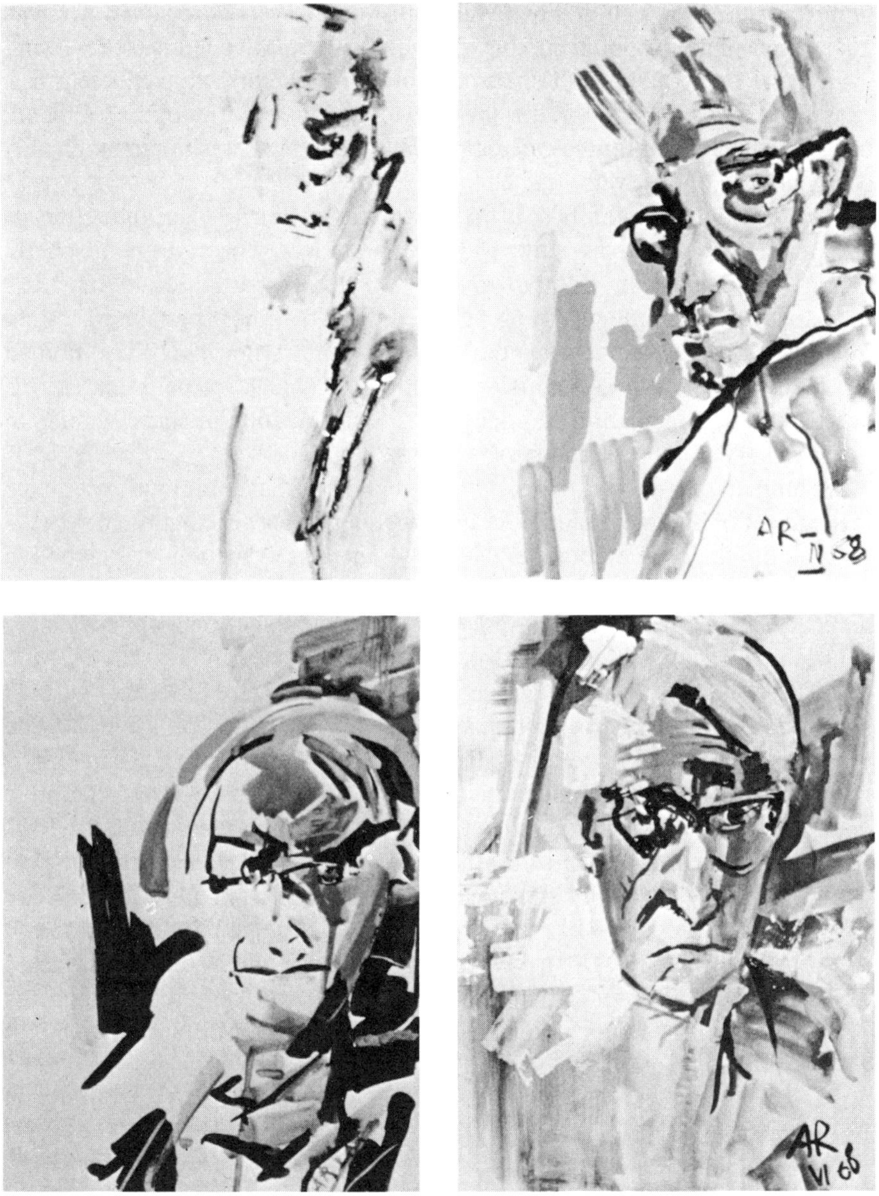

Physiological Constraints on the Visual Aesthetic Response 169

Fig. 1. Neglect of the left visual hemifield in self-portraits of an artist after a stroke in the posterior parietal region of the right cerebral hemisphere (*above left:* 2 months, *below left:* 3 1/2 months, *above right:* 6 months, *below right:* 9 months after the stroke). In the first portrait, only the right side of the picture is painted. With increasing time from disease onset, the neglect is gradually compensated (reproduced from Jung[20]).

to draw again, he was urged by his therapist to draw his home town. He was not yet able to use his left hand to perfection, but he succeeded in representing the village fairly well, with space and proportions correctly rendered. Encouraged by this experience, the artist developed the abilities of his left hand, and within a few months, he had regained his former mastership, including his personal style of drawing.

The case histories of these artists illustrate the functional asymmetries of the cerebral hemispheres quite well (see Part IV). The right-hemispheric damage suffered by the German painter resulted in a partial loss of his artistic competence, with the most pronounced disturbance of spatial perception. Yet this patient was not impaired in his verbal competence. The French caricaturist, by contrast, lost his ability to communicate verbally but not his artistic abilities, indicating an undisturbed representation of space within the intact right cerebral hemisphere.

Summarizing these findings, we may conclude that conscious experience is the result of the interaction of many functionally specific neuronal subsystems within the two cerebral hemispheres. The loss of the related perceptive or cognitive functions seemingly remains unnoticed if the neuronal subsystems underlying these functions are no longer available. This implies that the concept of an indivisible mental world is untenable.

The results summarized above also imply that many different neuronal subsystems[22,23] must interact before any aesthetic evaluation can be made. The mechanisms of this cooperative interaction are still unknown. Hence, it is premature to evaluate their specific contributions to perception and cognitive experience. It is, however, possible to demonstrate neuronal correlates to different visual qualities, such as brightness, darkness, color, depth, and movement in terms of the results of studies of single neurons in the visual system. Some of these properties can be explained by the functional organization of the visual pathways.[24-30] Up to now, most correlates found have been restricted to the activity in afferent pathways from the eyes to the cerebral hemispheres or to the early cortical processing areas. These sites are far from where it might be assumed that perception and cognition take place. Nevertheless, the related functional properties must be reflected in integrated brain functions, as demonstrated by defects in color vision or the characteristics of color naming (see chapter 6).

A common misconception about visual processing is the assumption of passive filtering of incoming retinal signals (see also chapter 8). A simple reconstruction of the retinal image at subsequent stages would only be redundant. The Gestalt psychologists provided many examples of how perception groups and organizes visual features according to inherent rules and fairly independent of physical conditions. Another indication for active information processing in vision is the construction of three-dimensional space out of the two-dimensional images of the two retinae. There are also the many so-called optical illusions that further suggest a lack of simple congruence between retinal images and their final, "mental" interpretation (Figs. 2 and 3). The interindividual constancy of illusory perceptions shows, however, that the brain processes the signals from the retina according to well-defined rules in its attempt to construct a dynamic neuronal model of the visual environment – a construct which we interpret as reality. Any possible perception must obey these rules, which have evolved to fit the needs and possibilities of the organism in its struggle for survival. Hence, the underlying neuronal mechanisms are designed to optimize adaptive behavior.

Next we have to consider the fact that visual processing is performed at several levels. The transformation of information begins in the retina, where the distribution of light across the receptors is converted into neuronal activity. This activity is organized by complex interactions among many morphologically and chemically classifiable nerve cells, depending on location, intensity, and color of the stimulus pattern. Thus, the retina is not a

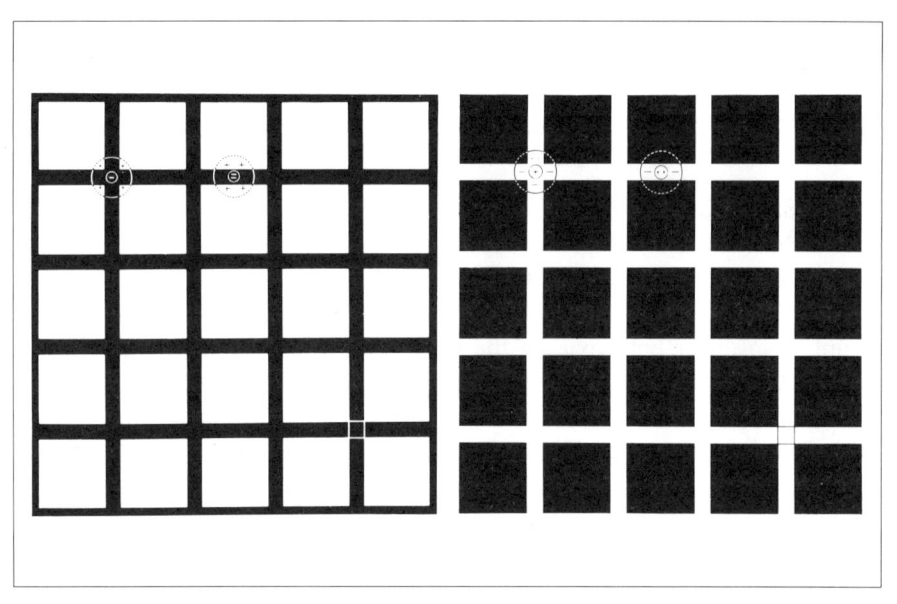

Fig. 2. Hermann's contrast illusion at black and white grids. The intersections of the black bars appear less dark and those of the white bars, less bright than the bars themselves. The illusion can be explained in terms of response properties of receptive fields of on- and off- center neurons located at the site of bars and their intersections (concentric circles: see Fig. 4). The illusion disappears if one fixates an intersection at reading distance. The latter phenomenon depends on the smaller size of receptive fields at the center of fixation. If the grid is dissected by adding the contour of a square to an intersection, the contrast illusion is also suppressed.

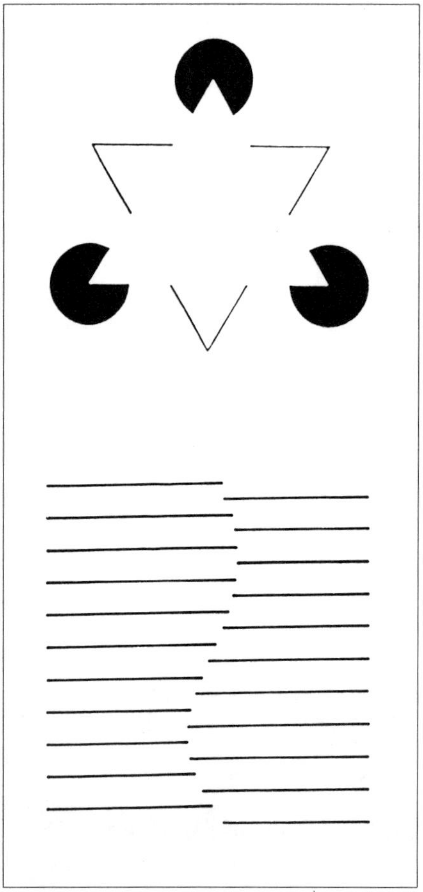

Fig. 3. Kanizsa illusory contours. A white triangle appears in front of three black discs and an outlined inverted triangle. An illusory contour is also preceived between two offset series of thin parallel lines.

simple transducer but a part of the brain, and it is able to transfer the signals of 10^8 photoreceptors via 10^6 ganglion cells without a loss of information. The enhancement of intensity gradients and the initiation of contrast, as well as brightness constancy, already take place at the level of the retinal ganglion cells. With some simplification, one may state that light increments or decrements are transferred beyond the retina by two distinct groups of ganglion cells (see chapter 8). One group responds to the appearance of a light stimulus with increased electric activity and to its disappearance with a decrease in activity (i.e., inhibition), whereas the other group reacts with inhibition to light-on and activation after light-off. The receptive fields of these cells (i.e., the areas of the retina from which their activity can be modified; see also Fig. 3, p. 153) are organized in an inverse fashion. Light-activated cells are excited from the center of their receptive field and inhibited from their surround. These neurons in the visual pathway are called

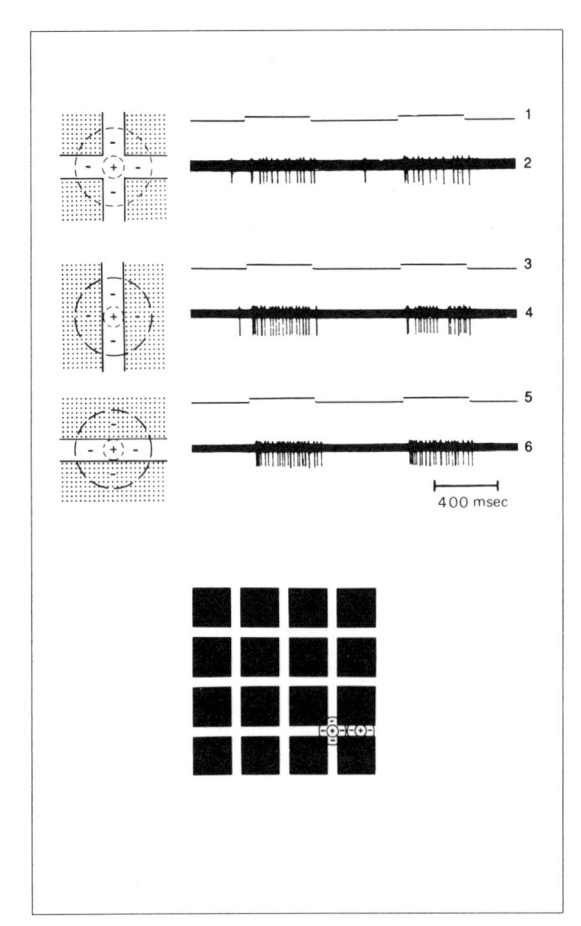

Fig. 4. Neuronal correspondence of the Hermann grid illusion observed at an on-center neuron in the cat's primary visual cortex. The scheme at the *top left* shows the respective position of the receptive field within the grid shown at the bottom. Corresponding discharge patterns of the neuron are plotted at the *right*. Lines 1, 3, and 5 represent records of a photocell (line elevation indicates light pattern on). Lines 2, 4, and 6 show action potentials of the cell (downwards strokes) caused by pattern stimulation. For understanding the differences in neuronal discharge patterns (i.e., the reduced number of action potentials in the first condition), it is important to note the extent of the activating field center (+) and the inhibitory surround (−). If centered in the intersection, the neuron is less activated than in the vertical or in the horizontal bar region due to increased inhibition from the periphery of its receptive field. The former condition corresponds to the diminished appearance of brightness at the intersections.

on-center cells. Correspondingly, the dark-activated neurons are called off-center cells and are inhibited by illumination of the center and excited by illumination of the surround. The dominant response in on- and off-center neurons is always the excitation of the receptive field center. These cells respond, therefore, to diffuse illumination.

The functional significance of the activation of on-center cells is the indication of brighter; activation of off-center cells indicates darker within the center of the receptive field. Such an arrangement of receptive fields is especially suited to provide the achromatic border contrast and, thereby, the enhancement of contours. The intensity gradient at an edge within the retinal image reduces inhibition of the on- center cells in the region of higher intensity and of the off-center cells in the region of lower intensity, thus leading to a stronger activation of both types of cells. An analogous organization is found in the first central station, the lateral geniculate body of the thalamus, and in layer 4 of the first cortical receiving area. The consequences of this organization on an on-center neuron is illustrated in Fig. 4.

We have, then, to consider the functional organization of the cerebral cortex, where the receptive fields of visual neurons are reorganized.[27,28] Thereby, they lose their concentric configuration and become arranged along an axis. Within a piece of cortical tissue, this has the shape of a column and extends perpendicularly to the cortical surface; all cells have receptive fields with the same orientation. The orientation of the axes of the receptive fields changes gradually from column to column. After a shift of about 800 um across the cortical surface, the original orientation recurs together with a small displacement of the receptive field location in the retina. The excitatory and inhibitory regions of the cortical receptive fields are balanced. As a result of this, such cells do not respond to diffuse illumination. They are only activated by light or dark bars or edges of appropriate orientation and localization. Many subgroups of cells with preferred stimulus orientation exist that respond exclusively to specific features.

The problem of what type of information these cortical cells encode remains unresolved. Yet it seems clear that cells with such properties prepare field contrast and the analysis of form. Under the contrast situations depicted in Fig. 5, the whole surface appears brighter or darker depending on whether the intensity gradients at the border correspond to an increase or decrease of intensity. Afferent neurons (i.e., neurons that carry information to the brain) whose concentric receptive fields are located within the homogeneously illuminated regions of the stimulus patterns do not react differently to the two conditions of contrast. Cortical neurons with oriented receptive fields within the homogenous surface do not respond at all. The neurons at the border respond as indicated in the figure. Thus, we can assume that the field contrast is brought about by an extrapolation of the activity of cortical cells in a radial direction from border to border. If this were true, a reversal of the contrast gradients on opposite borders should reduce the effect to one half. This is, indeed, the case, as can be seen in the lower inset of Fig. 5.

The contrast effect demonstrated in Fig. 5 is an example of cooperation among spatially separated neurons to promote form perception and field contrast. In one dimension, such cooperation was first demonstrated by the physiologists David Hubel and Torsten Wiesel in 1977.[27] They used a method which enables the local metabolism rate of nerve cells to be measured. In their experiments, they stimulated monkeys for minutes with light patterns of vertical stripes. By subsequent neuroanatomical analysis they found that the metabolism was selectively augmented in cell columns activated by vertically oriented stripes. Since such columns are spatially separated in the brain, a

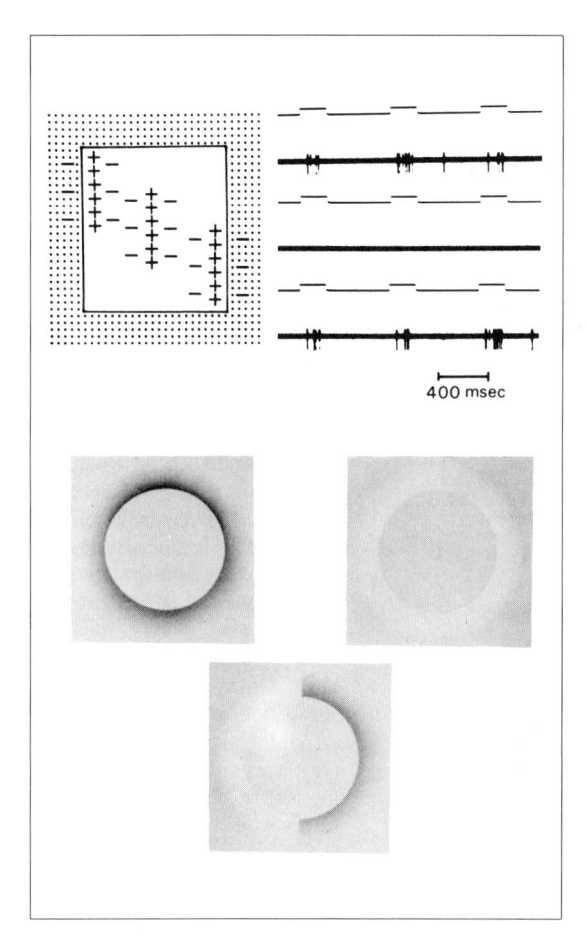

Fig. 5. The Craik-Cornsweet illusion of areal contrast and the response of simple field neurons of the cat's primary cortex. The activating (+) and inhibiting (−) zones of the elongated receptive fields are balanced in their contributions to the cells' net activities. Thus, only those neurons respond whose receptive fields are located at the border between homogeneously illuminated surfaces (*upper* and *lower* cases). The two discs in the *middle* are equal in diameter and luminance, but the *left* appears brighter and larger. Assuming that the area contrast observed in the discs is induced by the direction of the sudden step of luminance at their border, it should be reduced by a reversal of the contrast gradient on opposite sides. This is actually the case (bottom).

continuous line in external space is represented by the activity of spatially separated neurons in cell columns with the same receptive field orientation.

An even higher degree of organization has to be expected for the mechanisms responsible for the generation of illusory contours.[30] This phenomenon, illustrated in Figs. 3 and 4, consists of the generation of reproducible illusions, such as a triangle, bar, etc., by the appropriate arrangement of a few pattern components. The stimulation of single neurons within the first cortical receiving area (called V1) with an illusory bar does not elicit any response. However, cells in V2, which respond to a physical white or black bar, are also frequently activated by an illusory one (Fig. 6).[31,32] These findings demonstrate that the visual system is organized to construct the visual scenery with the utmost economy by processing a minimum of stimulus characteristics.

It is also interesting to note that the mechanisms responsible for optical illusions offer a key to the understanding of the functional organization of the

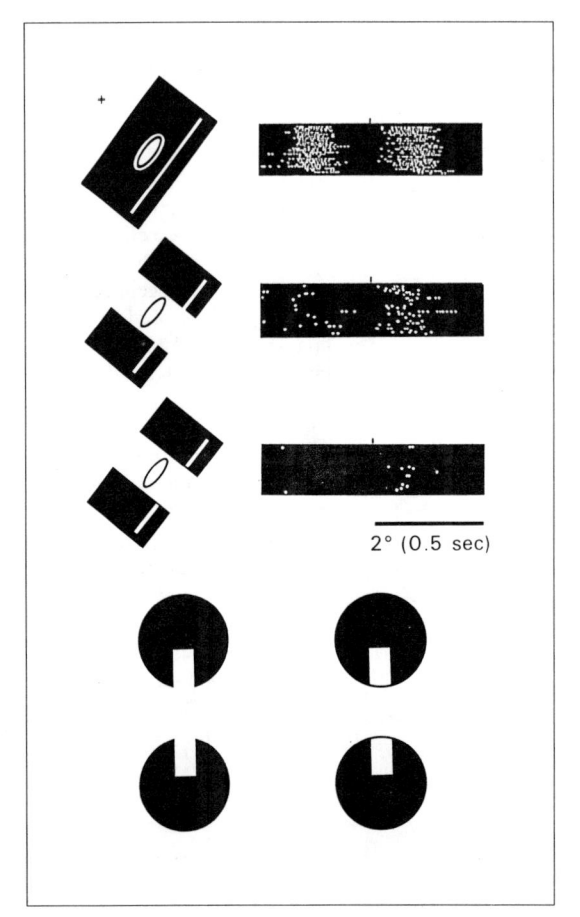

Fig. 6. Neuron of the monkey's second visual area in response to a real and an illusory bright bar. On the *right*: Dot display of neuronal activity (every bright spot indicates a neuronal discharge, and every line of dots corresponds to a back-and-forth movement of a stimulus). On the *left* is a visual pattern. The oval-shaped region corresponds to the receptive fields and the orientation as it has been measured with bright bars of different length and optimal orientation. The first display shows the response to a real bar moving across the receptive field with a movement amplitude of 2° and a cycle time of 0.5 s. The second display corresponds to the stimulation with an illusory figure by moving synchronously only the two notches within the black region. The third display shows the strongly diminished response after closing the notches, a manipulation of the stimulus pattern that abolishes the illusory white bar (see the patterns at the bottom).

visual system. Illusory phenomena are usually hidden within the familiar structure of the visual environment that they generate. As mechanisms for the enhancement of contours or the effect of shading, they are of great importance in drawing.[29] Illusions and contrast effects were also extensively used in op (optical) art (Fig. 7).[33]

This is not to say that visual processing is completed in the cortical area V2. The retina is represented several times in the cortical areas defined as V1, V2, V3, etc. The functions of these areas are different. In simplification, one could say that shape is processed in the columnar modules of V1 and V2, depth in V2, color in V4, and motion in the visual field in V5.[34] This would imply that different qualities of vision are processed by neuronal populations located in different areas in the cerebral cortex. One has to assume that extensive neuronal interaction is necessary to construct a complete visual scene. This may help us to understand the many peculiar defects of visual perception after

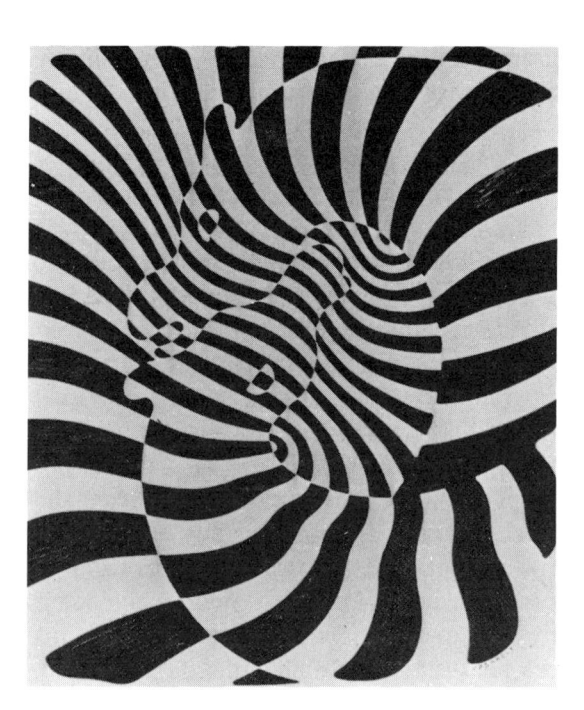

Fig. 7. Two zebras perceived by anomalous contours as shown in the line pattern of Fig. 3 (reproduced from Vasarely[33])

circumscribed brain lesions. If we learn more about the characteristics of these neuronal interactions, we may even discover the reason for some forms of aesthetic preference.

In higher processing areas, visual neurons were found that show a clear preference for face stimuli or for stimuli representing parts of a face.[35,36] The response of these neurons does not depend on the color, the angular orientation, the size, or the location of the face stimulus. Thus, it seems that neurons of this kind are incapable of detecting a specific face in a defined position in space. Yet we are strongly dependent on performing this task. Consequently, we have to assume that the different features of a given face are encoded and processed by different and separately located neuronal populations. The so-called face neurons may just add the index "face" to a complex and widely distributed neuronal activity. In other words, the visual system seemingly does not present a fixed and invariant solution to the problem of visual representation. It is more likely that the visual environment is represented in the brain by means of the dynamic pattern of activity of many spatially distributed cells. It is also important to note that these cells are not only localized in the cerebral cortex, but cooperate with neurons in deeper structures of the brain (e.g., basal ganglia, thalamus) as well.

All this leads us to assume that stimuli are preferred whose properties are favored by the internal mechanisms of visual processing. This could also imply that such types of stimuli constitute positive aesthetic events – a possibility reminiscent of Kant's statement that form is judged beautiful if it facilitates the process of perception.[37] The visual system may thus reward a simple solution to a problem in much the same way as a clear verbal description of a complicated subject is more appealing than a confusing essay, even if it offers more information.

If this seemingly "mechanical" interpretation of the visual aesthetic response is appropriate, why do the conventions of aesthetics vary from culture to culture and even from individual to individual? This seems to be a consequence of the plasticity of the brain. We know, for instance, that the cortical circuitry is not completely preprogrammed genetically but depends on visual exposure in early postnatal life for its final wiring. Yet this cannot explain the continuous modification of our aesthetic judgements during the course of our lives. Plasticity, or learning, remains one of the most important features of the central nervous system. Moreover, learning seems especially enduring in cerebral areas of polymodal convergence, i.e., in substructures where signals from different sensory channels come together. These regions and their polymodal cells are probably involved in cognition. It is probably the enduring learning capacity of such neuronal structures that underlies the individual, the intracultural, and the intercultural variability of aesthetic judgement (see chapter 2). The physiologically determined decrease in learning capacity with age may likewise underly the aesthetic conservatism of the elderly.

We also face the problem of the biological significance of aesthetic experience when we suggest that there are physiological constraints on the aesthetic. Thereby, we may assume that aesthetic events can be termed as biologically rewarding since they are positive. Everyone knows that rewarding stimuli are preferred. The aesthetic can be both intellectually and emotionally rewarding, and both modes are coupled – again, an idea already expressed by Kant.[37] Emotional parameters seem to depend strongly on the activity of cortical areas called the limbic system, a part of the brain surrounding the brainstem and lying beneath the neocortex. Phylogenetically, the limbic system is a primitive cortical structure. Connections between visual and limbic structures exist; hence the possibility that the latter are influential for aesthetic judgement.

In conclusion, we may note that the functional organization of the visual system leads to a representation of the environment in dynamic patterns of neuronal activity. This representation embodies our concept of reality, which allows us to successfully interact with the physical world. What we consider as beautiful, or pleasing, may be a type of visual input that corresponds optimally to the processing rules of the central nervous system. These rules are, to some extent, genetically predetermined. However, the wealth of visual experiences, as well as the enduring learning processes, make aesthetic preferences subject to change. This adaptability is probably the reason why any static theory of aesthetics is unsatisfactory. There is little reason to believe that a more complete understanding of these rules of internal processing of information will improve this situation. The complexity of the application of these rules is so extreme that aesthetic evaluation may never be predictable.

References

1. Eigen M, Schuster P (1979) The hypercycle. Springer, Berlin
2. Murdoch I (1980) Structure in the novel. In: Medawar P, Shelley J (eds) Structures in science and art. Excerpta Medica, Amsterdam, pp 95–103
3. Fechner GT (1860) Elemente der Psychophysik. Breitkopf und Härtel, Leipzig
4. Mach E (1914) The analysis of sensation and the relation of the physical to the psychical. The Open Court, Chicago. Translation of: Die Analyse der Empfindungen – und das Verhältnis des Physischen zum Psychischen, 6th edn. G. Fischer, Jena
5. Stevens SS (1961) The psychophysics of sensory functions. In: WC Rosenblith (ed) Sensory Communication. MIT Press, Cambridge, pp 1–33
6. Hering E (1874) Grundriß einer Theorie des Farbensinnes. Sber Akad Wiss Wien math-nat Kl III 70: 169–204
7. Leonardo da Vinci (1651) Trattato della Pittura di Leonardo da Vinci. Scritta da Raeffaelle du Fresne. Langlois, Paris
8. Homer WI (1964) Seurat and the science of painting. MIT Press, Cambridge
9. Köhler W (1938) The place of value in a world of facts. Liveright, New York
10. Köhler W (1969) The task of Gestalt psychology. Princeton University Press, Princeton
11. Koffka K (1930) Psychologie der optischen Wahrnehmung. In: Bethe A, Bergmann GV, Embden G, Ellinger A (eds) Handbuch der normalen und pathologischen physiologie, vol 12. Springer, Berlin, pp 1215–1271
12. Wertheimer MC (1923) Untersuchungen zur Lehre von der Gestalt. Psychol Forschung 4: 176
13. Geschwind N (1974) Selected papers on language and the brain. D Reidel, Dordrecht
14. Hecaen H, Albert ML (1978) Human neuropsychology. John Wiley and Sons, New York
15. Luria AR (1973) The working brain. Basic Books, New York
16. Lassen NA, Ingvar DH (1972) Radioisotopic assessment of regional blood flow. Progr Nucl Med 1: 346–409
17. Mazziotta JC, Phelps ME, Carson RE, Kuhl DE (1982) Tomographic mapping of human cerebral metabolism: Auditory stimulation. Neurology 32: 921–937
18. Roland PE (1985) Cortical organization of voluntary behavior in man. Human Neurobiol 4: 155–167
19. Brown WS, Lehman D (1979) Verb and noun meanings of homophone words activate different cortical generators: A topographic study of evoked potential fields. Exp Brain Res Suppl 2:159–168
20. Jung R (1974) Neuropsychologie und Neurophysiogie des Kontur- und Formsehens in Zeichung und Malerei. In: Wieck HH (ed) Psychopathologie musischer Gestaltungen. Schattauer, Stuttgart, pp 30–88
21. Sabadel (1980) L'homme qui ne savait plus parler. Nouvelle Editions Baudiniere
22. Creutzfeldt OD (1983) Cortex cerebri. Springer, Berlin
23. Edelman GM, Mountcastle VB (1978) The mindful brain. MIT Press, Cambridge

24. Kuffler SW (1953) Discharge patterns and functional organization of mammalian retina. J Neurophysiol 14: 37–69
25. Baumgartner G (1961) Die Reaktionen des zentralen visuellen Systems der Katze im simultanen Helligkeitskontrast. In: Jung R, Kornhuber HH (eds) Neurophysiologie und Psychophysik des visuellen Systems. Springer, Berlin, pp 296–313
26. Grüsser O-J (1978) Visual function of the inferotemporal cortex. In: Schindler S, Gilor WK (eds) Informatik-Fachberichte, vol 16. Springer, Berlin, pp 234–273
27. Hubel DH, Wiesel TN (1977) Functional architecture of macaque monkey visual cortex. Proc Roy Soc B 198: 1–59
28. Hubel DH, Wiesel TN, Stryker MP (1977) Orientation columns in macaque monkey visual cortex demonstrated by the 2-desoxyglucose autoradiographic technique. Nature 269: 328–330
29. Jung R (1974) Neuropsychologie und Neurophysiologie des Kontur- und Formensehens in Zeichung und Malerei. In: Wieck HH (ed) Psychopathologie musischer Gestaltungen. FK Schattauer, Stuttgart, pp 27–88
30. Kanisza G (1979) Organization in vision. Praeger, New York
31. Peterhans E, Von der Heydt R, Baumgartner G (1986) Neuronal reponses to illusory contour reveal stages of visual cortical processing. In: Pettigrew JD, Sanderson KJ, Lewick WR (eds) Visual neurosciences. Cambridge University Press, Cambridge, pp 343–351
32. Von der Heydt R, Peterhans E, Baumgartner G (1984) Illusory contours and cortical neuron responses. Science 224: 1260–1262
33. Vasarely V (1969) Vasarely. Editions Du Griffon, Neuchatel
34. Zeki S (1983) The distribution of wavelength and orientation selective cells in different areas of monkey visual cortex. Proc Roy Soc B 217: 449–470
35. Gross C G (1973) Visual functions of inferotemporal cortex. In: Jung R (ed) Handbook of sensory physiology, vol VII, part 3B. Springer, Berlin, pp 451–482
36. Perret DI, Smith PAJ, Potter DD, Mistlin AJ, Head AS, Milner AD, Jeaves MA (1984) Neurons responsive to faces in the temporal cortex: Studies of functional organization, sensitivity to identity and relation to perception. Human Neurobiol 3: 197–208
37. Kant I (1799) Kritik der Urteilskraft, 3rd edn., part I, Kritik der ästhetischen Urteilskraft, paragr. 15. Berlin

Focusing in on Art*

Ingo Rentschler
Institute of Medical Psychology, Goethestrasse 31, 8000 München 2, Federal Republic of Germany

Terry Caelli
Department of Psychology, Queen's University, Kingston, Ontario, Canada K7L 3N6

Lamberto Maffei
Istituto di Neurofisiologia del Consiglio Nazionale delle Ricerche, Via S. Zeno 51, 56100 Pisa, Italy

Attitudes toward and evaluations of aesthetics have varied over the ages, and sometimes rather quickly. As an illustration of this, consider the positions of the scientist, Hermann von Helmholtz, and the artist, Wassily Kandinsky, on the relationship between art and music. Preceding the modern schools, von Helmholtz[1] argued that art and music are fundamentally different insofar as the role of the painter was to replicate, reflect, or interpret visible nature. Music, in contrast, is not derived from an equivalent auditory nature, but emanates totally from the composer's creative mind. In his book *Concerning the Spiritual in Art,* published in 1912, Kandinsky[2] shared this understanding of music but contended that a painter who finds no satisfaction in mere representation seeks to apply the methods of music to his art. He saw the modern desire for rhythm in painting, for mathematical construction, for repeated notes of color, and for setting color in motion as a result of this.

More radical was the aesthetics of "suprematism" conceived by the Russian artist, Kazimir Malevich,[3] only a few years later:

"The utilitarian constructions of technology, which develop out of the skillful pitting of one natural force against another, have in them no trace of

---
* dedicated to Piero Dorazio

an 'artistic' imitation of natural forms; they are new creations of human culture.

A work by a realistic artist reproduces nature as it is and represents it as a harmonious, organic whole. In such a reproduction of nature no creative element can be discerned because the creative element is not to be found in the unchanging synthesis of nature as such but, rather, in the variable synthesis of its interpretation.

An artist who creates rather than imitates expresses himself; his works are not reflections of nature but, instead, new realities, which are no less significant than the realities of nature itself.

The inventive engineer, the creative artist and the professional 'copyist' thus represent three possible forms of productive activity, of which the work of both the inventive engineer and the original artist expresses the creative, while the imitator, as reproducing agent, serves the existing.

The basis of this diversity in activity, in my opinion, resides in the fact that our conceptions of things around us, transmitted mechanically by our senses, with the co-operation of one brain center or another, can turn out to be different from each other."

Two points raised by Malevich are particularly interesting. First, for him the creative element resulted from the changeable character of the artist's interpretation of nature and did not depend on the distinction between nature and mind. Second, he contended that the different interpretations of nature arise from the activation of different states of brain activity. Thus, it appears that the positions of Kandinsky and Malevich were separated by a watershed in the development of epistemology. Kandinsky's ideas were still consistent with Kant's distinction between sensibility and understanding, that is, the mind's capacity to be affected by things as they are and its faculty of acting on the sensibility.[4] For Kandinsky, representational art expressed the former, whereas nonrepresentational art reflected the latter. More recently, perceptions have been seen essentially as interpretations of the world of objects in terms of knowledge represented in the brain. This led Gregory[5] to conceive of the mind as "consisting of hypotheses of perception and understanding," with "the private hypotheses of perception and the shared hypotheses of conception making up our reality." Seen within the context of this epistemology, Malevich's aesthetics seems to imply that the creative element in art depends on the potential to provide us with new forms of reality rather than on the dissimilarity between works of art and physical objects. Below we will attempt to show that recently acquired knowledge of the function and coding properties of the perceiving brain and, in particular, of the human visual system supports this remarkable idea.

Perception as a Mental Construct

To go into the subject more deeply, it is evidently necessary to better understand the nature of perception. Thereby, it is most important to note that modern theories emphasize the active nature of perception as being mediated by processes searching for the best interpretation of the signals conveyed by the afferent nervous pathways.[5] This renaissance of the Kantian notion of perception is a rather recent event. In the nineteenth century, von Helmholtz, although aware of the influence of unconscious inferences on our perception of physical objects, stressed the analogy between the eye and a camera. The assumption of a passive and unbiased transmission of physical stimuli was typical for the empiricists' approach to the problem of perception. Perceived objects were thought to impose their structure upon the mind to an extent determined by previous exposure. Consistent with this view was the idea that ensuing percepts consisted of a summation of sensations and ideas, the latter being copies of previous sensations. This "perceptual atomism" was apparently supported by the success of the concept of atomism in the physical and chemical sciences.[6]

A radically different view was held by Immanuel Kant.[7] He argued that the physical world offers only the substance of sensations, while the mind actively organizes this substance in space and time and provides the concepts to interpret experience. The Kantian position influenced Goethe with his color theory ("Farbenlehre"), which was based on the idea that the eye is an active agent rather than a passive recipient. Otherwise, it had little impact on psychological theories of perception with the exception of Gestalt psychology, which evolved from the writings of Christian von Ehrenfels[8] in the late nineteenth century. According to von Ehrenfels, the percept of form surpassed the percepts of the individual elements composing the whole. Authors like Max Wertheimer, Wolfgang Köhler, and Kurt Koffka even suggested that the very nature of elements of perception is determined by the organization of the whole.[9]

Largely due to the failure of Gestalt psychology to conceive a viable model of how figure-ground relationships and properties like "good continuation" and "enclosedness" could be quantitatively evaluated, its ideas have been neglected by subsequent researchers in the field of perception. In contrast, psychophysics, conceived in the nineteenth century by the physicist, Gustav Theodor Fechner[10], became mainly concerned with the measurement of sensory thresholds as the hypothetical elements of perception. In much the same way, neurophysiologists considered receptive fields as innate and invariant templates subserving the extraction of stimulus properties critical for object recognition.

Psychologists were becoming increasingly aware of the role that the active modification of afferent signals plays in cognition. There are, for instance, the effects of selective attention, as evident in the "cocktail party effect," where the voice of a particular person can be listened to in a room that is buzzing from many people talking at the same time. Other popular examples of this are ambiguous figures[11], such as Jastrow's duck-rabbit or the Necker cube (Fig. 1). Common to such images is that either one or another figure is seen but not both simultaneously. The animal drawing is either a duck or a rabbit; the cube is a box seen either from above or from below.

Nevertheless, the notion of perception as an active process was more substantially supported by the technical disciplines. Aristotle taught that the world consists of objects provided with numerous properties. He used the term "es-

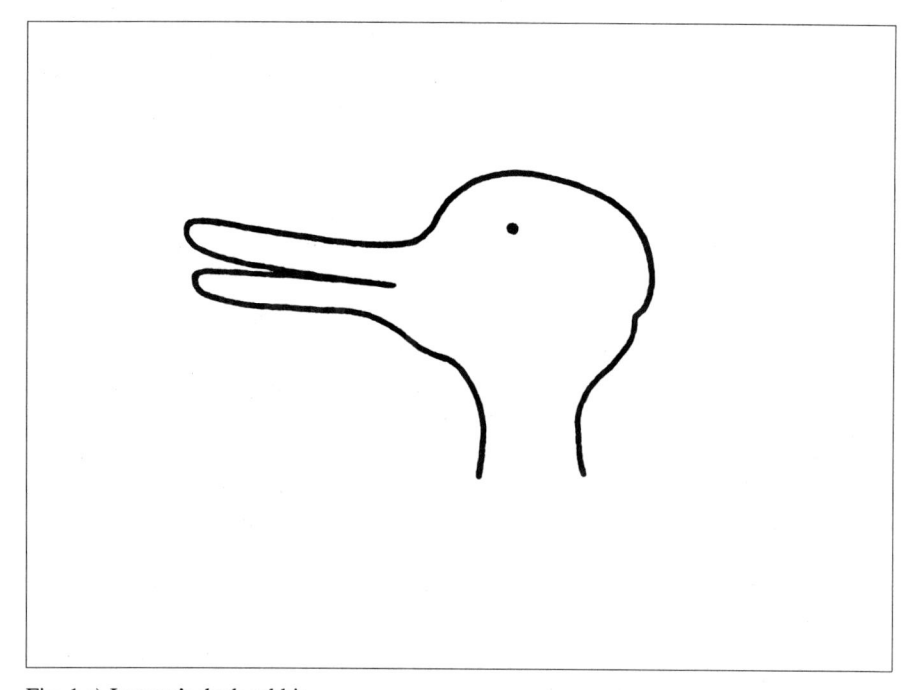

Fig. 1.a) Jastrow's duck-rabbit

sence" for those properties, without which an object would cease to be itself and, equally important, to belong to a certain category. A category then, is defined by its essence.[12] In the language of communication engineering, the task of assigning a category or a class to an object is essentially the task of pattern recognition. Therefore, it is not difficult to understand that perception can be equated with pattern recognition. Watanabe[13], in his detailed discussion of

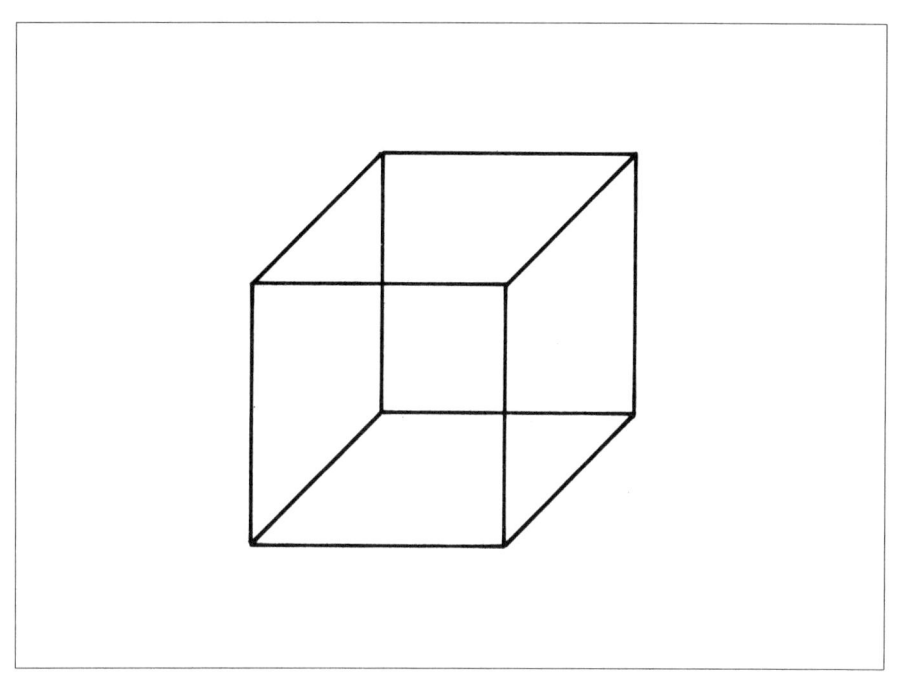

1.b) Necker cube

the principles underlying pattern recognition, illustrated this with Wittgenstein's comment about "seeing something$_1$ as something$_2$." According to the latter, the verb "see" has two usages, such as, "I see this picture" and "I see this picture as a rabbit." Something$_2$ corresponds to a percept, whereas something$_1$ refers to a physical reality. This led Watanabe to characterize "seeing-one-in-many" or "one-in-two," as in the duck-rabbit example, as one important kind of pattern recognition.

One gains more insight into the definition of seeing as a classification process by considering how pattern recognition is performed by automata.[13] The process begins with the observation of a large number of variables, e.g., the number of picture elements ("pixels") determined by the raster available for image reproduction. The process ends with a single binary decision as to whether or not the pattern belongs to a given class. In sharp contrast to the requirements for passive image transmission, the reduction of information is essential for solving a pattern recognition problem. This is usually performed by seeking a symbolic representation common to all class samples. Thereby, the original occurrence with its many variables is represented by a much smaller number of substitute patterns, or features, that are (1) simpler than the original and (2) can be associated with it.[14]

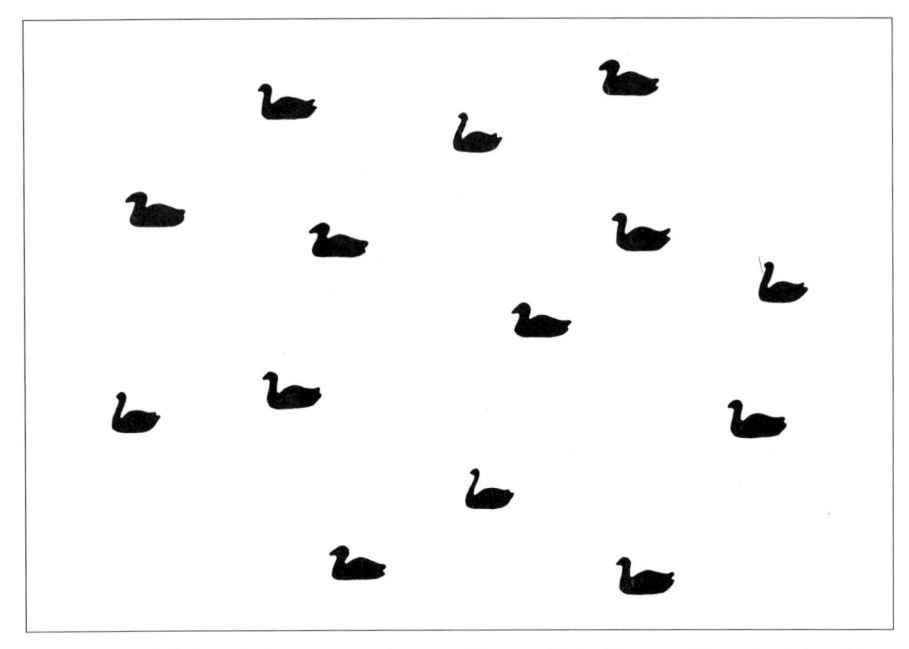

Fig. 2. Seeing birds as ducks, geese, and swans. Thomas Kuhn illustrated the principles of pattern recognition with the example of teaching a child to recognize such water birds (reprinted with permission from ref. 16).

a) Whenever one of them occurs, the father would not only tell his little son which type of bird it is. He would also help the child by pointing out that ducks have short and bent necks, that those of geese are longer and relatively straight, and that swans have even longer necks that are less straight.

Figure 2 shows an example of such a symbolic representation, and further examples will be considered below. At the classification stage of pattern recognition, the similarity of a given pattern and the samples of each class is evaluated in terms of their symbolic representation, and a decision is made as to which class the pattern resembles most.

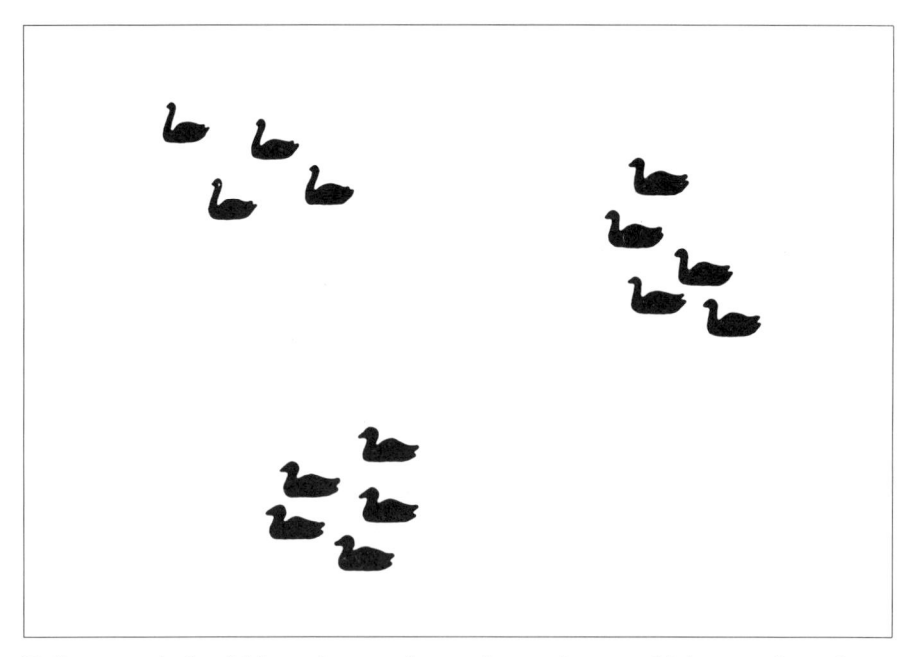

b) Consequently the child may learn to place each occurring water bird onto an internal map with the coordinates of neck length and curvature. Such a symbolic representation is suitable for solving the task of object (or pattern) recognition if it results in object clusters, or classes, having relatively low within-variance and higher between-variance.

Revolutionary Changes of World View

In much the same way as perception has been considered as an accumulation of sensations, scientific knowledge is commonly thought of as being embodied in a set of rules and theories. Thomas Kuhn[15], in his famous book *The Structure of Scientific Revolutions*, argued that this is not the case. He stressed the role that exemplary past achievements, or paradigms[16], play in the professional judgement of scientific communities. According to Kuhn, students do not primarily gain practice in the application of rules when they are solving problems. Rather they learn to see similarity relationships between physical situations, and this ability is the prerequisite for successfully applying laws and theories. For instance, the student of mechanics adopts the view of Galileo Galilei when he learns to handle the equation of motion for a pendulum. After translating the concept to the formalism of quantum mechanics, this paradigm can be used for understanding more complex situations in terms of superimposed, harmonic oscillations. Thus the use of scientific paradigms is the same as in pattern recognition – having been provided with paradigms of a class of situations, one becomes capable of deciding whether or not a new situation belongs to the same class.

It is now conceivable that Kuhn saw scientific progress as the result of revolutionary changes in paradigms. Following a new paradigm, scientists may regard things as distinctly different that were considered similar before. One of Kuhn's examples of this is the relationship between the sun and the moon before and after Copernicus. Hence, scientific concepts of reality are mental constructs in much the same way as has been argued above for perceptions. Kuhn illustrated this with the following words: "It is as elementary prototypes for these transformations of the scientists' world that the familiar demonstrations of a switch in visual gestalt prove so suggestive. What were ducks in the scientists' world before the revolution are rabbits afterwards. The man who first saw the exterior of the box later sees its interior from below."[17]

This view of the nature of scientific progress is related to what the psychiatrist and biographer of Sigmund Freud, Ernest Jones, wrote in 1916 on the relationships between symbols and the more general development of civilization: "The progress of the human mind when considered genetically, is seen to consist, not – as is commonly thought – merely of a number of accretions, added from without, but the following two processes: on the one hand the extension or transference of interest and understanding from earlier, simpler, and more primitive ideas etc., to more difficult and complex ones, which in a certain sense are continuations of and symbolize the former; and on the other hand the constant unmasking of previous symbolism, the recognition that these, though previously thought to be literally true, were really only aspects or representations of the truth, the only ones of which our minds were – for either affective or intellectual reasons – at the time capable".[18]

Jones evidently used the word "symbol" in a wider sense than was referred to above in the context of pattern recognition. Nevertheless, he characterized its meaning by essentials, the most important of which are congruent with the more technical definition quoted from Kohonen: "1. A symbol is representative or substitute of some other idea...," and "2. It represents the primary element through having something in common with it."[19] As Jones was concerned with the role that symbols play in psychoanalysis, he added that they are typically sensorial and concrete, whereas the idea represented may be abstract and more complex. According to Jones, symbolic modes of thought are also more primitive, both ontogenetically and phylogenetically; hence the idea that the development of civilization depends upon the replacement of more primitive ideas by more complex ones.

Sir Ernst Gombrich[20], in his essay "Psycho-Analysis and the History of Art," related Ernest Jones' views on the relationships between symbols and thought to the evolution of modes of pictorial representation. We owe much to his ideas, but we shall abstain from arguing in psychoanalytical terms. Consistent with Malevich's concept of the creative element in art, we shall consider the variable interpretation of nature within the context of more recent theories of perception.

Information Aesthetics

An extreme form of symbolic representation is a code, as defined in Shannon's theory of communication.[21] The latter is concerned with the task of reconstructing at some point a message selected at another point. A major issue of this theory is whether the output of a communication channel is constructed by the signal (as in photography or in television) or selected from a set of predetermined symbols (as in telegraphy), that is, by using a code. To illustrate the efficiency of using an optimal code, one need only to consider the task of transmitting a page of printed text. If a video technique is used, one frame consists of, say, 512x512=262.144 elementary signals or pixels. Telegraphy, by comparison, requires far fewer signals to simply transmit the instructions for selecting the required sequence of alphanumeric characters.

In information aesthetics, as developed about two decades ago by Abraham Moles[22] and Max Bense[23], the ideas of communication theory were applied to the analysis of structure in music, in language, and to certain developments in the visual arts. One extensive example of this is provided by Leonard Meyer's book, *Music, the Arts and Ideas*.[24] Another example discussed by Moles (and others) is op art, with its preference for geometrical and highly periodic structures. In general, the concept behind visual information aesthetics is that the painter and the observer enter into a transmitter-receiver relationship. The painter extracts structure from the environment that, by definition, reduces uncertainty. This information has to fit between quantitative bounds in order for the observer to process the image as intended by the artist.

One important achievement of information aesthetics was the discovery of the role redundancy plays in aesthetic experience. It depends upon the fact that aspects of form, or "gute gestalt," can be captured in terms of pattern redundancy in the sense of Shannon's theory.[25] A complex message or pattern in either the temporal or spatial domain is viewed here as consisting of a sequence of parts whose properties occur with specific frequencies or probabilities. Having received some parts of the message, an observer can make better guesses about the remainder, the more regular the properties of the parts of the message are distributed. For instance, rhythm makes some parts of a piece of music highly predictable, and this is also true for the symmetrical properties of an image. Such parts are called redundant, or uninformative. The properties of other parts of a message are less predictable and, therefore, convey a great deal of information.

However, the problem of applying communication theory to painting or to images in general is the fact that it is impossible to determine such parts by merely considering the physical properties of an image. How, for instance, should image redundancy be determined for a painting by Claude Monet? The reason for this difficulty is the lack of a generally acceptable set of image features. For the analysis of speech, this difficulty does not exist, as speech contains a variety of features that can be measured, such as volume, pitch, and spectral energy. Speech can also be characterized by a universally accepted set of symbols called phonemes. The sound of "d" in the word "dog," for example, is a phoneme. By using phonemes it is, in principle, possible to obtain a complete representation of an utterance. Thus, the symbolic description of speech consists of describing phonemes in terms of such features.

For visual perception, we do not have an acceptable set of image symbols and probably never shall have such a system, since visual processing seems so adaptive to the type of objects and tasks. On similar grounds, Neisser[26] has already denied the usefulness of applying information theory to psychology in general, and Epstein[27] questioned whether describing the perception of music in terms of information theory is a paraphrase of other existing theories or whether it affords a truly higher level of abstraction.

Visual Representations in the Brain

From our inability to verify the existence of an explicit "brain code" for image information arises the question as to the nature of internal representations of the visual world. Here the most conspicuous result of research is the finding that there is a high degree of functional specificity associated with the location of neural responses in the brain. First, there is a specialization of brain areas onto which the major sensory modalities (vision, audition, somatosensation) project, and such a specialization is also found for various forms of action (e.g., speech and motor functions) (Fig.3). Within each of the major sensory systems, a number of cortical areas have been identified that provide representations for different purposes. At this stage, we know of no less than seven somatosensory areas, four auditory ones, at least twelve visual areas, and a variety of maps that also exist in lower structures of the brain.[28]

For visual information processing, some of the cortical maps are retinotopically organized and others are not. In retinotopic maps, the visual field (i.e., the two-dimensional projection of the world onto the retina) is rep-

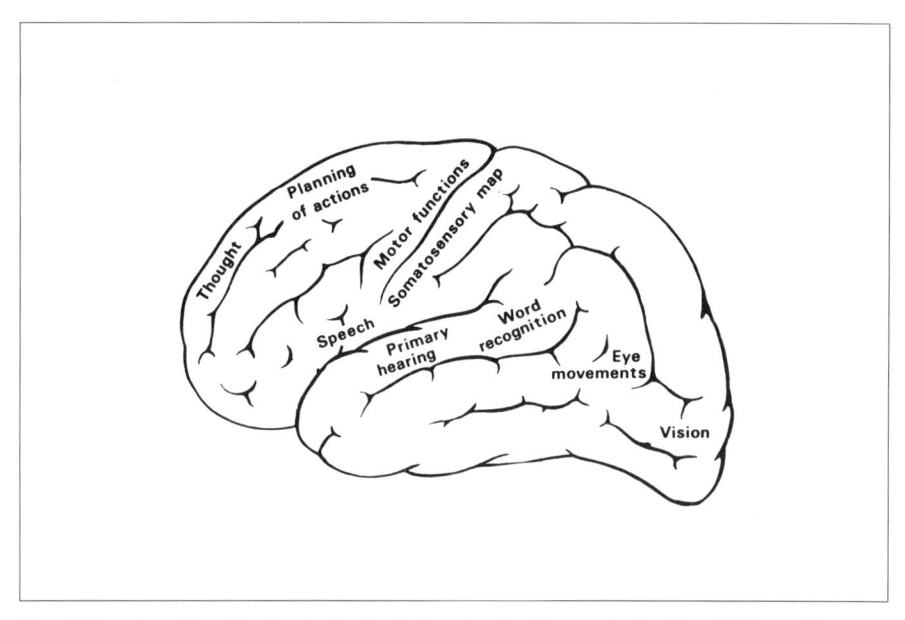

Fig. 3. Functional localization in the brain (reprinted with permission from Kohonen[14])

resented in spatial order, whereas nonretinotopic maps impose further abstractions and syntheses upon the information they receive. The functional differences between these maps are the result of successive transformations and convergences along different neural pathways in the brain. The origin of these differences was a mystery until recently, when the study of processes of self-organization suggested that, both in simple physical systems and in the brain, the representation of knowledge in specific categories of things might assume the form of feature maps.[29]

We have no reason to believe that there exists an area in the visual system onto which these divergent elements of representation converge to produce localized neural correlates of perception. It seems, instead, that our holistic world views are incorporated in the dynamic patterns of activity within the neural network, consisting of the linked cortical areas. Most of the evidence supporting this idea is anatomical in nature, but there are also clinical observations suggesting that the synchronization of information from several visual maps is not always possible: fever, drugs, migraines, or brain damage may produce bizarre symptoms, like fragmentation, selective fading, doubling of contours, jerky movements of objects, brief inversion of parts of the visual world, and dissociation of color and form.[30]

Adding to the reports in the clinical literature is the powerful description of drug-related alterations of visual perception in the personal experiences of the well-known author, Aldous Huxley. In his book, *The Doors of Perception*, he suggests that "what the rest of us see only under the influence of mescalin, the artist is congenitally equipped to see all the time."[31] Taking into account the more recently acquired knowledge of brain function, this (rather exaggerated) claim made by Huxley, nevertheless, supports the idea that the artist may be able to emphasize the selected information contained in specific visual maps in the brain more than is evident in normal observations. This view is clearly consistent with Malevich's, who wrote that "with the co-operation of one brain center or another" the artist may choose his own "conception of things" around him.[3] Shifts of attention to a particular type of visual representation may be brought about by emotional, intellectual, or cultural factors in the painter and result in "style."

We may summarize these considerations by suggesting that when Malevich sees the creative element in art as dependent on a change in the cooperation among brain centers, this may well be related to what has been discovered about the multiple visual representations in the cerebral cortex. In other words, we assume that art can be evaluated along similar dimensions of internal visual representations, although various schools are differentiated by emphases among and within these maps. This concept may be characterized as the "equality of dimensions and plurality of attention."

As the issue of pictorial representation in art is concerned, it is important to note that some visual areas in the brain deal with common features, such as elements of contour, color, and movement, whereas the function of others is still obscure. The former property is more easily understood if one considers the fact that the first primitive type of visual representation involves the retinal receptor mosaic (rods and cones) as a two-dimensional, point-by-point array. However, already within the retina neural responses are determined by the interaction between signals from cells beyond this primary level of encoding[32] – via the complex neural network of bipolar, horizontal, amacrine, and ganglion cells. For example, as a result of the inhibitory character of one type of coupling between such cells, the response from one receptor is counteracted by the responses of its neighboring receptors to result in a "receptive field." The latter determines the type of spatial structures a given cell is specifically sensitive (or "tuned") to (see chapters 6 and 7). Thus, we see that the specific internal organization within the brain determines what physical properties of the world are perceivable. Regardless of whether it be color, spatial, or motion "mappings" of the sensory input onto the perception of the physical world, the vehicles of such encoding processes seem to be units, or functional subgroups of nerve cells in the brain. These units relate localized physical events with feature maps covering a certain range of physical properties and parameters common to the categories to which these events are associated.

Such units are usually represented as filters specifically tuned to the mapping parameters.

More commonly known examples of such filters are the red, green, and blue mechanisms of color vision, which are roughly analogous to the channels used for communicating signals on color television. Isaac Newton demonstrated that the corresponding color components are related to the ranges of relatively long, middle, and short wavelengths or low, middle, and high frequencies of light. Similarly, we can characterize images in terms of levels of detail analogous to the low- to high- frequency ranges which, together, compose complex sound patterns. The range of (spatial) frequencies meaningful for vision is obviously restricted by visual resolution thresholds. If this is a 30-second visual angle, then a spatial frequency of 60 cycles (light and dark stripes) per degree of visual angle (cpd) is just resolvable. This corresponds to an apparent width of 10^{-1} mm for one light and one dark stripe at a viewing distance of about 30 cm. The wavelength of light is between 10^{-4} and 10^{-5} mm. Thus, the order of magnitude of spatial frequencies across an image (being inversely related to spatial wavelengths) is rather different from the optical frequencies of light waves.

By accumulating the responses from subgroups of receptive fields differing in average size, one obtains the type of image representation illustrated in Fig. 4. The larger the receptive fields, the lower the image resolution qualities ("region-like" spatial information), while smaller receptive fields offer finer details, like edges and clarity ("boundary-like"). Consequently, the image corresponding to the large receptive field size *(top right)* shows essentially the light and dark regions of the image, whereas the smallest receptive field size *(bottom right)* reproduces mainly the contours present in the original. These images were computer generated by filtering the input image *(top left)* with a given filter size, a process called convolution.[33] Each of the filtered images contains only a limited band of spatial frequencies; hence the name band-pass versions of the input image.

Although these filter operations were conducted in the physical domain, the physiologist, Fergus Campbell, has suggested that similar results may be achieved perceptually by shifting attention between the outputs from variously sized spatial filters.[34] Indeed, at a cocktail party we may enjoy quite different perceptual experiences when switching attention from the appreciation of the texture of a lady's dress (high spatial frequency information) to the more general outlines of her appearance (low spatial frequency information). Campbell's idea is supported by the finding that there are substructures in the visual cortex that selectively respond to limited ranges of spatial frequency.[35] David Marr, however, pointed out if one can inspect the world independently in different bands of spatial frequencies, one should also be able to recognize

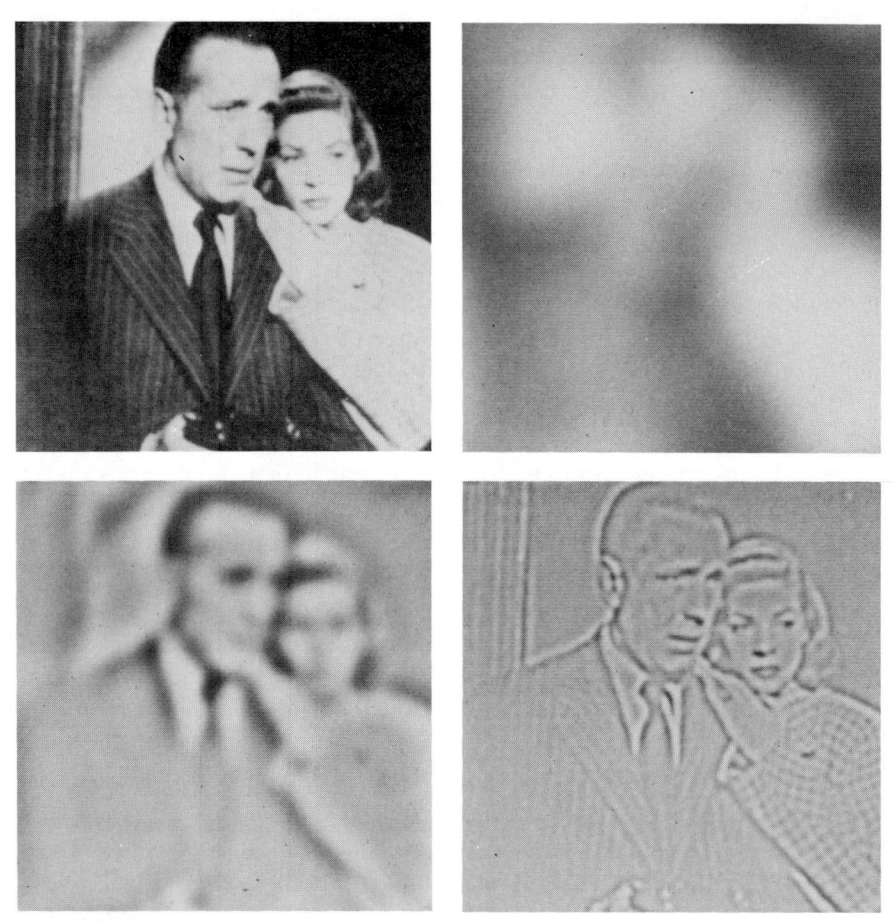

Fig. 4. Original scene and three band-pass filtered versions thereof (Bogart-Bacall photograph copyright AGI SYDNEY)

objects in block-quantized images.[36] This is not the case, as can be seen in Fig. 5, where Bogart and Bacall are hidden by the checkerboard contours that result from the block quantization of their portrait. The actors can only be seen by physically blurring the image (e.g., by squinting or by sufficiently increasing the viewing distance).

This led Marr[37] to suggest that it is not the individual bands of spatial frequencies that constitute the "early" visual representation (before further processing), but special combinations thereof. He considered these combinations to be the result of spatial coincidence between zero-crossings (i.e., the places where the luminance values pass from above to below the mean luminance) from different frequency bands, and this allowed him to construct edge-only versions of physical objects. For the present purpose, we adopted the idea of combining information from different frequency bands but, unlike Marr, we found it essential to use nonlinear filter operations.

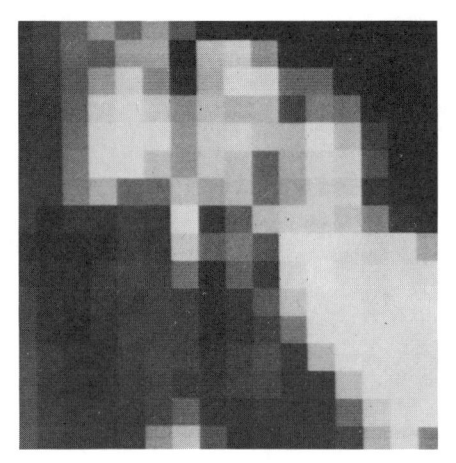

Fig. 5. Block-quantized version of Bogart-Bacall scene. To recognize the actors, squint or increase viewing distance.

In Fig. 6 we show the zero-crossings[38] of the two band-pass images in the bottom row of Fig. 4. The images in the top row of Fig. 7 were generated by "coloring" the areas enclosed by zero-crossings in black and white, depending on whether the corresponding regions in the band- pass image were darker or lighter than the mean value. The image at the bottom left of Fig. 7 resulted

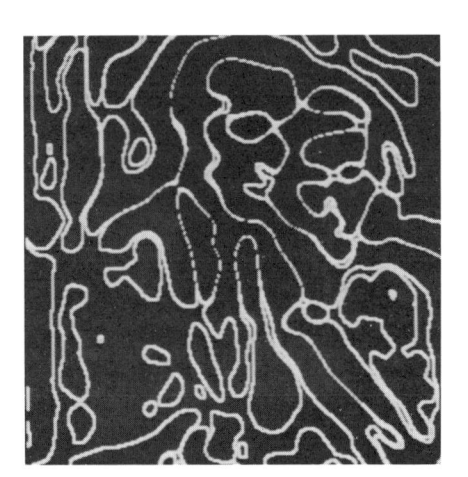

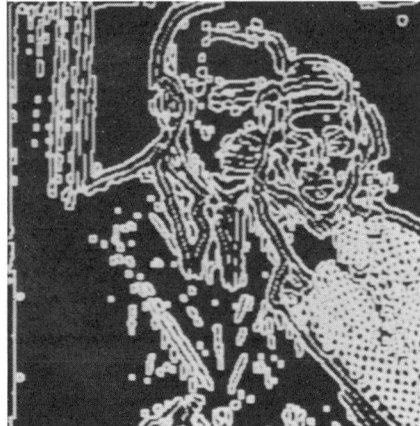

Fig. 6. Zero-crossings of the two band-pass images shown in the bottom row of Fig. 4

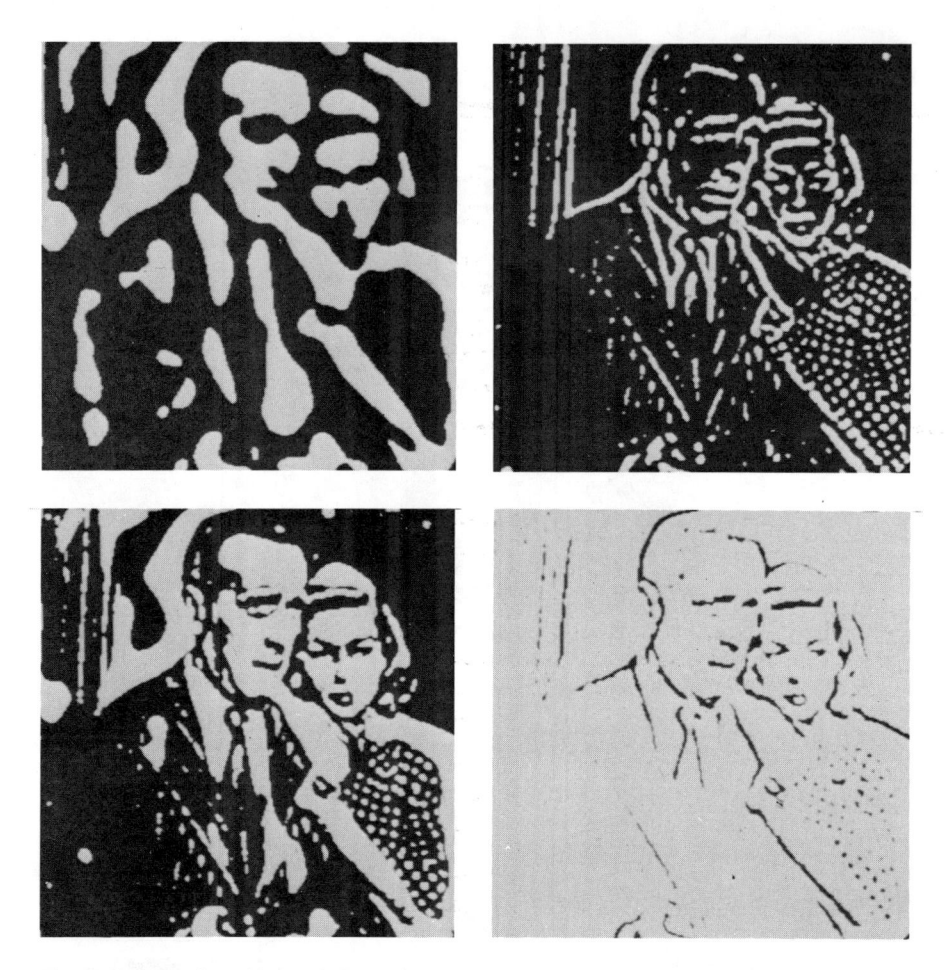

Fig. 7. Combination of image information contained in individual bands of spatial frequency. *Top*: zero-crossing versions of Fig. 6 "colored" black and white; *Bottom left*: images from top row combined; *Bottom right*: same process but somewhat different thresholds used for converting high-pass image into binary version

from combining the two pictures in the top row. Thereby we applied the rule that the compound image is white wherever at least one of the component pictures is white. The same procedure was used for generating the image at the bottom right of Fig. 7; the difference in appearance depends on a slight departure from the former conditions that led to the coloring of the component image with the finer details. This demonstrates that the combination of information from different frequency bands results in more interesting representations of the input image than is possible by using individual frequency bands only.

Reducing Image Information by Filtering

It is now time to illustrate the points made above by actual examples. In Fig. 8, we demonstrate how the filtering out of high-spatial-frequency information renders a painting of the Sienese School by Duccio di Buoninsegna more similar to a Renaissance painting by Leonardo da Vinci. In comparison to the work by Duccio, there is less high frequency information in the painting by Leonardo, corresponding to a preponderance of surfaces and less distinctly marked features, a peculiarity of style called "sfumato." The correlations between the style of paintings and the ways in which image features are captured within various ranges of spatial frequencies have been investigated more quantitatively by T. Caelli and W. Kelly (1988, What determines an artist's uniqueness – and to whom: A conjecture?, unpublished work). Paintings from the classical, the impressionist, the cubist, and the surrealist periods were ex-

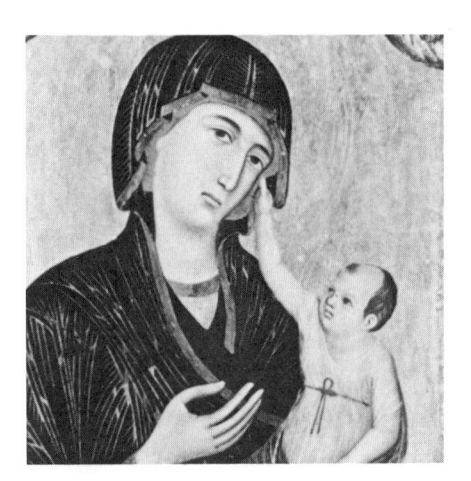

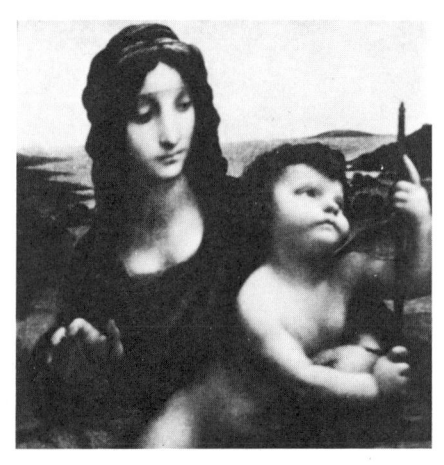

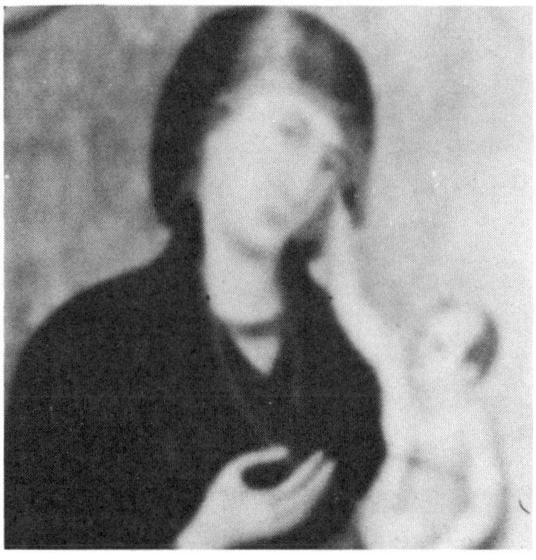

Fig. 8. Details from "Madonna di Crevole" by Duccio di Buoninsegna *(above)* and Leonardo da Vinci's "Madonna with the Yarnwinder" *(below right)*. *Below left*, low-pass filtered version of Duccio's work

amined. The results indicated that the ability to group photographs of paintings into their correct schools is not a function of art education or of the subject matter of the picture. Instead, similarity of style could be assessed according to similarities in texture, brushstroke, quality of light and dark, and spatial qualities. These image features were statistically captured by what is

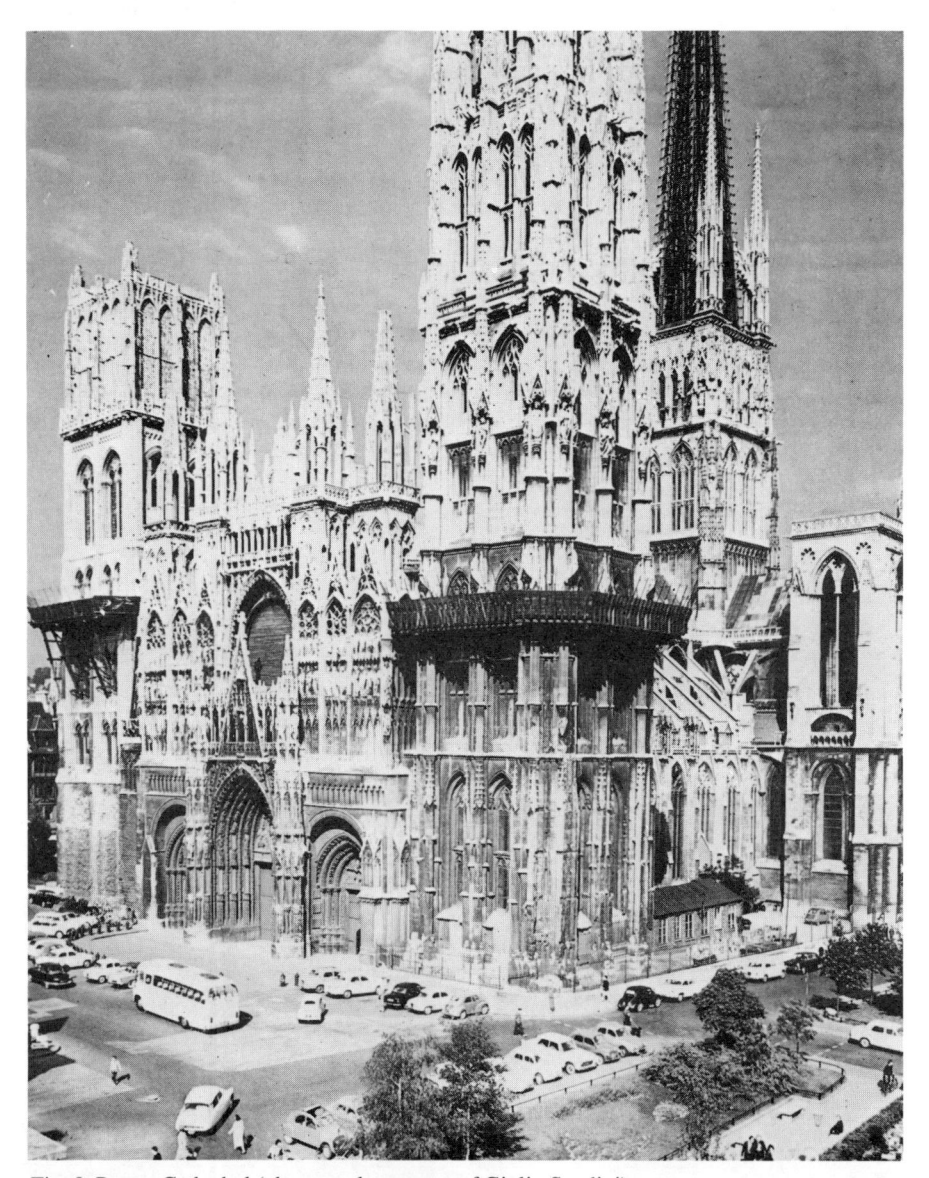

Fig. 9. Rouen Cathedral (photograph courtesy of Giulio Sandini)

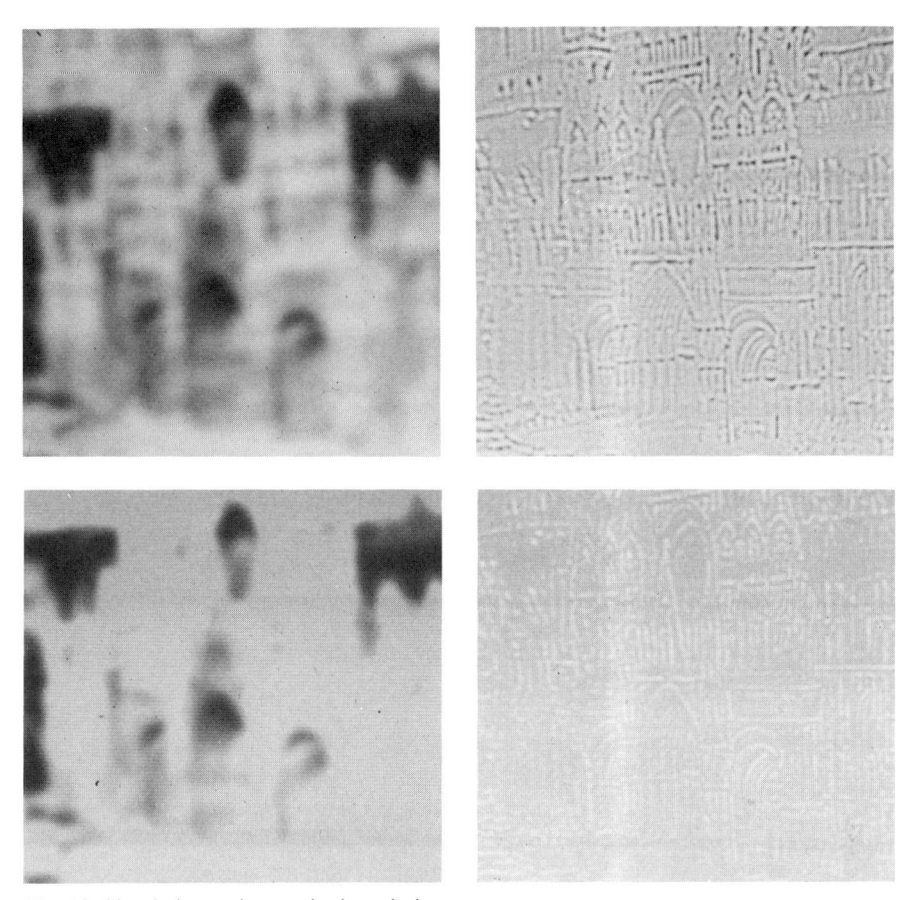

Fig. 10. Simulating an impressionist painting
a) Low- and high-pass filtered detail of photograph of Rouen Cathedral (*top*), as well as dark and light image components thereof (*bottom*)

termed the "power spectrum" of the image, which corresponds to the strengths (amplitude or power) of various frequency components over the image.

The filtering processes considered so far imply the selective reduction of image information within a certain range of spatial frequencies, whereby we suggest that the artist becomes creative not by adding something to the conventional view of the world but rather by depriving it of information irrelevant to his concept of reality. This perspective of the creative act in painting seems to contradict what Malevich[3] called the "additional element" determining the creative quality of a work of art. There is, however, a more general class of

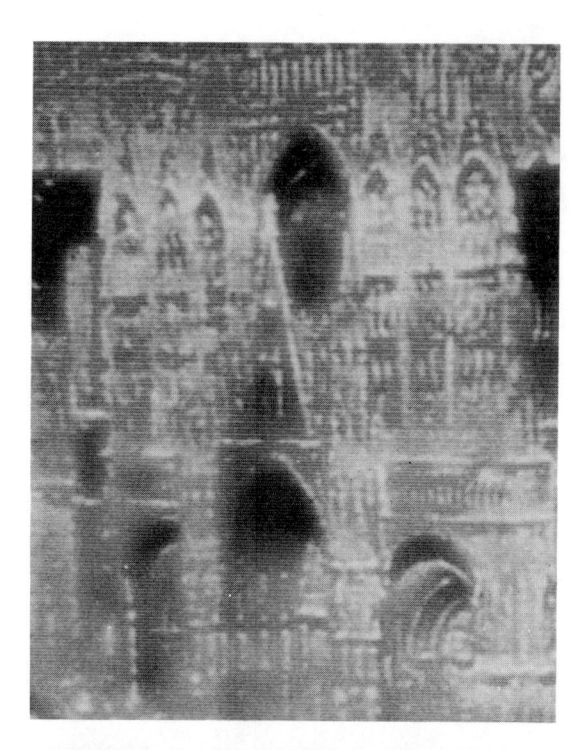

Fig. 10.b) Combination of the images in the bottom row of a)

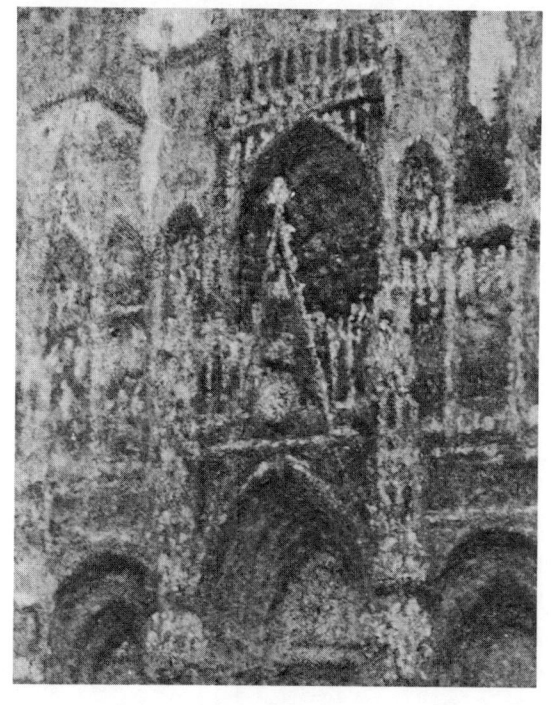

c) Claude Monet's Rouen Cathedral (1894) The portal, dull weather (reproduced with permission of Musée d'Orsay, Paris)

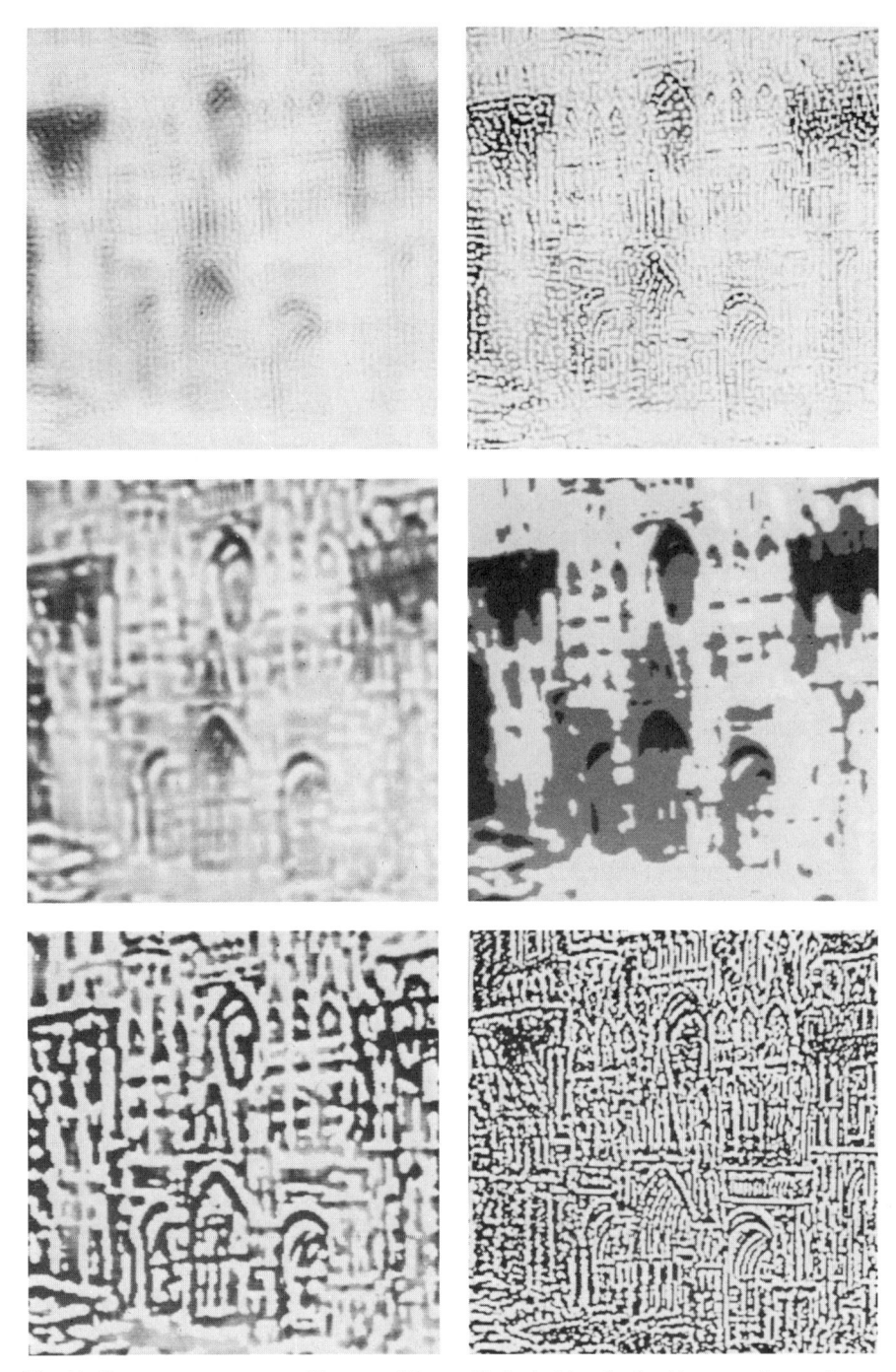

Fig. 11. Six computer-generated images of Rouen Cathedral (as obtained by excerting nonlinear operations on band-pass versions of the original photograph and by subsequent recombination of the resulting images)

filtering operations, which seemingly embrace Malevich's use of the term additional. Consider, for instance, the (nonlinear) selective enhancement and recombination of image components demonstrated in Figs. 6 and 7. We used a detail of a photograph of the Cathedral of Rouen in France (Fig. 9) and generated two band-pass versions thereof (Fig. 10a, *top row*). Of these images, only the gray levels below (Fig. 10a, *lower left*) and above the average (Fig. 10a, *lower right*) were recovered, respectively, and subsequently recombined to result in Fig. 10b. This operation is biologically plausible because the receptive fields underlying the process of band-pass filtering exist in the visual system in two polarities, namely "on-center" and "off-center" units (see chapter 7). The information conveyed in the resulting "brightness" and "darkness" channels" is kept separate for further processing.[39]

The comparison of Fig. 10b with one of Monet's paintings of the same subject (La Cathedrale de Rouen, temps gris [1894]) is revealing (Fig. 10c). However, there is nothing unique about this particular type of rendering, as we can generate variations of the same theme by selecting and differentially emphasizing various image components (for some examples, see Fig. 11), and

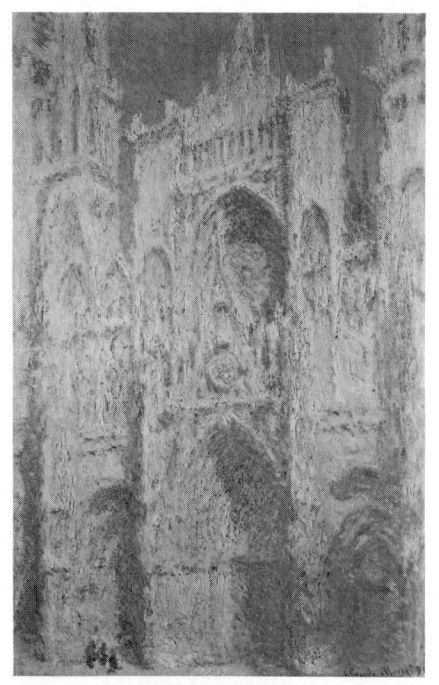

Fig. 12.a–d) Rouen Cathedral
a) Claude Monet (1893) The Portal and the Tower Saint Romain, Full Sunlight (reproduced with permission of Musée d'Orsay, Paris)

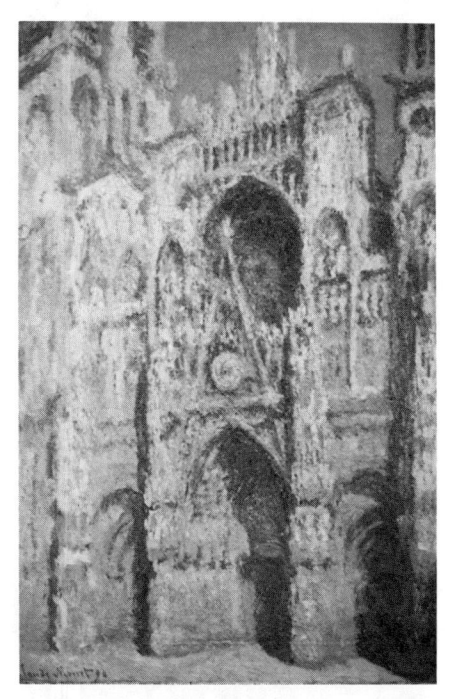

12.b) Claude Monet (1893) The Portal, Morning Sun, Harmony in Blue (reproduced with permission of Musée d'Orsay, Paris)

so, apparently, do the artists (e.g. Fig. 12). Within the same conceptual framework, it is also possible, as we have already seen in Fig. 7 *(bottom right)*, to produce "edge only" versions of an original scene (Fig. 13). It is conceivable that such a strategy of information processing may underlie the human ability to sketch a scene.[40]

Having shown that styles of painting from the Middle Ages up to neoimpressionism can be characterized by the preservation of the structure of physical images rendered through different types of spatial filters, we may proceed to more difficult interpretations, such as cubism and abstract art. Typical for such styles is the loosening or disruption of the physical structure of objects. One way to obtain alterations of structure depends on the reduction of information along the orientation (e.g., vertical, horizontal, or oblique) in the image domain. In images with an energy distribution varying along two dimensions, orientation information is represented by the distribution of amplitude values (contrast) along specific orientations. This is illustrated in Fig. 14a, where the original photograph of the Cathedral of Rouen is filtered by using a number of orientation-specific filters. Again, this filter operation is biologically

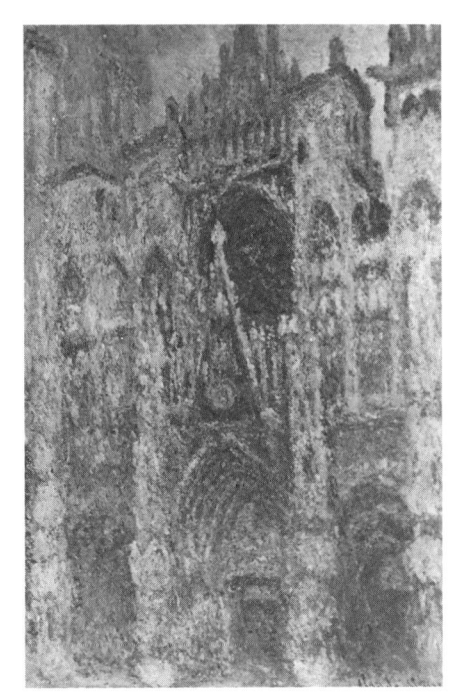

12.c) Claude Monet (1894) Rouen Cathedral, West Facade, Sunlight. National Gallery of Art, Washington, D.C., Chester Dale Collection (reproduced with permission)

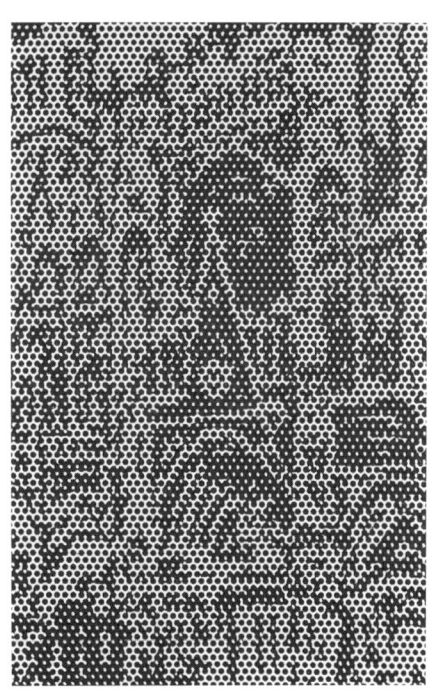

12.d) Roy Lichtenstein (1969) Cathedral #3 (one color lithograph, Gemini)

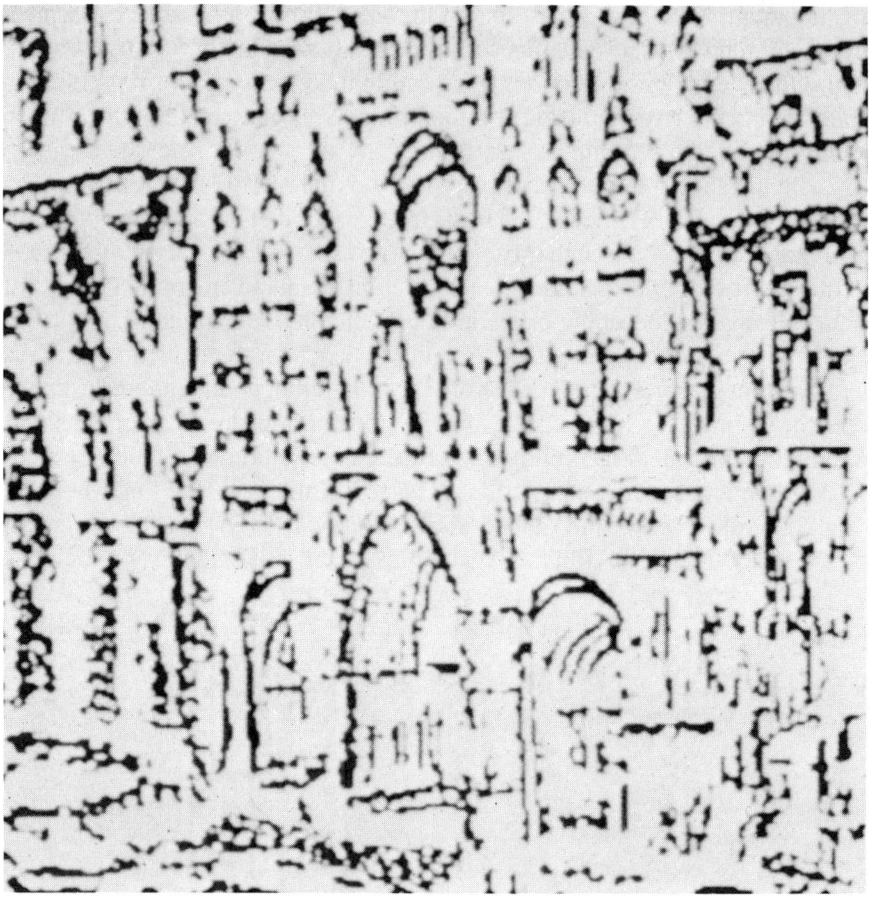

Fig. 13. Edge-only version of Rouen Cathedral (obtained from photograph)

plausible, as orientational selectivity is the most important characteristic of receptive fields in the visual cortex (see chapter 6). For comparison, we add a reproduction of Lyonel Feininger's painting showing the "Marktkirche von Halle" (Fig. 14b).

Another example of orientation filtering is provided in Fig. 15, where the original portrait is filtered by discarding 20% of the amplitude information within evenly spaced, orientation-specific filters. As the percentage of suppressed orientation information is increased to 80%, the appearance of the image is dramatically altered. The new image, in an interpretive sense, provides an aesthetically more interesting experience than the original portrait.

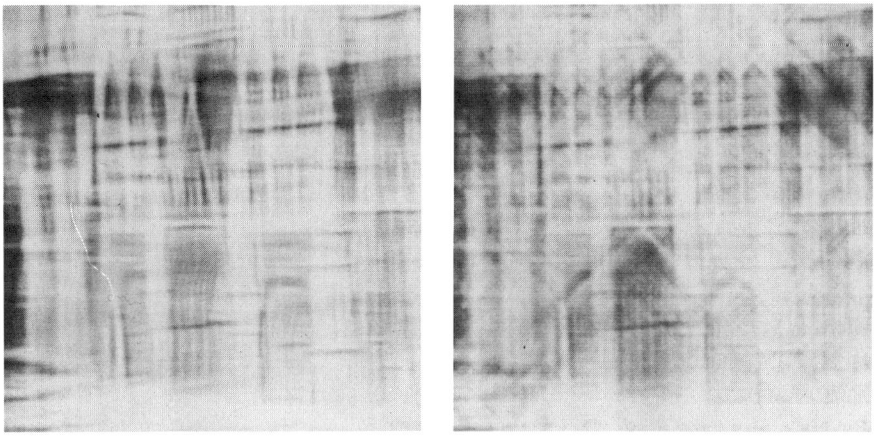

Fig. 14.a) Rouen Cathedral: Results of orientation-selective filtering

While the filtering operations considered so far cause significant alterations of image structure, they are not appropriate for reproducing the type of contour fragmentation common in cubist paintings. In this sense, cubist image representation seems to be more focused upon the shifting of object

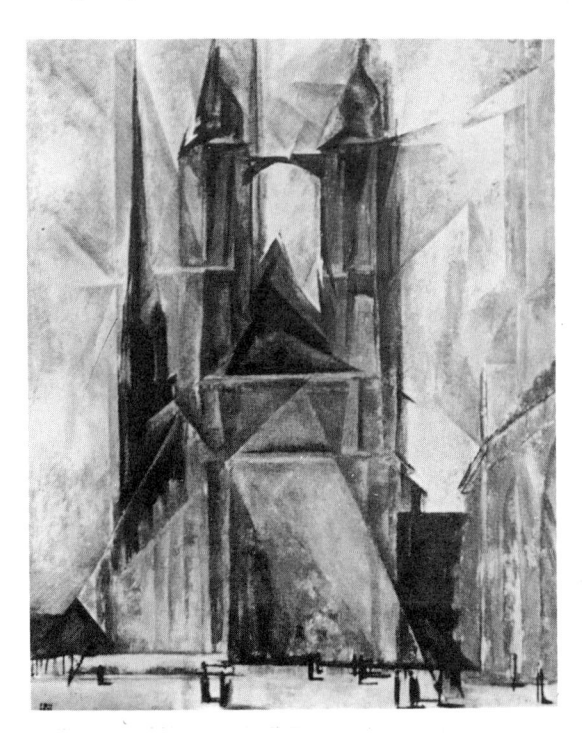

b) Lyonel Feininger (1931) Marktkirche von Halle (reproduced with permission of the Staatsgalerie Moderner Kunst, München)

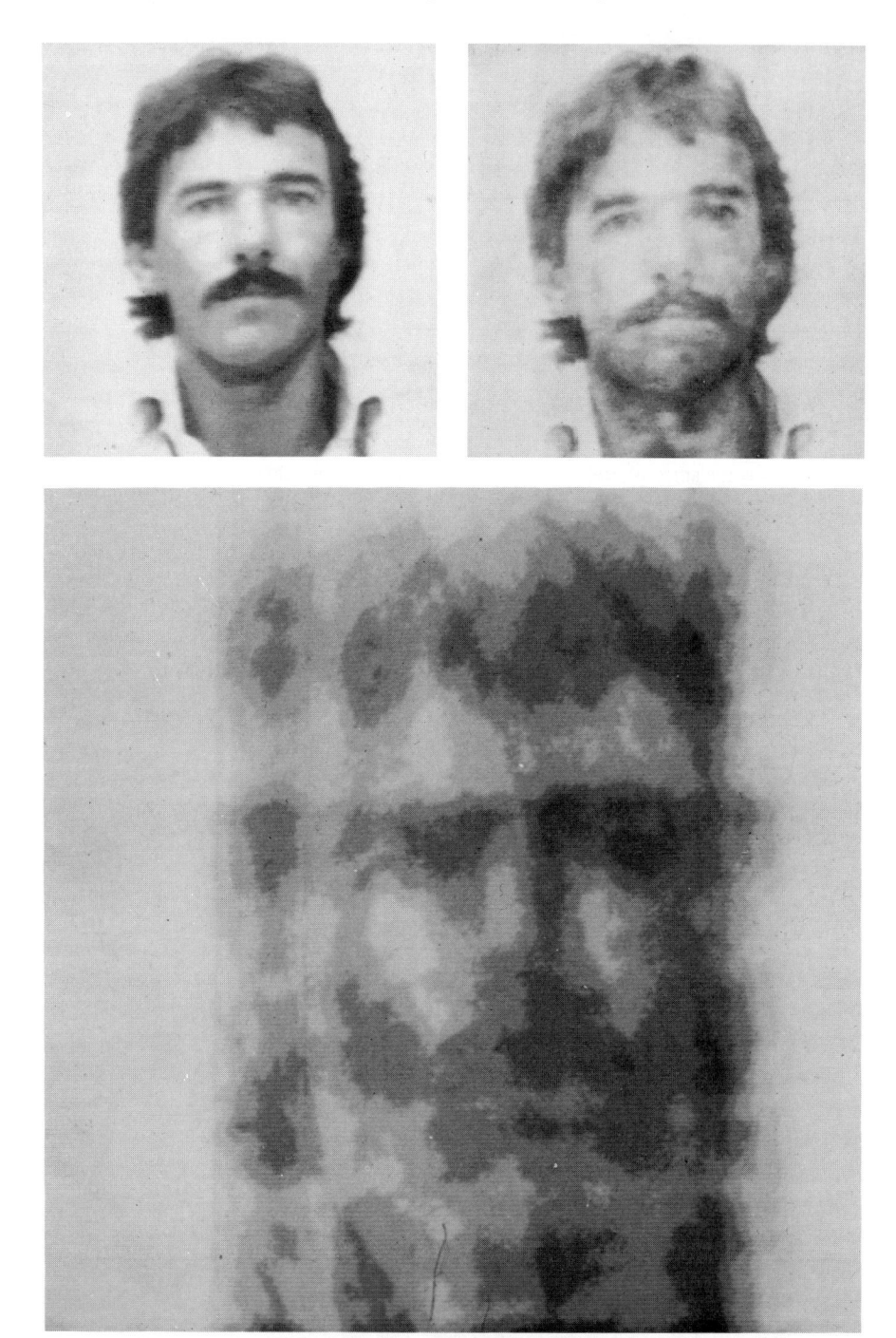

Fig.15. "Harry" – The effect of orientation-selective filtering on a portrait

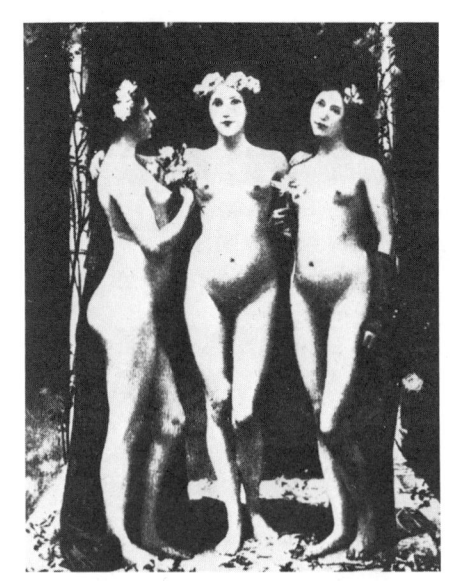

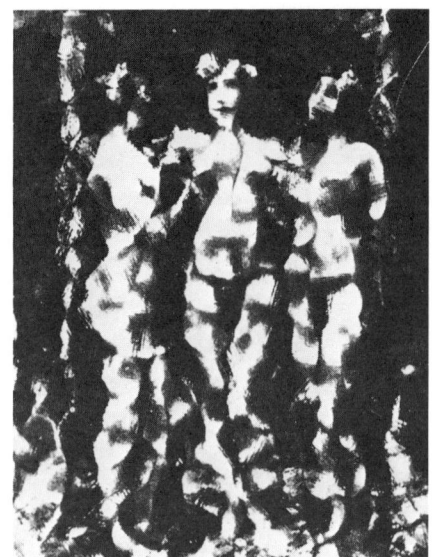

Fig. 16. Bonnencontre (about 1900) Three Graces. Original and painting seen through wobbly glass (reproduced with permission from Gombrich[20])

relationships in the creative process. To illustrate the possible effects of such a transition to disorder, we reproduced a painting by Bonnencontre unaltered and seen through wobbly glass (Fig. 16). These images have been produced by Gombrich[20] to demonstrate how the artificial degradation of a painting of French nineteenth-century "art officiel" can make it quite interesting.

If, as is maintained here, art can be evaluated along dimensions of internal image representation, various schools of painting, or styles, may be characterized by shifts of attention among and within these dimensions or "maps." The existence of such degrees of freedom has been called plurality of attention. However, we are not suggesting that the artist is using only a particular filter characteristic once he has sufficiently elaborated his skills of painting. A more appropriate perspective would be that he creatively "zooms" across various modes of pictorial representation in much the same way that a biologist changes the focus of his microscope to examine various layers of tissue. We feel that such a process of shifting the focus of attention during the creation of a major work of art is beautifully documented by a series of drawings and paintings by the French cubist Robert Delauney (Fig. 17), which were brought to our attention by Walter Siegfried . They all constitute representations of the "Three Graces," which evolved from the photographic reproduction of a fresco from Pompei found in the artist's atelier. The final version (Fig. 17, *center*)

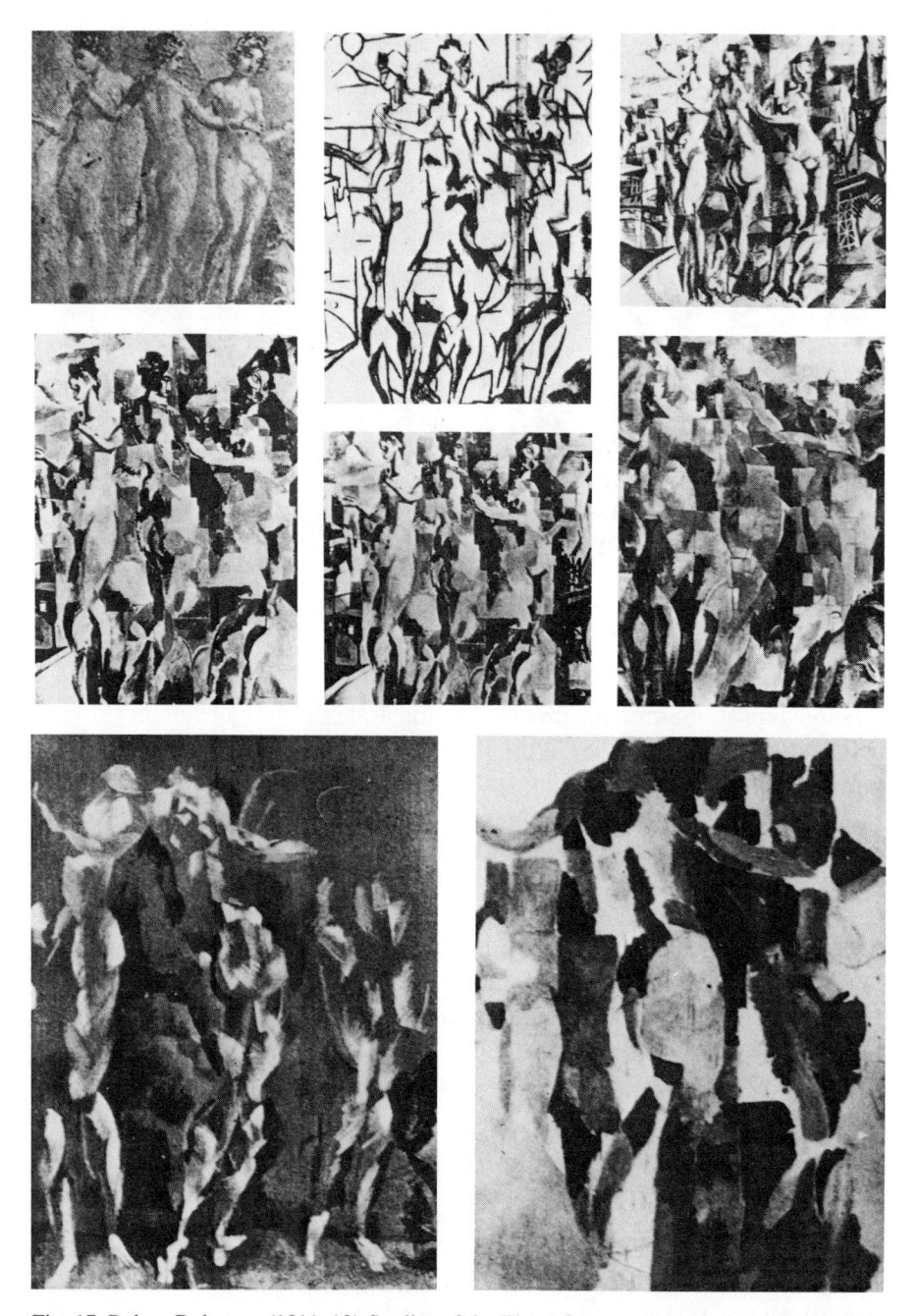

Fig. 17. Robert Delauney (1911–12) Studies of the Three Graces, after a fresco from Pompei (*top left*)

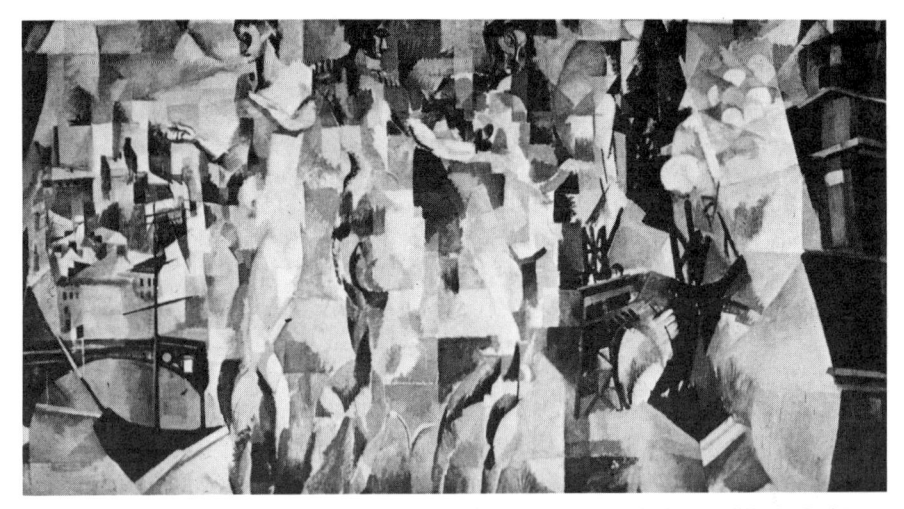

Fig. 18. Robert Delauney (1912) La Ville de Paris (Museé d'Art Moderne, Ville de Paris)

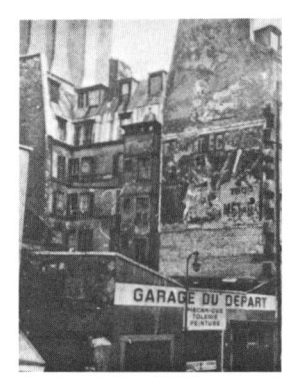

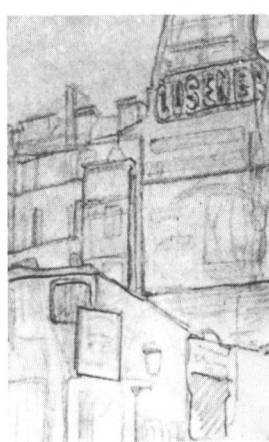

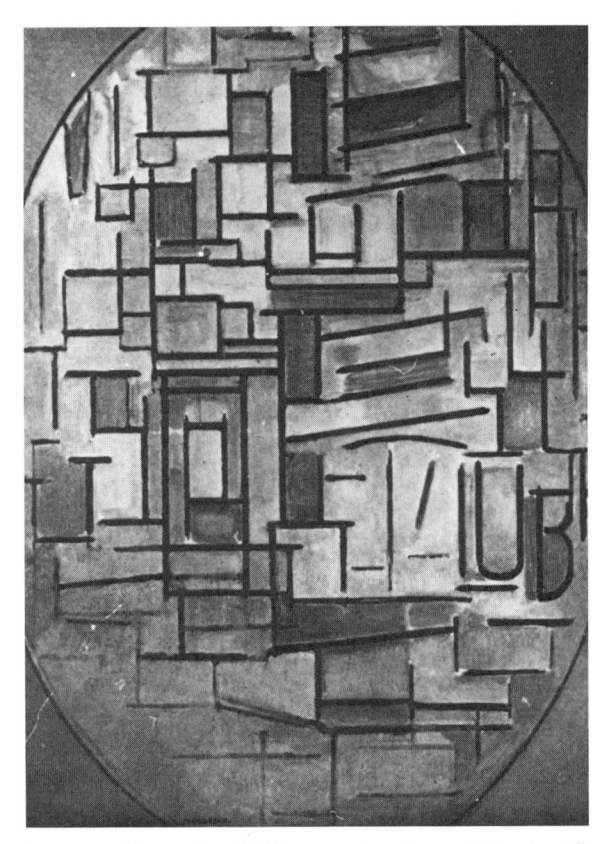

Fig. 19. Piet Mondrian (1913–14) Composition in Oval KUB (reproduced from Wijsenbeek[42])

became the centerpart of Delauney's famous painting "La Ville de Paris"[41] (Fig. 18). Another possible example of increasing abstraction may be seen in a series of three pictures (Fig. 19) that are related to the view from Piet Mondrian's study in the Rue du Depart 26 in Paris. The photograph taken from this study shows an advertisement painted on a wall. In Mondrian's rather naturalistic drawing of the scene, the advertisement is for "KUB" soup cubes, and the three letters are still visible in the cubist "Composition in Oval KUB," which the Dutch artist created from this view.[42]

Nonrepresentational Art

As the list of art styles considered above is evidently not complete, we shall next discuss the development of nonrepresentational art. In 1885, the French physiologist, Charles Henry, published a book entitled *Introduction à une Esthétique Scientifique*.[43] Based on his knowledge of aesthetics and mathematics, he advanced the hypothesis that correlations exist between the directions of movement (up and down, left and right) and their emotional significance. In subsequent publications, and especially in *Cercle Chromatique* (1888), Henry presented a more elaborate version of his theory and discussed the respective roles of line, tonality, and color as basic elements of pictorial representation. His most important idea was that the emotional impact of these elements is independent of their function in representing a particular object. George Seurat, the key figure in the French school of neoimpressionism, was deeply influenced by Henry's theories, as can be seen from his famous "Aesthetics," a text contained in a letter to Beaubourg written August 28, 1890: "Art is harmony. Harmony is analogy of differences, analogy of the similar, of tonality, colour, and the line in serene, calm, or sad combinations...."[44] Thus the interaction of these two minds strongly influenced the development of nonrepresentational art.[45]

The triad of line, tonality, and color played again a key role in the "General System of Pictorial Media," on which Paul Klee[46] lectured at the Bauhaus in the winter of 1923/24. It has been noted that, for the development of his theoretical position, Klee made use of principles and patterns elaborated earlier by the Gestalt psychologists.[47] This, however, cannot necessarily be taken as evidence for a causal effect of scientific research on art, as Klee anticipated other important results that were obtained in the laboratory only decades later. The most striking example of this is his illustration, well *before* the physiologists, of the principle of contour enhancement.[48] Klee and Henry conceived of the line as an abstract thing, which came into being through perceived motion or intersecting planes in visual space. Similarly, Kandinsky considered "the line an invisible thing ...created by movement."[49] Nevertheless, besides point and plane, Klee's colleague at the Bauhaus viewed the line as a "basic element without which a work in any particular art cannot even come into existence."[50]

The physiologist, Charles Sherrington, went one step further. Where Klee[51] was intrigued by "the open question of (the line's) reality," the former contended: "When we hear that Nature has no such thing as a line, vision answers that all contours are lines. That every contact of fields of light or colours is sharpened and stressed into a line – a psychological line. 'Contrast' develops a 'line' at any contact between abruptly distinguishable areas." But to Sherrington, it was still the *mind* whose "thinking largely accepts 'lines' and manufactures them."[52]

Almost a century after Henry's discovery of the line, the situation changed dramatically. In the early sixties, the neurophysiologists, David Hubel and Torsten Wiesel[53], discovered in the mammalian brain neurons responding selectively to elongated objects of particular orientation in the visual field (see chapter 7). This indicated that the early visual processing stages of the brain contain an arsenal of feature detectors tuned to lines and edges of varying width and orientation. This notion received support from psychophysical measurements of visual sensitivities to contrast and orientation of line segments as well as their mutual spatial interactions.[54] Related developments revealed that the brain is equally well equipped with mechanisms for the perception of tonality and color.[55] These results imply that lines, tonality, and color are not only the basic elements of pictorial representation in art but also in the brain. This supports the proposed relationship between visual information-processing characteristics and the evolution of style.

Conclusions

The main thesis of our paper is that the evolution of style in art is related to shifts in the focus of attention between multiple visual representations in the brain. Some evidence from visual research and art history seems to support this notion. First, recent results from the disciplines of pattern recognition and cognitive psychology suggest that perception is not uniquely determined by the physical properties of nature, but is an active process of constructing interpretations thereof. Second, it seems that brain function, with its adaptivity through learning, is the basis of such interpretive activity. Third, there are many similarities between image representations developed in art history and research in visual image processing. Clearly, more systematic experimental work should be done to explore how far the latter correlations can be confirmed within the framework of the present or any future perspective on visual information processing.

If we accept the notion that art is concerned with the variability of interpretations of nature, we are left with the question of what determines aesthetic preference with respect to different representations of reality. As can be inferred from the theory of symbolism of Ernest Jones[18], there is no unique solution to this problem. On the one hand, the progress of the human mind depends on the replacement of more primitive ideas, or symbolisms, by more difficult and complex ones. From this, one might expect that representations based on a richer set of features or aspects of reality are preferred. On the other hand, the human mind also seeks the unmasking of previous symbols as mere aspects of the truth, and this is possibly related to the role simplicity plays in aesthetics and epistemology.[56] This ambiguity would explain why both the evolution of art from prehistoric times[57] to realism in the European nineteenth century and the development of human artistic skills from early childhood to mastership begin with simple line drawings and lead to "realistic" painting. But once the skills of rendering nature are sufficiently developed to compete with the photographic process, their products are discerned as mere reproductions of nature lacking the creative element.[3] From this, we may conclude that it is not the physical characteristics of pictorial representation as such that determine aesthetic preference but rather their potential to change internalized symbolic renderings of the world, which actually structure what is perceived.

Another way of looking at the ambiguities in the relationship between biological determinants and aesthetic preference results from Eibl-Eibesfeldt's view of three levels of aesthetic evaluation (chapter 2). According to Eibl-Eibesfeldt, aesthetic responses may be elicited at the level of basic perceptual mechanisms that man shares with other higher vertebrates, next are species-specific processes of encoding sensory signals, and, finally, there are culturally determined patterns of response. It is conceivable that what is aesthetically preferred on the basis of responses at one level may be ignored when evaluated at another level of encoding. Depending on his or her personal history, an individual who visits the Chicago Art Institute may either adore the paintings by Monet in the room of the impressionists or the "Sledge" by Joseph Beuys in the neighboring department.

This dynamic understanding of aesthetic preference is nicely illustrated by the explanation Gombrich[20] offered for the increase in aesthetic value of Bonnencontre's "Three Graces" seen through wobbly glass (Fig. 16). It depends on the distinction between the ritualistic and the aesthetic attitude toward painting, as has been invoked by Ernst Kris. The ritualistic attitude relates to the origin of art in prehistoric times, when a work of art was an object of worship. The evolution of symbols, as conceived by Ernest Jones[18], however, put increasing demands on the imagination of the beholder of a piece of art. As a result of this development, the beholder must take part in the creative process by recreating the artist's conception of things in his/her own mind, thus assuming what Kris called the aesthetic attitude. Clearly, this view is shared by artists themselves, as can be seen from the ideas expressed by Malevich and by a statement made by the Dutch artist, Theo van Doesburg: "The aesthetic comprehension of an exactly creative piece of art is only possible if the beholder has aesthetic relationships to pieces of art in general. That is, when the beholder looks at a piece of art, he must be able to re-create it in his consciousness."[58]

The transition from the ritualistic to the aesthetic attitude toward pictorial art is reminiscent of another revolution that has taken place in the relationship between man and nature. In quantum physics, the measuring device used to observe nature is itself a physical system subject to the same laws and principles as the system under observation. The process of observation actually consists, therefore, of an interaction between the instrument of observation and the observed. This insight ended the belief that the observer can remain aloof from the observed. The physicist concludes that "... through man nature can observe itself."[59] Regarding the evolution of pictorial representation in painting, we may paraphrase this statement by saying that through art, one can observe his/her reflections of reality in the brain.

Acknowledgement

The present authors are indebted to Professor Semir Zeki for stimulating discussions of the problems at issue. The Deutsche Forschungsgemeinschaft supported this study by grant Re 337/4 to I.R. and a guest-professorship Mu 93/103 to T.C.

References and Notes

1. Helmholtz H von (1962) On the physiological causes of harmony in music. In: Kline M (ed) Popular scientifique lectures. Dover, New York, pp 22–23. Translation of: Über die physiologischen Ursachen der musikalischen Harmonie. Vorlesung gehalten in Bonn (1857) In: Vorträge und Reden, 5th edn. Friedrich Vieweg und Sohn, Braunschweig, 1903, pp 119–155
2. Kandinsky W (1977) Concerning the spiritual in art. Dover, New York, p 19. Translation of: Über das Geistige in der Kunst. Piper, München, 1912
3. Malevich K (1959) The non-objective world. Paul Theobald, Chicago, pp 13–14. Translation of: Die gegenstandslose Welt. Bauhausbuch 11. Albert Langen, München, 1927
4. Strawson PF (1987) Kant's philosophy of the mind. In Gregory RL (ed) The Oxford companion to the mind. Oxford University Press, Oxford, pp 406–408
5. Gregory RL (1987) Perception as hypotheses. In: Gregory RL (ed) The Oxford companion to the mind. Oxford University Press, Oxford, pp 608–611

6. Wertheimer M (1974) The problem of perceptual structure. In: Carterette EC, Friedman MP (eds) Handbook of perception, Historical and philosophical roots of perception, vol I. Academic, New York, pp 75–91
7. Kant I (1965) Critique of pure reason. St. Martin's, New York. Translation of: Die Kritik der reinen Vernunft. In: Kants gesammelte Schriften. Ausgabe der Preussischen Akademie der Wissenschaften, vol 3, Berlin 1904
8. Ehrenfels C von (1890) Über Gestaltqualitäten. Vierteljahresschrift für wissenschaftliche Philosophie 14: 249–292
9. For a survey of Gestalt psychology, see: Koffka K (1935) Principles of Gestalt psychology. Harcourt, Brace and World, New York
10. Fechner GT (1860) Elemente der Psychophysik. Breitkopf und Härtel, Leipzig
11. Fisher GH (1968) Ambiguity of form: Old and new. Perception and Psychophysics 4: 189–192
12. Russell B (1946) History of Western philosophy – and its connection with political and social circumstances from the earliest times to the present day, chap XIX. George Allen and Unwin, London
13. Watanabe S (1985) Pattern recognition. Human and mechanical. John Wiley, New York
14. Kohonen T (1988) Self-organization and associative memory, 2nd edn. Springer, Berlin, p 24; see also Watanabe, ibid, chap 2
15. Kuhn TS (1970) The structure of scientific revolutions, 2nd edn. University of Chicago Press, Chicago
16. Kuhn TS (1974) Second thoughts on paradigms. In: Suppe F (ed) The structure of scientifique theories. University of Illinois Press, Urbana, pp 459–482
17. Kuhn, op cit 15, p 111
18. Jones E (1916) The theory of symbolism. In: Jones E, Papers on psycho-analysis, 5th edn. Maresfield Reprints, London, p 87
19. Jones E, ibid, p 89
20. Gombrich EH (1978) Psychoanalysis and the history of art. In: Meditations on a hobbyhorse, 3rd edn. Phaidon, London, pp 30–44
21. Shannon CE (1948) A mathematical theory of communication. Bell System Technical Journal 27 (July) 379–423, (October) 623–656
22. Moles AA (1966) Information and esthetic perception. University of Illinois Press, Urbana. Translation of: Théorie de l'information et perception esthétique. Flammarion, Paris, 1958
23. Bense M (1960) Programmierung des Schönen. Ägis, Baden-Baden
24. Meyer L (1967) Music, the arts, and ideas. University of Chicago Press, Chicago
25. Attneave F (1954) Some informational aspects of visual perception. Psychol Rev 61: 183–193
26. Neisser U (1960) Cognitive psychology. Appleton-Century-Croft, New York, chap 1
27. Epstein D (1979) Beyond Orpheus. Studies in musical time. MIT Press, Cambridge, pp 14–15
28. Zeki S (1978) Functional specialisaton in the visual cortex of the rhesus monkey. Nature 274: 423–428; Cowey A (1979) Cortical maps and visual perception. The Grindley Memorial Lecture. Q J exp Psychol 31: 1–17; for a recent review, see: Van Essen DC (1985) Functional organization of primate visual vortex. In: Peters A, Jones EG (eds) Cerebral cortex. Visual cortex, vol 3. Plenum, New York
29. Kohonen, op cit 14, chap 5
30. Critchley M (1949) Metamorphopsia of central origin. Trans Ophthalmol Soc UK 69: 11–121; Klee A, Willanger R (1966) Disturbances of visual perception in migraine. Acta Neurol Skandinav 42: 400–414; Milner B, Teuber HL (1968) Alterations of

perception and memory in man. In: Weiskrantz L (ed) The analysis of behavioural change. Harper and Row, New York, pp 268–375; Kölmel HW (1984) Coloured patterns in hemianopic fields. Brain 107: 155–167

31. Huxley A (1954) The doors of perception. Perennial Library P 171. Harper and Row, New York, p 33
32. In the context of sensory physiology, encoding simply means the mapping of stimulus properties onto patterns of neural activity; for further discussion, see: Uttal W (1974) The psychobiology of sensory coding. Harper and Row, New York
33. Caelli T (1981) Visual Perception. Pergamon, Oxford, chap 3
34. Campbell FW (1980) The physics of visual perception. Phil Trans R Soc Lond B 290: 5–9
35. Maffei L (1978) Spatial frequency channels: Neural mechanisms. In: Held R, Leibowitz HW, Teuber HL (eds) Handbook of Sensory Perception, vol VIII. Springer, Berlin pp 39–66
36. Marr D (1980) In: Campbell, op cit 34, p 9 (discussion)
37. Marr D (1976) Early processing of visual information. Proc Royal Soc 275: 483–519; Marr D (1982) Vision. Freeman, San Francisco
38. The idea that intensity changes are the physiologically relevant components of an image and can be detected as zero-crossings of the second derivative (Laplacian operator) of the intensity distribution dates back to the physicist Ernst Mach in the nineteenth century. Marr applied this concept to a set of blurred versions of an image that were obtained by using Gaussian point-spread functions as convolution kernels at different scales. We determined the zero- crossings of band-pass versions of an image. The equivalence of these two techniques is readily shown by taking advantage of the properties of the Fourier transform of a derivative.
39. The physiologist Ewald Hering contended that brightness and darkness are distinct sensations. Evidence of separated neural pathways subserving these sensations has been provided by Schiller P (1982) Central connections of the retinal ON and OFF pathways. Nature 297: 580–583; and Schiller P, Sandell JH, Maunsell JHR (1986) Functions of the ON and OFF channels of the visual system. Nature 322: 824–825
40. Jung R (1971) Kontrastsehen, Konturbetonung und Künstlerzeichnung. Studium Generale 24: 1536–1565
41. Dorival B (1975) Robert Delauney 1885–1941 (Catalogue). Jacques Damase, Paris, pp 30–35; Robert Delauney (Ausstellungkatalog). Staatliche Kunsthalle, Baden-Baden 1976, p 106, pp 121–124
42. Wijsenbeek LJF (1968) Piet Mondrian. Aurel Bongers, Recklinghausen, pp 67–72
43. Herbert RL (1970) Die Theorien Seurats und des Neoimpressionismus. In: Sutter J (ed) Die Neoimpressionisten. Rembrandt, Berlin, p 34
44. Sutter, ibid, p 223
45. Herbert, op cit 43, pp 35–36
46. Klee P (1973) Notebooks, vol 2. The nature of nature. Lund Humphries, London. Translation of: Unendliche Naturgeschichte. Schwabe, Basel, 1970
47. Teuber ML (1976) Blue Night by Paul Klee. In: Henle M (ed) Vision and artifact. Springer, New York; Vitz PC, Glimcher AB (1984) Modern art and modern science. Praeger, New York, chap 4
48. Klee P (1970), op cit 46, pp 303–307: Here Klee interpreted contrast as the result of antagonistic interactions between the poles of light and dark. Although this idea can be related to the earlier writings of Ernst Mach, the artist illustrated his concept with a graph ("mexican-hat function") that preempted later physiological findings on lateral spatial interactions in the visual system.

49. Kandinsky W (1979) Point and line to plane. Dover, New York , p 10. Translation of: Punkt und Linie zur Fläche. Bauhausbuch 6. Albert Langen, München, 1926
50. Kandinsky, ibid, p 20
51. Klee, op cit 46, p 229
52. Sherrington C (1975) Man on his nature. The Gifford Lectures, Edinburgh 1937–38. Reprinted paperback edn., Cambridge University Press, Cambridge, pp 254–255
53. Hubel DH, Wiesel TN (1962) Receptive fields, binocular interaction and functional architecture in the cat's visual cortex. J Physiol (Lond) 160: 106–154
54. For references, see: Rentschler I, Hilz R, Sütterlin C, Noguchi K (1981) Illusions of filled lateral and angular extent. Exp Brain Res 44: 154–158
55. Land EH (1959) Color vision and the natural image, Part I. Proc Nat Acad Sciences 45: 115–129; Land EH (1959) Color vision and the natural image, Part II. Proc Nat Acad Sciences 45: 636–644; a more popular description of these ideas is given by Land EH (1977) The retinex theory of colour vision. Scientific American 237: 108–128. Physiological evidence supporting Land's concept of tonality and color is provided by Zeki S (1980) The representation of colours in the cerebral cortex. Nature 284: 412–418; and Livingstone MS, Hubel DH (1984) Anatomy and physiology of a colour system in the primate visual cortex. J Neurosci 4: 309–356
56. Popper KR (1959) The logic of scientific discovery, chap IV. Hutchinson, London
57. Giedion S (1962) The eternal present: The beginning of art. A contribution on constancy and change. Bollingen Foundation, New York – Pantheon Books, New York. Translation of: Ewige Gegenwart – Die Entstehung der Kunst. DuMont Schauberg, Köln, 1964
58. Doesburg T van (1925) Grundbegriffe der Neuen Gestaltenden Kunst, Bauhausbuch 6. Albert Langen, München.
59. Rohrlich F (1983) Facing quantum mechanical reality. Science 221: 1251–1255
60. After finishing this manuscript, we read a recent study by Margaret S. Livingstone (1988) Art, illusion and the visual system. Scientific American 258:68–75. Obviously, we concur with her idea that visual aesthetics is closely interrelated with the multipartite character of visual processing in the brain. It is fortunate that this author elaborated on the role that color plays in art and science – an aspect that has been neglected in the present work.

Part IV
Two Brains – One Mind?

Cerebral Asymmetry and Aesthetic Experience

Jerre Levy
Department of Behavioral Sciences, University of Chicago, Chicago, Illinois 60637, USA

>The world is shadowed plays of light,
>Modelled, stripped, reformed, and lined,
>Bounded, bordered by the mind,
>Redone into an inner sight,
>
>Created worlds of shape and hue,
>Music, meaning, rhythm, time,
>Configurations made sublime,
>Constructions of an inner view.

I wrote the above quatrains for Professor Frederick Turner (see chapter 3), our poet at Bad Homburg, during the last meeting of the study group on The Biology of Aesthetics to summarize my own perspective concerning the essential nature of aesthetic experience and of aesthetic creation. They are meant to convey three deeply interrelated aspects of the apprehension of beauty. First is the external world and its properties. Second are the operations of the brains that reconstruct these properties into new forms, configurations, and orders that did not exist in the universe until minds came into being. Finally, there is the utterly mysterious process, incorporated in the spatiotemporal organization of neuronal action, that experiences its own creations as beautiful. I further suggest that this experience is the mind's self-reward for apprehending and constructing order, that it reinforces, promotes, and compels the constructive effort, and in so doing, binds us to our memories, shapes our dreams, and opens windows of the imagination. The building of a mental universe requires an impulsion to do so, and what better way can this be assured than through an inherent exaltation from the mind's own creations?

Quite conceivably, a computer program might be written that could derive the same ordered forms and constancies that are built by brains, but it could not experience the aesthetic values of its constructions, the sense of the beautiful, unless it contained emotion and a deep integration between its cognitive and affective operations. Perhaps someday this can actually be done, but at the current time, we know nothing regarding the necessary and sufficient conditions of the spatiotemporal organization of mechanistic systems that generate love, hate, joy, grief, or the sense of beauty. Some have argued that this mystery is so beyond conception that we must reject the materialistic hypothesis. But I believe that hidden in the many billions of neuronal interactions and relations are the secrets of a consciousness that finds fulfillment, awe, and beauty in the forms and configurations it makes. From this perspective, the generation of the aesthetic experience or creation depends both on the cognitive and the affective processes of brains and a close intertwining between the two.

Obviously, none of the foregoing would make sense if, as many philosophers have proposed in the past, the properties of the external world are simply passively impressed on the mind, like images on photographic film. However, psychologists have known and emphasized for years that there is no such thing as passive sensory experience, much less complex perceptions. The mind constructs its world of the senses, as much as it constructs its conceptions and ideas, and the construction is active, intelligent, and rule governed. This has been dramatically highlighted in studies of split-brain patients in whom the bridges of fibers interconnecting the two cerebral hemispheres (corpus callosum) have been surgically severed as a control for intractable epilepsy.

Perceptual Construction in Split-Brain Patients

Because of the anatomy of the visual system, visual information to the left of a fixation point is projected (through both eyes) to the right side of the brain and vice versa for visual information to the right of a fixation point. Thus, if a split-brain patient focuses on some point, a stimulus in the left visual field (LVF) is seen only by the right hemisphere, and a stimulus in the right visual field (RVF) is seen only by the left hemisphere (see p. 246). Voluntary refixations of the eyes take about 1/5 second, so if stimuli are rapidly flashed for a period less than this, they will have disappeared by the time a patient may have shifted fixation. In normal people, both sides of the brain have access to information on both sides of space since the interconnecting bridges between the two hemispheres are intact and support a constant communication: what one hemisphere sees is, within a few milliseconds (ms), known by the other.

In the split-brain patient, the hemispheres are both anatomically and mentally separated so that each side of the brain is in contact with only half a world of sensory experience.[1] Yet the world is whole, and brains evolved in this un-

unsplit universe. Their rules and programs evolved to generate perceptions and to build models of this world as it is. We may, therefore, wonder what kinds of percepts and concepts are derived by an isolated hemisphere when it receives information from half a face or half a word or half a picture. Figure 1 illustrates one of the tasks that has been presented to split-brain patients.[2]

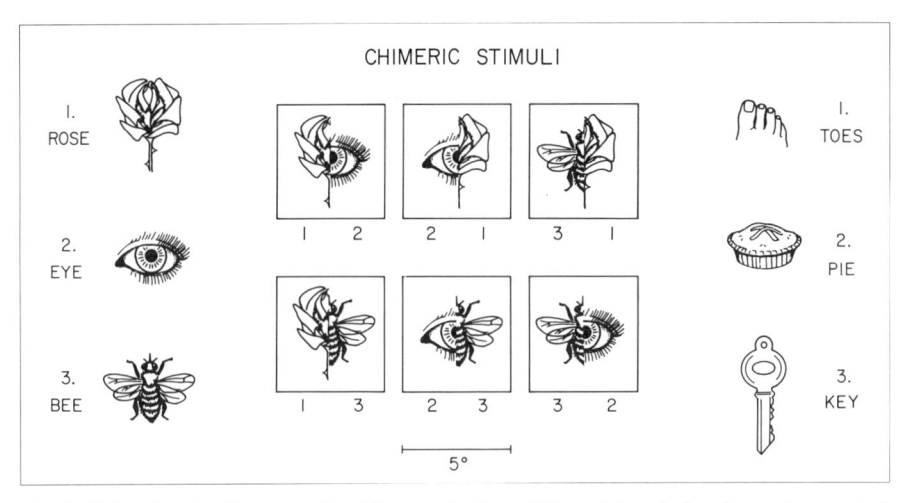

Fig. 1. Chimeric stimuli presented tachistoscopically and free-vision choices in a task presented to split-brain patients. When asked to name the picture seen, patients named the object on the right half of the chimera and were not aware that only half a figure had been presented. When asked to match the picture with choices in free vision, the left half of the chimeras was matched, and there was no awareness that only a half-figure had been presented. Matches to rhyming objects were based on the right half of chimeras, indicating the predominance of the left hemisphere for phonetic representation.[2]

The split, chimeric pictures are rapidly flashed as patients focus on a fixation point (see p. 244). Under these conditions, each hemisphere receives half a stimulus, different from that projected to the other hemisphere. When patients were asked to name what they saw, they named the object on the right half of the chimera that was seen by the left hemisphere. Speech, in the vast majority of right-handers, is confined to the left side of the brain, so it was not surprising that it was the right half-object that was named. However, the speaking left hemisphere was totally unaware that it had been presented with only a half-stimulus. Its *perception* was of a whole eye, bee, or rose.

When whole pictures of the objects were placed in free vision and patients were told to point to what they saw,[3] they made essentially perfect matches, but they matched the half-stimulus presented to the LVF and seen by the right half of the brain. Although the right hemisphere cannot speak, it displayed nonverbal evidence that it also perceived the half-stimulus as a whole object.

Normal people, when tested under similar conditions, immediately see the strange composite nature of the stimuli.

In one final test with these split pictures, pictures of rhyming objects were placed in free vision, and patients were asked to match the stimulus according to a rhyming name (i. e., rose with toes, eye with pie, bee with key). In this case, they matched the right half of chimeras, indicating the predominance of the left hemisphere for phonetic analysis and representation.

A variety of other tasks with split faces, nonsense shapes,[3] words,[2] and colors[4] revealed similar results. Only one hemisphere gained a percept on any given trial; the controlling hemisphere depended on the nature of the task demanded,[5] and regardless of which hemisphere dominated, its perception was of a whole and complete stimulus.

These observations demonstrate two things. First, adequate stimulus input is insufficient to guarantee a perception (since the nonresponding hemisphere behaved as if it had seen nothing at all), and second, depleted stimulus information does not imply a similarly depleted perception. The responding hemisphere interpreted a whole image, although only half an image had been presented. The model-building rules of the brain are evidently such that they make sense of the world. They do not accept the impossible situation of two different images being present in the same place at the same time, and they do not allow the world to be split in half.

The programs for world construction recognize that the world is whole. When information from that world is available (as in the normal person), it is used to construct the model, but when it is not available (as in the split-brain patient), a whole-world model is built anyway, based on the actual information present, memories, motivations, beliefs, conceptions, and a rich knowledge of the nature of the universe gleaned from millions of years of evolution and stored in the organizational pattern of the brain. It is the rules of world construction that bring us color and pattern, meaning and feeling, configurations in time and space that, on occasion, are experienced as beautiful.

These studies not only illustrate the elaborate model-building activities of brains, but they also illustrate that the left and right hemispheres are functionally asymmetric, not merely in their competencies for various processes, but in their tendencies to dominate mentation. In one of our tasks, patients were asked, in one run of trials, to match pictures according to visual similarity (e. g., a hat with a brim and a cake on a cakeplate), and in another run of trials, to match pictures according to functional association (e. g., a hat and gloves).[5] The right hemisphere dominated with visual-similarity instructions, and the left hemisphere dominated with functional-association instructions, yet the stimuli and the set of available choices remained invariant over the two instructional conditions. The aspects of stimuli that are perceived differ for the two sides of the brain, and as will be discussed, their models and representations of reality have different characteristics and different emotional implications. Could it be that one hemisphere, more than the other, generates those representations and emotional responses that are critical for aesthetic experience, or alternatively, is it the integration between the processes of the two hemispheres that makes aesthetic creation possible?

Cognitive Specializations of the Left and Right Hemispheres

Although there is considerable agreement among researchers regarding relative competencies of the two hemispheres for various tasks, there is much less consensus with respect to the nature of fundamental characteristics responsible for these differences.[6, 7] I emphasize, therefore, that the interpretations I offer reflect my own particular perspective, which may differ from that of others.

There can be little argument that the left hemisphere is predominant in the formal operations of language, which include speech, syntactical analysis, and phonetic representation. Thus, the right hemisphere of the split-brain patient suffers from an almost complete expressive aphasia,[1, 8] cannot discriminate tenses and plural from singular,[9] shows radical disorders of comprehension for sentences with complex syntax or that place a significant load on verbal short-term memory,[10] and is incapable of phonetic representation.[2, 11] However, it knows a word when it hears it and shows good capacity for deriving associative meaning for single spoken or written words,[12] a capacity that is shared by many avian and mammalian species.[13] The special abilities that are unique to the human left hemisphere involve a high-level sequential programming of the articulatory apparatus and refined programs for the discrimination of the temporal order of phonemic segments and causal relations as specified by syntactical rules.

The right hemisphere has been found to be superior to the left in discriminating line orientations,[14, 15] curvature,[16, 17] randomly shaped polygons,[18] vertical or horizontal alignments of dot matrices,[19] position in space of visual signals,[20-22] depth from stereoscopic cues,[23] the exclusion or inclusion of geometric or topological figures from sets sharing an unspecified invariant,[24] the similarity or dissimilarity between unified and fragmented shapes,[25] and at a variety of other tasks requiring imagistic representation, mental transformations of spatial relations, or integration and synthesis of global form.

I believe that the various differences in hemispheric capacities are likely to relate to a bias for the left hemisphere to order and program events in time and for the right hemisphere to represent and construct relations in space, regardless of whether the actual stimulus input is acoustico-temporal or visuo-spatial in its superficial characteristics. In terms of pure sensory function, the left hemisphere responds faster to auditory signals than the right hemisphere[26-28] when uncertainty exists whether a signal will appear at the left or right ear, whereas the right hemisphere responds faster than the left hemisphere to simple visual signals.[29-31] The opposite hemispheric superiorities for the auditory and visual modalities may be a primitive reflection of the left hemisphere's representation in a temporal domain and the right hemisphere's representation in a spatial domain.

Patients with left-hemispheric lesions require unusually long temporal separations between a pair of events before they can discriminate their order of occurrence, whereas patients with right-hemispheric lesions typically display the same threshold of temporal separation as normal people.[32-35] Normative studies show that it is the left hemisphere that performs temporal-order discriminations, even when one signal is initially projected to the right hemisphere and the other signal is initially projected to the left hemisphere.[36, 37] When pairs of acoustic signals are played to the right ear, responses are faster to identify a target sequence than when pairs of signals are played to the left ear[38] if the temporal separation between members of the pair is within the threshold range (10–75 ms).

The foregoing observations should not be taken to mean that the right hemisphere is incapable of discriminating one sequence from its opposite (e. g., a high-low tone sequence from a low-high tone sequence). At a 0.1-ms separation, the right hemisphere discriminates target sequences faster than the left hemisphere,[38] but it does so on the basis of differences in sound quality between target sequences and their opposite, not by an actual discrimination of which of two signals occurred first. Also, for ordered events that occur repeatedly with relatively long separations between events, the right hemisphere can learn to preserve the order by a remapping into a spatial domain and does so better than the left hemisphere. Cremonini et al.,[39] in an examination of unilaterally brain-damaged patients, found that those with an intact left hemisphere were superior at pointing in succession to a series of pictures in the same order in which they had just been presented, whereas those with an intact right hemisphere were superior in learning, over a series of trials, to arrange a set of pictures in a spatial order that matched the temporal order of presentation that was invariant on every trial. Thus, for closely spaced temporal events, the right hemisphere can use sensory quality to discriminate one sequence from another and, for widely spaced temporal events, can learn and retain the order by a spatial remapping.

These findings emphasize the point that sensory events that are superficially temporal in nature are not necessarily treated as such by the processing system. In certain cases, these can be represented imagistically or spatially more accurately than by direct temporal representation, and in this case, the right hemisphere is superior to the left. Buchtel et al.[40] found a clear right-hemispheric superiority in discriminating the duration of tones. It is probably relevant that in English, French, German, Hungarian, Arabic, Japanese, and almost certainly other languages as well, words for "long" and "short" can be equally applied to temporal duration and to spatial extent. This cross-modal equivalence in language usage probably derives from an inherent cross-modal equivalence in mental representations. At constant velocity, the spatial distance between two points is linear with respect to the elapse of time in moving from one point to the other, and it makes sense that the brain would have evolved to appreciate the equivalence.

Interestingly, there are no hemispheric asymmetries for discriminating the duration of visual signals.[41] Except for the appearance and disappearance of lights, it is ecologically meaningless to speak of the "duration" of visual objects. These may move in and out of view, but in contrast to acoustic signals, duration is not one of their fundamental properties, and, indeed, the deer which believes that a lion has ceased to exist when it has moved from sight would not survive to transmit its genes to future generations. As Bertoloni et al. suggest, there may simply have been no evolutionary pressure towards hemispheric specialization for judging the duration of visual events. In contrast, there would be strong adaptive demands for judging velocity, and Bertoloni et al. found a strong right-hemispheric superiority for velocity evaluation.[41]

Just as the right hemisphere is superior to the left in processing certain types of information involving the time dimension, the left hemisphere is superior to the right for some aspects of the visuo-spatial dimension. Patterson and Bradshaw[42] constructed pairs of cartoon faces that differed either in a single feature or in three features. Although the right hemisphere was superior at discriminating faces differing in three features, the left hemisphere was superior when discrimination depended on detection of a single-feature variation. Umiltà et al.[43] found a right-hemispheric superiority for processing complex shapes and figures, but a left-hemispheric superiority for simple shapes and figures. The authors suggested that the left hemisphere predominates when the task depends on extracting a few, clear-cut details, whereas the right predominates when complex configurational characteristics must be integrated.

This distinction is congruent with findings that patients with unilateral brain damage show defects in drawing that differ in nature depending on whether the lesion is in the left or the right hemisphere.[44, 45] With right-hemispheric lesions, drawings lose configurational integrity. Basic form characteristics are missing or so distorted that they are barely recognizable. However, with left-hemispheric brain damage, although the basic configuration is usually retained, drawings are impoverished with respect to detail.

In brief, the "spatial" right hemisphere and the "temporal" left hemisphere both have capacities that allow them to make important contributions to performance in most realms of activity. The left hemisphere seems to have a temporal and auditory bias, and the right hemisphere seems to have a spatial and visual bias. Theses biases may promote a tendency for the left hemisphere to note details and label them so that strict categorical boundaries may define separable events that can be ordered in time, whereas for the right hemisphere, the simultaneity of spatial forms and features may encourage a search for integrative relations and configurations. If the foregoing interpretations are valid, they suggest that each hemisphere treats identical input differently and reformulates sensory stimuli in terms of its special representational strategies. The complementarity of the specialized functions of the left and right hemispheres almost certainly means that the models of reality constructed by normal brains are qualitatively distinct from any mere summation of the types of representational strategies characteristic of each hemisphere alone.

Emotion and the Cerebral Hemispheres

There is a great deal of evidence that the right hemisphere is predominant in the experience, expression, and discrimination of emotion. In studies of normal people, there is a LVF (right-hemispheric) advantage in discriminating emotional expressions on faces,[46-49] a left-ear (right-hemispheric) advantage in discriminating emotional tones of voice,[50-52] emotional human sounds, such as laughing and crying,[53] and the emotional tone of musical passages,[54] and a left-face advantage in the intensity of emotional expression.[47, 48, 55-57]

Patients with right-hemispheric brain damage often lose emotional intonation in speech,[58] whereas with left-hemispheric brain damage and aphasia, the intact right hemisphere can discriminate emotional intonation.[59] Right-hemispheric lesions produce serious impairments in the appreciation of humor[60] and in the comprehension of affective speech.[61]

The emotional disorders arising from right-hemispheric damage are closely related to general arousal functions. Left-side neglect is common in cases of right-hemispheric lesions, and Heilman et al. have related this to hypoarousal.[62] Heilman and Van Den Abell showed that, in normal people, the right hemisphere is dominant for mediating cerebral activation. Thus, reaction times to simple sensory signals are greatly reduced when the signal is preceded by a warning cue, and warning cues presented to the right hemisphere are more effective than those presented to the left hemisphere, even for right-hand responses.[63] Any form of stimulation (sensory or cognitive) generates a selective increase in regional metabolism in the parietal and mesiotemporal cortex of the right hemisphere (A. D. Rosen et al. 1981, Mapping attentional functions in humans using positron emission tomography, unpublished work).

Tucker[64] has proposed that the tendency of the right hemisphere to synthesize and integrate multiple complex input into a global configurational form plays a critical role in the elaboration and stimulation of emotional experience and that the left hemisphere's tendency to analyze experiences into discrete, time-ordered, and strictly bounded details serves to modulate and reduce emotional reactions. From this perspective, the cognitive and emotional characteristics of the two hemispheres are closely related, and the two hemispheres are as complementary in their regulation of emotion as they are in cognitive specializations. It has been known for many years that there is a quadratic relation between performance and arousal:[65] Performance improves as arousal increases up to some optimum and then starts to deteriorate as arousal becomes excessive. From an adaptive standpoint, it is clear that regulatory systems are needed both for the enhancement of arousal and emotional intensity and for their control and modulation. By implication, the mental construction of forms, relations, images, and abstractions in time and space is optimized when the emotions are engaged (prior to disruptive hyperarousal), and, presumably, it is at this optimum when aesthetic creations occur.

Aesthetic Experience and Cerebral Asymmetry

In music and the visual arts, in prose and poetry, it seems clear that the specialized cognitive and emotional processes associated with both hemispheres must be integrated into a unified representation. There must be form and detail, images and abstractions, relations in space and orders in time, and these must be synthesized, tested, and judged within an emotional framework in which the mental construction yields the experience of the beautiful. Indeed, for the creative mathematician or scientist, models of the universe are also conditioned by their aesthetic appeal and elegance. Einstein's belief in and search for a unified field theory held him in thrall until the end of his life, not because any experimental evidence demanded a conclusion that the forces of physics could be unified, but rather because the conception was, to him, of sublime beauty.

> Poincaré says,
> "The scientist does not study nature because it is useful; he studies it because he delights in it, and he delights in it because it is beautiful. If nature were not beautiful, it would not be worth knowing, and if nature were not worth knowing, life would not be worth living . . . . I mean that profounder beauty which comes from the harmonious order of the parts and which a pure intelligence can grasp . . . . It is, therefore, the quest of this especial beauty, the sense of harmony of the cosmos, which makes us choose the facts most fitting to contribute to this har-

mony, just as the artist chooses from among the features of his model those which perfect the picture and give it character and life."[66]

Thus, both for the artist and scientist, it is the search for those constructions of the mind that possess harmony and beauty that defines the central effort, and, indeed, I believe that even in the most mundane activities of life, it is this same motivation that guides the building of our models of reality.

We know little or nothing, however, regarding the processes by which the special functions of the two sides of the brain become integrated into a whole, harmonious, and aesthetic mental construction. There is no homunculus that sits astride the corpus callosum and whose responsibility it is to unify the processing activities of the left and right hemispheres. Nor is it obvious how either side of the brain manages to interpret and incorporate the communications from the other, communications that are transmitted in a different language from its own. How does speech, whose mechanical aspects are so centrally dependent on left-hemispheric processes, come to have its prosody and emotional intonation, which is differentially dependent on the right hemisphere?[58] Or how do we come to understand the metaphorical meaning of language when its phonetic and syntactic decoding depends on the left hemisphere, but when the escape from the literal depends on the right hemisphere?[67]

How does the normal person manage to render drawings with appropriate global form that, at the same time, include well-ordered and appropriately placed details? We are enraptured by the Mona Lisa precisely because the finest detail of a line is so perfectly integrated into the total configuration, because we simultaneously analyze and synthesize its elements, because our intellect and emotions are both aroused in constant reformulations of meaning. In music, there is a great deal of evidence that the right hemisphere is predominant in the representation of chords,[68] intensity, timbre,[69–71] and in the detection of errors in familiar tunes.[72] Yet rhythm is processed predominantly by the left hemisphere,[73] and the left hemisphere is superior in detecting that two unfamiliar tunes differ by a single note.[74] How are the separate contributions of the two hemispheres integrated to yield either an appreciation or production of musical creations?

It seems apparent that the mental constructions that characterize aesthetic experience must require intimate collaboration between the two sides of the brain, and it is not unreasonable to imagine that the artist may be distinguished from ordinary people by a superior capacity for interhemispheric integration. Perhaps those processes essential for artistic creation are more bilaterally represented in the artist so that the two hemispheres have more common ground for intercommunications.

Hemispheric Organization in the Artist

Given the defects in drawings observed in neurological patients following damage to either the left or right hemisphere, it might be expected that similar defects would be observed in talented painters with brain damage. Yet, this is not so. Although Lovis Corinth showed a radical change in style following right-hemispheric damage, in which his art became bolder and more expressive, he still manifested a high level of talent that was not inferior to his premorbid productions. There was no loss of configurational integrity. Similarly, Anton Räderscheidt, following a right-hemispheric stroke, continued to paint with considerable brilliance. At first, the left half of the canvas was ignored, but with time, this left-side neglect disappeared.[75] (See p. 169.)

With a left-hemispheric lesion and aphasia, a major French painter continued to paint with the same style and skill as premorbidly.[76] A Bulgarian artist, who was forced to switch to his left hand due to right hemiplegia following a left hemispheric stroke, regained his artistic skill but developed a completely new style.[77] Premorbidly, his paintings had been narrative in character, but postmorbidly, his paintings showed clearer colors and dream-like images. Winner[78] suggests, on the basis of these two cases, that the left hemisphere is less important in drawing and painting for the artist as compared to the nonartist, yet, by similar reasoning, the cases of Corinth and Räderscheidt suggest that the right hemisphere is less important!

I believe a more reasonable interpretation is that processes that are strongly laterally differentiated in ordinary people are more bilaterally represented in the artist. Over a lifetime of experience, this greater similarity in the two hemispheres of the artist would permit an especially intimate and close interhemispheric communication that would further promote symmetry of organization. The right hemisphere would develop to a high degree the representational strategies specialized to the left hemisphere, and the left hemisphere would develop to a high degree the representational strategies specialized to the right hemisphere. Each side of the brain would develop structures, forms, and methods necessary for artistic creation, and, in the face of unilateral brain damage suffered in adulthood, the intact hemisphere could sustain the artistic abilities inherent to it and that were developed over a lifetime in collaboration with the other hemisphere.

Studies of musicians also suggest that functions important for musical ability are more bilaterally represented than among nonmusicians or less talented musicians. Melody perception is, of course, complex since it involves both imagistic representations of pitches, intensities, and chords, as well as rhythm and tempo. The relative predominance of one or the other hemisphere would, at least in principle, depend on which aspects of melodies are processed and accorded priority. Further, highly familiar melodies can be encoded as a global gestalt, whereas unfamiliar melodies would require more analytic attention to component elements. Indeed, it has already been noted that the right hemisphere is superior for detecting errors in familiar tunes,[72] whereas the left hemisphere is superior in discriminating whether two unfamiliar melodies are identical or differ by a single note.[74] Differences between musicians and nonmusicians in melody perception could, therefore, have little to do with differences in hemispheric organization and could reflect, instead, differences in strategies of processing.

Nonetheless, it is of interest that nonmusicians show a left-ear (right-hemispheric) superiority for discriminating melodies, and that musicians show a right-ear (left-hemispheric) superiority.[79, 80] The authors interpreted the results in terms of strategy differences and argued that musicians listen for separate components of the melody and that nonmusicians respond to overall musical contour. Gordon found that among amateur musicians, better performance was correlated with a left hemispheric superiority, possibly suggesting that an analytic strategy in which separate and time-ordered notes are encoded is a superior method for melody discrimination as compared to a more global approach.[81]

Piano performance is highly dependent on a constant auditory feedback from the notes played and is greatly disrupted if feedback is artifically delayed through earphones placed on the pianist. Conforming with the difference in musicians and nonmusicians in melody perception, Bradshaw et al.[82] found that melody production was more disrupted by delayed auditory feedback played to the left ear (right hemisphere) of nonmusicians and to the right ear (left hemisphere) of musicians.

Possible strategy differences between musicians and nonmusicians for the perception and production of melodies do not, as discussed, necessarily mean that functions are differently lateralized in the two groups, but other investigations strongly suggest that they are. Gordon[68] examined hemispheric differences in chord perception in students in music high schools, members of kibbutz orchestras, music teachers who were taking courses in advanced musical study, conservatory students, and professional musicians who were members of two major Israeli symphony orchestras. The same groups were examined for hemispheric differences in word perception. For high school students, members of kibbutz orchestras, and music teachers, there was a left-ear (right-hemispheric) superiority for chord discrimination and a right-ear (left-hemispheric) superiority for word perception, but for conservatory students and professional musicians, there was no hemispheric asymmetry either for chord perception or for word perception. Gordon also concluded that the lack of hemispheric asymmetry for chord perception in the professional musicians was unlikely to be due to a capacity to verbally label the chords, since performance on this task was extremely poor.

The indication that there was greater left-hemispheric participation in chord perception for the more talented musicians (conservatory students and professional musicians) is particularly interesting in view of another observation that Gordon made. There is a musical illusion in which low notes are typically localized to the left side of space and high notes to the right side of space when the two are played simultaneously, regardless of which side projects which note.[83] Gordon compared music teachers and conservatory students for their ability to localize a high or low chord when the two were played simultaneously, one to each ear. Both groups showed the expected illusory effect, but for high-chord localization, music teachers showed a greater right-ear (left-hemispheric) superiority than conservatory students, and for low-chord localization, conservatory students showed a greater left-ear (right-hemispheric) superiority than music teachers. Thus, music teachers tended to be shifted toward a right-ear localization and conservatory students toward a left-ear localization.

Deutsch and Roll[84] found that for two pure tones, one octave apart and played simultaneously, one to each ear, the ear in which the high tone appeared controlled where subjects localized the single tone that they heard. However, with alternating high-low sequences that were 180° out of phase for the two ears, subjects perceived the alternation as being a low tone to the left ear alternating with a high tone to the right ear. In other words, if the high-tone appeared at the left ear and the low tone at the right ear, the perceived tone was localized to the left ear, but was perceived as the low tone. This suggests that music teachers in Gordon's study[68] were more controlled by the high-tone localization effect than were conservatory students. The illusion that high tones are localized to the right and the additional illusion that sounds are localized to the ear in which the high tone appears was exemplified by music teachers when they were asked to localize the ear in which the high chord appeared and disappeared when they were asked to localize the ear in which the low chord appeared. Possibly, the equality of the two hemispheres in conservatory students for chord discrimination relates to their greater independence from the high-tone localization effect. In any case, it seems unlikely that the differences Gordon found between conservatory students and professional musicians versus other groups of musicians for chord discrimination and localization are attributable to differences in musical training or differences in strategies. Rather, it seems more likely that they reflect differences in inherent hemispheric organization between less and more talented musicians.

Gaede et al.[74] examined four groups of subjects defined by the amount of their musical training (extensive or none) and by musical aptitude (high or low), as assessed from a standardized test, for hemispheric differences on two musical tasks. In the first task, subjects had to decide how many piano notes (1–6) made up a chord, and in the second, they had to decide whether two successively played tunes were identical or differed by a single note. If they differed, subjects had to identify which note differed. Overall, there was a left-ear (right-hemispheric) superiority for the chord test and a right-ear (left-hemispheric) superiority for the tune test. This was unaffected by the amount of musical training but was greatly affected by musical aptitude. For those with low musical aptitude, the hemispheric asymmetries were strong, but for those with high musical aptitude, there was no hemispheric asymmetry for either task, and performance was superior on both tasks for high-aptitude subjects.

In conjunction with Gordon's investigation,[68] that of Gaede et al.[74] strongly suggests that musical talent is associated with greater bilateral representation of musical abilities than is usually found in nonmusicians or in less talented musicians. Gordon[68] notes, however, that the lack of asymmetry in conservatory students and professional musicians for chord discrimination was more due to a bimodal distribution of hemispheric asymmetries in these groups than to a consistent lack of asymmetry in individual members of the groups. He did not, however, compare variances in hemispheric asymmetries between the more and less talented musicians, and this makes it impossible to know whether his interpretation is statistically valid or not. Gaede et al.[74] presented no variance measures for any groups.

Examinations of musicians with unilateral brain lesions indicate that, as among painters, abilities are retained to a much better degree than among ordinary people. Botez and Wertheim[85] described an accordion player with a right-hemispheric lesion who could still recognize pieces, could detect slight errors in music, and could criticize his own performance. He could still sing individual pitches, although he could not combine these into a song, and he had lost his ability to play the accordion. Judd et al. (1980, unpublished work) reported that a musician with right-hemispheric damage retained his ability to discriminate, produce, and compose music. He correctly judged that his postmorbid compositions lacked interest, although they were musically correct, but, in spite of his retained abilities, the right-hemispheric stroke greatly reduced his motivation to compose or to listen to music since it no longer had its former emotional impact. In these two cases, there were evident changes in musical competence, but the residual abilities were far greater than would be expected based on capacities of ordinary people with right-hemispheric damage and studies of hemispheric functions among normal subjects.

Shebalin, the Russian composer, continued to compose and teach music, with little evidence of impairment, after a left-hemispheric stroke had left him severely aphasic.[86] Similarly, an American composer, although somewhat impaired in his ability to read musical notation after a left-hemispheric stroke, continued to compose music of the same quality as premorbidly.[87] In contrast to these cases, Ravel suffered a left-hemispheric stroke in mid-career and lost the ability to compose or play the piano.[76] However, he could still recognize and evaluate music and retained his love for it.

Winner concludes that "right hemisphere damage is far more destructive to a musician than is left hemisphere damage."[78] I am unable to appreciate why this conclusion follows from the evidence available. The patient with right-hemispheric damage described by Judd et al.[87] retained good musical judgements and the ability to compose correctly, even if his compositions were uninspired. His major deficit seems to have been a serious reduction in his interest in music. Although Shebalin seemed to suffer few deficits after his left-hemispheric stroke,[86] Ravel,[76] in spite of retaining his love for music, completely lost his ability to compose or play the piano.

Investigations of ordinary people clearly show that different aspects of music are lateralized to different hemispheres and are selectively affected by unilateral brain damage. There is evidence, also, that nonmusicians tend to process melodies using a global strategy that is more dependent on the right hemisphere than on the left. It seems likely that for the nonmusician or the musically untalented or untrained, the right hemisphere plays a greater role than the left in most aspects of music, but I do not think this conclusion is warranted in the case of talented musicians, and, indeed, it may well be that as talent increases, so too does bilateral representation of musical abilities. Highly talented musicians may and probably do vary among themselves in the extent to which they approach music via left- or right-hemispheric specializations, but hemispheric differences in the perception of tones, intensities, pitches, chords, rhythm, and tempo seem to be considerably less among talented musicians than among others. I suggest that artists, whether musicians or painters, have an unusual degree of bilateral representation of artistic skills, which permits superior interhemispheric integration. Experience in the artistic endeavor further promotes a concordance of hemispheric representations and structures and collaboration between the two hemispheres.

Balance, Aesthetics, and Interhemispheric Integration in Ordinary People

If integration between hemispheric processes underlies aesthetic creation in the artist, it is likely that aesthetic mental constructions in ordinary people depend on similar integrative activities. Each hemisphere becomes selectively activated and aroused when a task is presented that is differentially dependent on its specialized capacities. This has been determined from studies of regional cerebral blood flow[88, 89] and investigations of asymmetric electrocortical activity.[90–94] Such asymmetric activation induces an attentional bias toward the contralateral side of space, so that even if stimuli themselves are symmetric, they are not perceived as such.

Figure 2 shows an example of an item from a face-processing task that selectively activates the right hemisphere. The two chimeric faces are exact

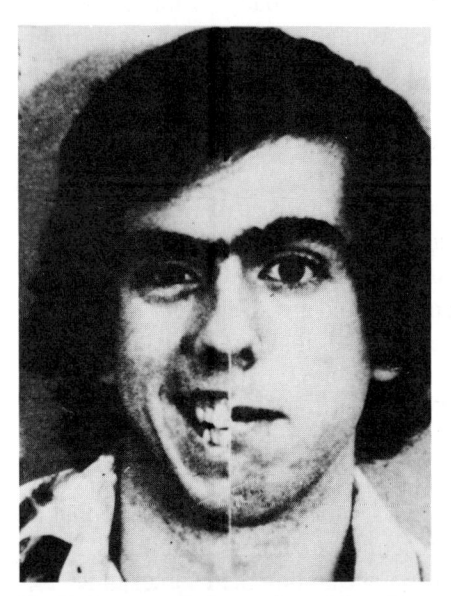

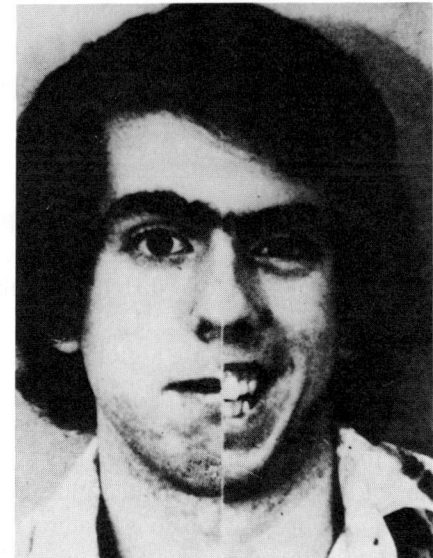

Fig. 2. An example from a free-vision, face-judgement task. The two chimeric faces are exact mirror images of each other, yet the majority of right-handers perceive the chimera with the smile to their left as being happier.

mirror images of each other, yet, for the majority of right-handers, they yield a very different impression of relative happiness. The chimeric face with the smile to the viewer's left is perceived as happier than the mirror-reversed chimera with the smile to the viewer's right. Greater attention is allocated to the left side of space so that the smile to the left has greater saliency than the smile to the right. For left-handers, who are diverse in hemispheric specialization, there is a similar diversity in the perceptual bias.

This same leftward attentional bias occurs when viewing scenes, random shapes, or many other types of nonverbal visual stimuli, and it would be ex-

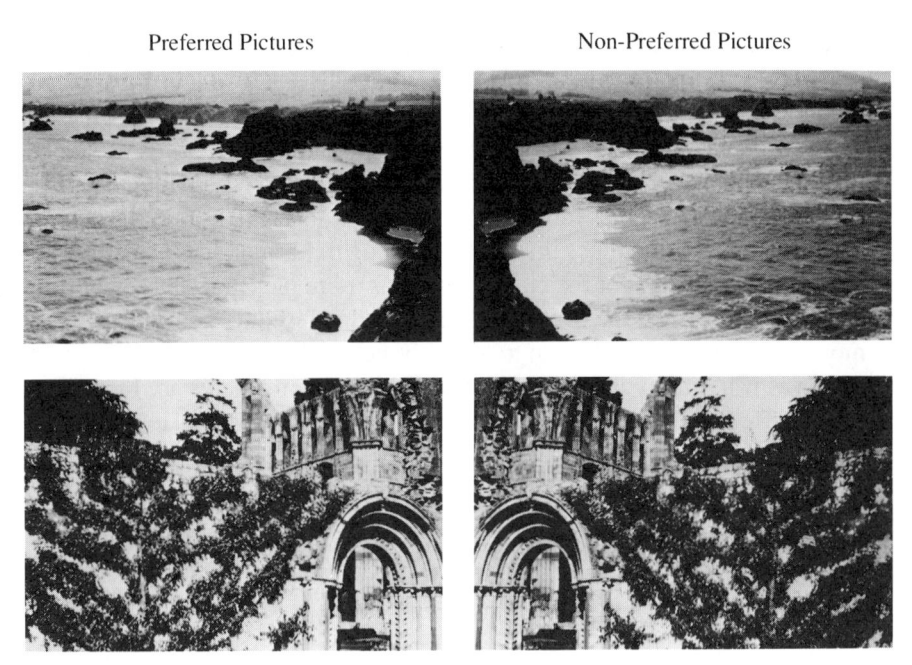

Fig. 3. Examples of pictures in which right-handers prefer the version in which the center of interest is displaced to their right[95]

pected to affect how pictures or their mirror reversals are perceived. To a right-handed viewer, one version of a picture looks quite different from its reversal, and the difference has aesthetic consequences. It might be thought that pictures would be preferred in which the center of interest is displaced to the left, since this would position the focal point in the field of greater attention and would be more available to the visuo-spatial right hemisphere. Perhaps this would be true in a split-brain patient, but it is not in the normal individual.

Right-handers manifest a clear preference for pictures in which the center of interest is displaced to the right (Fig. 3),[95] and this preference increases as a picture becomes more asymmetric. Thus, there is a minor preference for the right-displaced version when the degree of displacement is small and a large preference for the right-displaced version when the degree of displacement is large. When basically symmetric pictures elicit no preference for one version over the over, right-handed judges perceive pictures as having a very small leftward displacement, a judgement induced by their own attentional asymmetry and not by actual asymmetries in the stimuli.

Right-displaced versions of pictures are preferred because these appear to be more balanced. The stimulus asymmetry compensates for the inherent perceptual bias, whereas for left-displaced versions, stimulus and perceptual asymmetries combine to yield a perception in which the picture's content seems to be falling off the left edge. It is unaesthetic because it is unbalanced. But note what this means. Picture perception differentially activates the right hemisphere, resulting in an attentional bias toward the left, yet it is not merely the right hemisphere that determines the aesthetic response. Rather, the brain's own attentional bias forms a framework against which stimulus characteristics are placed, and those that yield a feeling of harmony and balance, because they compensate for the bias, are seen as more pleasing. This can be accomplished only when the center of interest is displaced to the right, where it is more available to the left than to the right hemisphere.

It is as if harmony is achieved when the two hemispheres are brought to the same effective level of interest and engagement. The right hemisphere is aroused by the visuo-spatial nature of the task, and the left hemisphere's interest is enhanced by placement of the center of interest in the contralateral hemispatial field. This is not to suggest that balance is the sole or even the major determinant of picture preference, but it does suggest that when other factors are controlled, it is a highly important factor and one that depends on interhemispheric integration.

Changes in asymmetric hemispheric arousal should, according to the foregoing interpretation, affect the placement of content in pictorial art. Conforming with suggestions in the literature, we obtained evidence from a study of right-handed adults that a dysphoric mood is associated with asymmetrically low right-hemispheric arousal and that an euphoric mood is associated with asymmetrically high right-hemispheric arousal.[96] Wendy Heller, as part of her dissertation research, has examined the placement of affective objects in the art of 48 eight-year-old children who were asked, on one occasion, to "make a happy picture" and on another, to "make a sad picture." If children have the same tendency as adults to integrate intrinsic perceptual biases with stimulus asymmetries, happy affective objects should have a relative displacement to the right (in compensation for a leftward perceptual bias due to asymmetrically high right-hemispheric arousal) compared to sad affective objects (when there would be a rightward perceptual bias due to asymmetrically low right-hemispheric arousal).

Figure 4 shows a typical example of happy and sad pictures for one of the children. For the vast majority of the 48 children, happy affective objects were displaced to the right compared to sad affective objects. The lateral placements of affective objects were correlated between sad and happy pictures, revealing individual differences among children in mean lateral placement, but, regardless of a child's mean placement, sad figures had a relative left displacement and happy figures had a relative right displacement.

Although a number of interpretations are possible for these lateral asym-

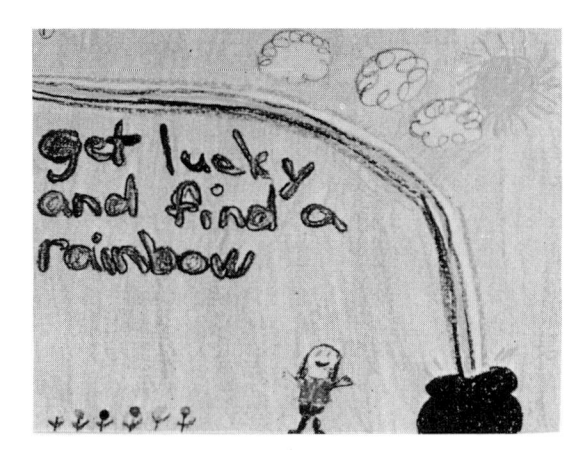

Fig. 4. Happy and sad pictures produced by an eight-year-old child. These exemplify observations that happy affective objects are displaced toward the right compared to sad affective objects for the large majority of children. (Photo: Dr. Wendy Heller)

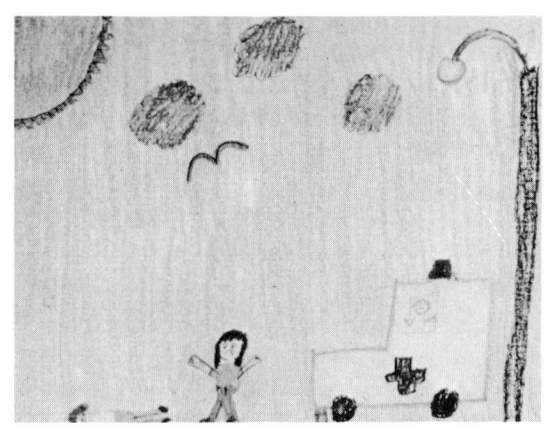

metries in children's art, they are fully consistent with the view that children, like adults, have an aesthetic sense that is determined in part by a balancing between intrinsic perceptual biases and asymmetries of stimuli in the external world, a balancing that implies bihemispheric participation in the experience and production of aesthetic creations.

Conclusion

Research extending over the last quarter century has demonstrated that the two cerebral hemispheres are complementary in their cognitive and emotional functions, and this complementarity means that the rich and unified mental representations of the brain and their emotional implications derive from an inseparable integration of the specialized processes of each side. Even in the most trivial and mundane of perceptual activities, the mind is an active, rule-guided, and motivated builder of models layed out in a four-dimensional, space-time continuum – models with color, configuration, rhythm, tempo, features, form, and all the other mental characteristics that entered the universe with the evolution of brains. The models are not merely useful, they are crucial, since they are the only reality we know, and our survival depends on the extent to which the relations they specify correlate with those in the external world. Neither hemisphere alone can capture the full richness of reality, either as it is experienced, as it is conceived, or as it might be in our imaginative dreams. Each has a remarkable capacity to use its specialized programs for adaptive behavior in most everyday activities, but in the face of challenge, when new insights are demanded, when complexity requires new structurings and new creations, these are built by the whole brain. When they are built well, the effort is rewarded by the experience of the beautiful. Poincaré recognized a profound truth when he said that "the longing for the beautiful leads us to the same choice as the longing for the useful."[66]

References

1. Sperry RW (1974) Lateral specialization in the surgically separated hemispheres. In: Schmitt FO, Worden FG (eds) The neurosciences: Third study program. The MIT Press, Cambridge, Mass.
2. Levy J, Trevarthen C (1977) Perceptual, semantic and phonetic aspects of elementary language processes in split-brain patients. Brain 100: 105–118
3. Levy J, Trevarthen C, Sperry RW (1972) Perception of bilateral chimeric figures following hemispheric deconnection. Brain 95: 61–78
4. Levy J, Trevarthen C (1981) Color-matching, color-naming, and color-memory in split-brain patients. Neuropsychologia 19: 523–541
5. Levy J, Trevarthen C (1976) Metacontrol of hemispheric function in human split-brain patients. J Exp Psychol: Human Perception and Performance 2: 299–312
6. Bogen JE (1969) The other side of the brain. II: An appositional mind. Bull Los Ang Neur Soc 34: 135–162
7. Bradshaw, JL, Nettleton NC (1983) Human cerebral asymmetry. Prentice Hall, Englewood Cliffs, New Jersey
8. Sperry RW, Gazzaniga MS, Bogen JE (1969) Interhemispheric relationships: The neocortical commissures; syndromes of hemisphere disconnection. In: Vinken PT, Bruyn GW (eds) Handbook of clinical neurology, IV. North Holland, Amsterdam
9. Hillyard SA, Gazzaniga MS (1971) Language and the capacity of the right hemisphere. Neuropsychologia 9: 273–280
10. Zaidel E (1977) Unilateral auditory language comprehension on the Token Test following cerebral commiussurotomy and hemispherectomy. Neuropsychologia 15: 1–18
11. Zaidel E (1976) Language, dichotic listening, and the disconnected hemispheres. In: Walter DO, Rogers L, Finzi-Fried JM (eds) Conference on Human Brain Function. Brain Information Service/BRI Publications Office, Los Angeles
12. Zaidel E (1976) Auditory vocabulary of the right hemisphere following brain bisection or hemidecortication. Cortex 12: 191–211

13. Levy J (1983) Language, cognition, and the right hemisphere: A response to Gazzaniza. Am Psychol May: 538–541
14. Atkinson J, Egeth H (1973) Right hemisphere superiority in visual orientation matching. Can J Psychol 27: 152–158
15. Umiltà C, Rizzolatti G, Marzi CA, Zamboni G, Franzini C, Camarda R, Berlucchi G (1974) Hemispheric differences in the discrimination of line orientation. Neuropsychologia 12: 165–174
16. Longden K, Ellis C, Iversen SD (1976) Hemispheric differences in the discrimination of curvature. Neuropsychologia 14: 195–202
17. Nebes RD (1971) Superiority of the minor hemisphere in commissurotomized man for the perception of part-whole relations. Cortex 7: 333–349
18. Hellige JB (1975) Hemispheric processing differences revealed by differential conditioning and reaction time performance. J exp Psychol: General 104: 309–326
19. Nebes RD (1973) Perception of spatial relationships by the right and left hemispheres in commissurotomized man. Neuropsychologia 3: 285–289
20. Kimura D (1969) Spatial localization in left and right visual fields. Can J Psychol 23: 445–458
21. Levy J, Reid M (1976) Variations in writing posture and cerebral organization. Science 194: 337–339
22. Robertshaw S, Sheldon M (1976) Laterality effects in judgement of the identity and position of letters: A signal detection analysis. Q J exp Psychol 28: 115–121
23. Durnford M, Kimura D (1971) Right hemisphere specialization for depth perception reflected in visual field differences. Nature 231: 394–395
24. Franco L, Sperry RW (1977) Hemisphere lateralization for cognitive processing of geometry. Neuropsychologia 15: 107–114
25. Nebes RD (1972) Dominance of the minor hemisphere in commissurotomized man in a test of figural unification. Brain 95: 633–638
26. Haydon SP, Spellacy FJ (1974) Monaural reaction time asymmetries for speech and non-speech sounds. Cortex 9: 288–294
27. Simon JR (1967) Ear preference in a simple reaction-time task. J exp Psychol 75: 49–55
28. Provins KA, Jeeves MA (1975) Hemisphere differences in response to simple auditory stimuli. Neuropsychologia 13: 207–211
29. Anzola GP, Bertoloni G, Buchtel HA, Rizzolatti G (1977) Spatial compatibility and anatomical factors in simple and choice reaction time. Neuropsychologia 15: 295–302
30. Bradshaw JL, Perriment AD (1970) Laterality effects and choice reaction time in a unimanual two-finger task. Percept Psychophys 7: 185–188
31. Jeeves MA, Dixon NF (1970) Hemisphere differences in response rates to visual stimuli. Psych Sci 20: 249–251
32. Belmont I, Handler A (1971) Delayed information processing and judgement of temporal order following cerebral damage. Journal of Nervous and Mental Diseases 152: 353–361
33. Edwards AE, Auger R (1965) The effect of aphasia on the perception of precedence. Proceedings of the 73rd Annual Convention of the American Psychological Association, pp 207–208
34. Lackner JR, Teuber HL (1973) Alterations in auditory fusion thresholds after cerebral injury in man. Neuropsychologia 11: 409–415
35. Swisher L, Hirsh IJ (1972) Brain damage and the ordering of two temporally successive stimuli. Neuropsychologia 10: 137–152

36. Efron R (1963) Effect of handedness on the perception of simultaneity and temporal order. Brain 86: 261–284
37. Mills L, Rollman GG (1980) Hemispheric asymmetry for auditory perception of temporal order. Neuropsychologia 18: 41–47
38. Leek MR, Brandt JF (1983) Lateralization of rapid auditory sequences. Neuropsychologia 21: 67–77
39. Cremonini W, De Renzi E, Faglioni P (1980) Contrasting performance of right- and left-hemisphere patients on short-term and long-term sequential visual memory. Neuropsychologia 18: 1–9
40. Buchtel HA, Rizzolatti G, Anzola GP, Bertoloni G (1978) Right hemispheric superiority in discrimination of brief acoustic duration. Neuropsychologia 16: 643–647
41. Bertoloni G, Anzola GP, Buchtel HA, Rizzolatti G (1978) Hemispheric differences in the discrimination of the velocity and duration of a simple visual stimulus. Neuropsychologia 16: 213–220
42. Patterson K, Bradshaw JL (1975) Differential hemispheric mediation on nonverbal visual stimuli. J exp Psychol: Human Perception and Performance 1: 246–252
43. Umiltà C, Bagnara S, Simion F (1978) Laterality effects for simple and complex geometrical figures and nonsense patterns. Neuropsychologia 16: 43–49
44. McFie J, Zangwill O (1960) Visual constructive disabilities associated with lesions of the right cerebral hemisphere. Brain 83: 243–260
45. Warrington EK, James M, Kinsbourne M (1966) Drawing disability in relation to laterality of lesion. Brain 89: 53–82
46. Buchtel HA, Campari F, De Risio C, Rota R (1978) Hemispheric differences in discriminative reaction time to facial expressions. Italian Journal of Psychology 5: 159–169
47. Campbell R (1978) Asymmetries in interpreting and expressing a posed facial expression. Cortex 14: 327–342
48. Heller W, Levy J (1981) Perception and expression of emotion in right-handers and left-handers. Neuropsychologia 19: 263–272
49. Safer MA (1981) Sex and hemisphere differences in access to codes for processing emotional expressions and faces. J exp Psychol: General 110: 86–100
50. Haggard MP, Parkinson AM (1971) Stimulus and task factors in the perceptual lateralization of speech signals. Quart J exp Psychol 23: 168–177
51. Ley RG, Bryden MP (1982) A dissociation of right and left hemispheric effects for recognizing emotional tone and verbal content. Brain and Cognition 1: 3–9
52. Safer MA, Leventhal H (1977) Ear differences in evaluating emotional tones of voice and verbal content. J exp Psychol: Human Perception and Performance 3: 75–82
53. Carmon A, Nachshon I (1973) Ear asymmetry in perception of emotional nonverbal stimuli. Acta psychol 37: 351–357
54. Bryden MP, Ley RG, Sugarman JH (1982) A left-ear advantage for identifying the emotional quality of tonal sequences. Neuropsychologia 20: 83–87
55. Borod JC, Caron HS (1980) Facedness and emotion related to lateral dominance, sex and expression type. Neuropsychologia 18: 237–241
56. Chaurasia BD, Goswami HK (1975) Functional asymmetry in the face. Acta ant 91: 154–160
57. Sackeim HA, Gur RC (1978) Lateral asymmetry in the intensity of emotional expression. Neuropsychologia 16: 473–481
58. Ross E, Mesulam MN (1979) Dominant language functions of the right hemisphere? Prosody and emotional gesturing. Arch Neur 36: 144–148

59. Cicone M, Wapner W, Gardner H (1980) Sensitivity to emotional expressions and situations in organic patients. Cortex 16: 145–158
60. Gardner H, Ling PK, Flamm L, Silverman J (1975) Comprehension and appreciation of humorous material following brain damage. Brain 98: 399–412
61. Heilman KM, Scholes R, Watson RT (1975) Auditory affective agnosia: Disturbed comprehension of affective speech. J Neurol Neuros Psychiat 38: 69–72
62. Heilman KM, Schwartz HD, Watson RT (1978) Hypoarousal in patients with the neglect syndrome and emotional indifference. Neurology 28: 229–232
63. Heilman KM, Van Den Abell T (1979) Right hemispheric dominance for mediating cerebral activation. Neuropsychologia 17: 315–321
64. Tucker DM (1981) Lateral brain function, emotion, and conceptualization. Psych Bull 89: 19–46
65. Yerkes RM, Dodson JD (1908) The relation of strength of stimulus to rapidity of habit formation. Journal of Comparative and Neurological Psychology 18: 459–482
66. Poincaré H (1913) The foundations of science. The Science Press, New York, pp 366–367
67. Winner E, Gardner H (1977) The comprehension of metaphor in brain-damaged patients. Brain 100: 719–727
68. Gordon HW (1980) Degree of ear asymmetries for perception of dichotic chords and for illusory chord localization in musicians of different levels of competence. J exp Psychol: Human Perception and Performance 6: 516–527
69. Best C, Hoffman H, Glanville BB (1982) Development of infant ear asymmetries for speech and music. Percept Psychophys 31: 75–85
70. Entus AK (1975/1977) Hemispheric asymmetries in processing of dichotically presented speech and non-speech sounds by infants. Society for Research in Child Development, Denver, Colorado, April, 1975. In: Segalowitz SJ, Gruber FA (eds) Language Development and Neurological Theory. Academic, New York
71. Milner B (1962) Laterality effects in audition. In: Mountcastle VB (ed) Interhemispheric relations and cerebral dominance. Johns Hopkins University Press, Baltimore
72. Shapiro B, Grossman M, Gardner H (1981) Selective musical processing deficits in brain-damaged patients. Neuropsychologia 19: 161–170
73. Gordon HW (1978) Left hemisphere dominance for rhythmic elements in dichotically presented melodies. Cortex 14: 58–70
74. Gaede SE, Parsons OA, Bertera JH (1978) Hemispheric differences in music perception: Aptitude vs experience. Neuropsychologia 16: 369–373
75. Jung R (1974) Neuropsychologie und Neurophysiologie des Kontur und Formsehens in Zeichnung und Malerei. In: Wieck HH (ed) Psychopathologie musischer Gestaltungen. Schattauer, Stuttgart, pp 30–88
76. Alajouanine T (1948) Aphasia and artistic realization. Brain 71: 229–241
77. Zaimov K, Kitov D, Kolev N (1969) Aphasie chez un peintre. Encephale 68: 377–417
78. Winner E (1982) Invented worlds, the psychology of the arts. Harvard University Press, Cambridge, Mass.
79. Bever, Chiarello R (1974) Cerebral dominance in musicians and nonmusicians. Science 185: 137–139
80. Kellar L, Bever T (1980) Hemispheric asymmetries in the perception of musical intervals as a function of musical experience and family handedness background. Brain and Language 10: 24–38
81. Gordon HW (1975) Hemispheric asymmetries and musical performance. Science 189: 68–69

82. Bradshaw JL, Nettleton NC, Geffen G (1971) Ear differences and delayed auditory feedback: Effects on a speech and music task. J exp Psychol 91: 85–92
83. Deutsch D (1974) An auditory illusion. Nature 251: 307–309
84. Deutsch D, Roll PL (1976) Separate "what" and "where" decision mechanisms in processing a dichotic tonal sequence. J exp Psychol: Human Perception and Performance 2: 23–29
85. Botez M, Wertheim N (1959) Expressive aphasia and amusia following right frontal lesion in a right-handed man. Brain 82: 186–201
86. Luria A, Tsvetkova L, Futer D (1965) Aphasia in a composer. Journal of Neurological Science 2: 288–292
87. Judd T, Gardner H, Geschwind N (1980) Alexia without agraphia in a composer. Project Zero Technical Report No. 15, Harvard Graduate School of Education, Cambridge
88. Gur RC, Reivich M (1980) Cognitive task effects on hemispheric blood flow in humans: Evidence for individual differences in hemispheric activation. Brain and Language 9: 78–92
89. Risberg J, Halsey JH, Blavenstein VW, Wilson EM, Wills EL (1975) Bilateral measurements of the rCBF during mental activation in normals and in dysphasic patients. In: Harper AM, Jennett WB, Miller JG, Brown JO (eds) Blood flow and metabolism in the brain. Churchill Livingstone, London
90. Amochaev A, Salamy A (1979) Stability of EEG laterality effects. Psychophysiology 16: 242–246
91. Ehrlichman H, Wiener MS (1979) Consistency of task-related EEG asymmetries. Psychophysiology 16: 247–252
92. Ehrlichman H, Wiener MS (1980) EEG asymmetry during covert mental activity. Psychophysiology 17: 228–235
93. Galin D, Ellis RR (1975) Asymmetry in evoked potentials as an index of lateralized cognitive processes: Relation to EEG alpha asymmetry. Neuropsychologia 13: 45–50
94. Morgan AH, McDonald PJ, MacDonald H (1971) Differences in bilateral alpha activity as a function of experimental task with a note on lateral eye movements and hypnotizability. Neuropsychologia 9: 459–469
95. Levy J (1976) Lateral dominance and aesthetic preference. Neuropsychologia 14: 431–445
96. Levy J, Heller W, Banich M, Burton L (1983) Are variations among right-handed individuals in perceptual asymmetries caused by characteristic arousal differences between hemispheres? J exp Psychol: Human Perception and Performance 9: 329–359

Beauty May Differ in Each Half of the Eye of the Beholder

Marianne Regard and Theodor Landis
Neurology Department, University Hospital, 8091 Zürich, Switzerland

The perception of what we regard or ought to regard as aesthetic depends on the zeitgeist. Aesthetics was, thus, not an issue in neuropsychology until cognitive psychology revived, leading to a more dynamic conception of brain function. Moreover, interpretations of the aesthetic experience depend on the philosophical viewpoint towards mind and body, i.e., on whether one defends a holistic concept or considers physical and mental processes to be separate entities. Despite changing views on beauty, we believe that rules regarding aesthetic perception in relation to hemispheric processing can be investigated. A purely hierarchical view of mental processes from sensation to perception to cognition does not provide a suitable framework for investigating the underlying hemispheric mechanisms of aesthetic preference. Less hierarchical views permit the reintroduction of two classical, seemingly contradictory approaches to the judgement of beauty: the objective approach, i.e., the notion that beauty is inherent to the object or the subjective approach, which claims that beauty lies in the eye of the beholder.

David Hume believed that logic underlies the judgement of art. This could be true for any visual stimulus. Numerous studies with the tachistoscope (an apparatus for fast picture projections, in which information can be presented to the right or left cerebral hemisphere only) have produced results demonstrating that the type of visual information presented and the hemisphere stimulated influence the quality of perception.

From these so-called visual half-field studies with the tachistoscope, we learned that the two hemispheres treat visual information differently – as if we had two separate cognitive beings in our mind. We also learned that there is an objective factor to perception, since the visual field advantage, i.e. the hemispheric advantage, varies with different types of stimuli. Some years ago, results were reported demonstrating that hemispheric processing also varies with the emotional quality of the information presented.[1,2] The interaction of

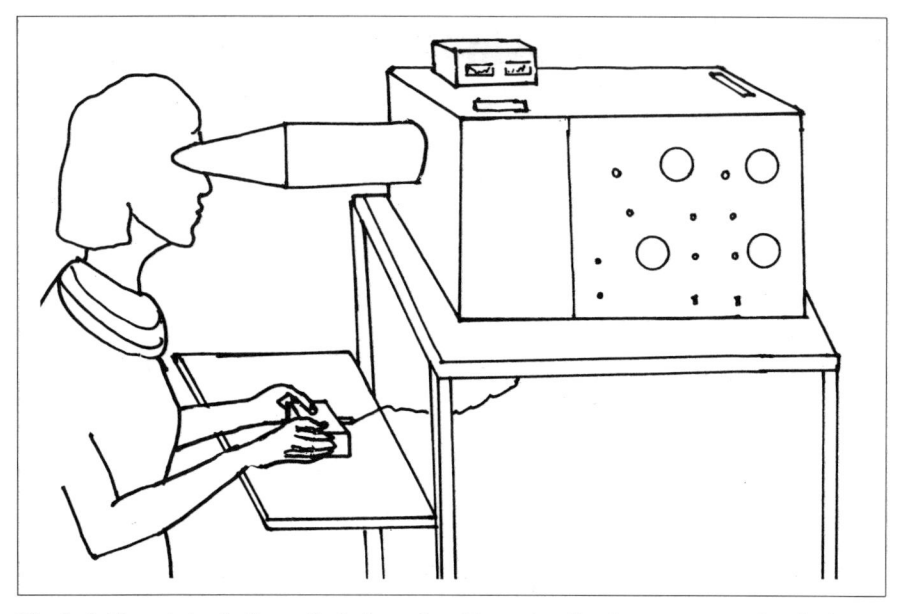

Fig. 1. Subject sitting in front of a 2-channel tachistoscope fixating on a center dot. An image is then flashed to the right or to the left of the fixation point for a very short time. The subject is asked to press the response buttons according to a given instruction.

stimulus qualities, such as form, content, and emotional appeal, to the perceiving subject was one of the basic concepts of the Gestalt school of psychology. Visual perception has been regarded as a complex process of subject/object interaction, resulting in simplification and reduction of the visual stimuli perceived.[3] For some of the laws of perception postulated by the "gestaltists," electro- or neurophysiological correlates have been found. Landis et al.[4] found specific changes in the electrical response of the brain to a picture seen as a man or the same picture seen as a meaningless composite, and von der Heydt et al.[5] monitored single cells in the visual cortex of the monkey that responded to illusory contours (see chapter 7).

Despite only minor anatomical differences between the two visual cortices of the human brain[6], consistent differences in perceiving and processing visual information became evident in studies of patients with brain lesions limited to one hemisphere or of patients after surgical separation of the two hemispheres (see chapter 9). Comparable results come from tachistoscopic studies with healthy subjects.[1] Moreover, the two hemispheres seem to differ in their evaluation of the emotional content of visually presented stimuli.[2]

There exists an inherent difficulty in the study of aesthetic preference in relation to hemispheric laterality because we are often not aware of an aesthetic sensation, and, if we are, we are not necessarily able to report on it. Thus, the "unconscious," a concept basic to most psychological and neuropsychological theories, needs to be externalized experimentally. Verbal awareness, the ability to report on one's actions verbally, may only be one kind of process in decision making.[7,8] Landis et al.[9] were able to show that the verbal awareness of the correctness of motor responses was high when stimuli reached the speech-dominant, left hemisphere and that verbal awareness was low, despite correct motor reactions, when stimuli reached the non-speech-dominant, right hemisphere.

Another approach to the investigation of aesthetic preference is documented in numerous studies concerning unconscious perception. The so-called subliminal exposure of stimuli, i.e., extremely short exposure times allowing no verbally conscious perception, remains controversial. The controversy whether such short exposures are subconscious at all and in what way they influence conscious perception has recently been discussed at length.[10,11] Kunst-Wilson and Zajonc[12] reported a study in which they subliminally presented geometric figures. Under these conditions, subjects were only able to report flashes. Subsequently, subjects were shown pairs of geometric figures, one of which had been previously presented subliminally, and they had to indicate which of the two figures they preferred. The result of the study was that the previously presented but not consciously seen figure was significantly more often preferred than the new figure. The same subjects were also asked which of the two figures they thought they had previously seen. This condition showed no significant effects of subliminal perception. Zajonc[10] concluded that feeling precedes cognition, a challenging hypothesis.

For a long time, the study of aesthetics was identical to the study of sensory experience. Aesthetics then became a synonym for beauty when the two approaches – the subjective and the objective approach – evolved. In our attempt to investigate hemispheric differences in aesthetic preference, we conducted studies involving both approaches. On the one hand, we were interested in the stimulus, i.e., what are the criteria of a visual stimulus that influence our "conscious" (supraliminal) and "unconscious" (subliminal) preferences. On the other hand, our experiments were set up to elucidate the ways in which the left and the right cerebral hemisphere of an observer differ in the aesthetic judgement of visual stimuli. We discuss three experiments, which we conducted with healthy subjects. All three are lateralized tachistoscopic experiments, allowing the visual stimulation to reach each hemisphere separately. As Fig. 2 illustrates, subjects had to fixate a point in the center of the display. Due to the crossing of the optic nerve, a stimulus presented to the left of fixation first reaches the visual cortex of the right hemisphere, where

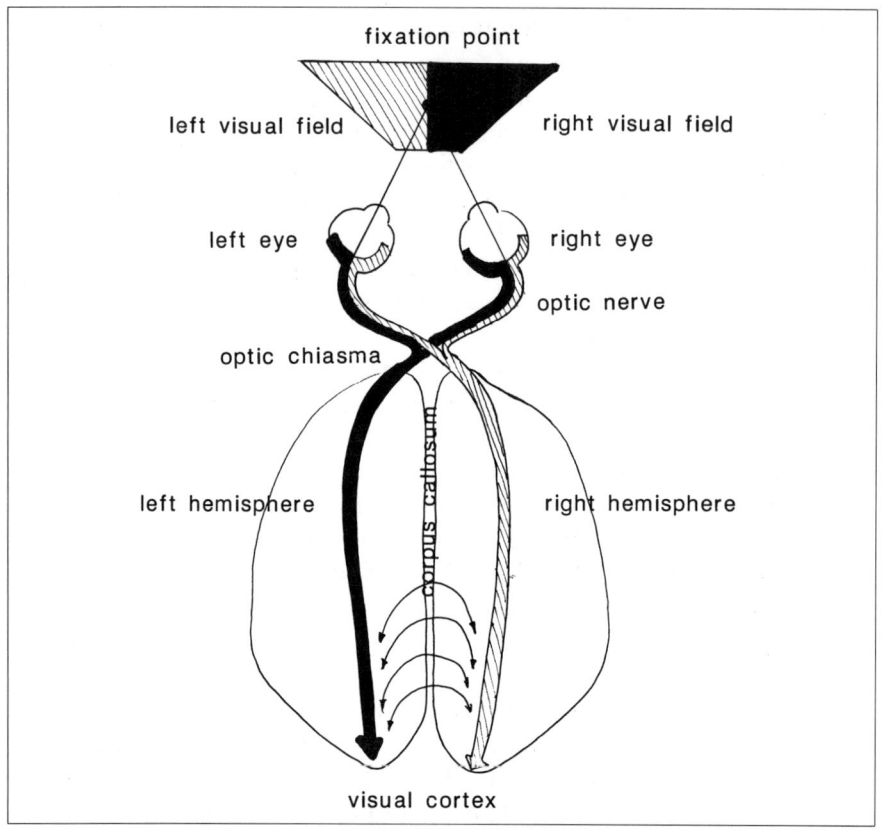

Fig. 2. The visual stimulus is transferred from the left visual field to the right visual cortex via the chiasma opticum along the visual pathway, and a stimulus in the right visual field is transferred to the left visual cortex. Severing the corpus callosum, as in split-brain patients, prevents information from passing from one cerebral hemisphere to the other.

primary perceptual processing takes place. A stimulus presented to the right of the fixation point first reaches the left hemisphere.

Affective Choices of Geometric Figures

Twenty male and 20 female, right-handed subjects were shown pairs of the Breskin figure test[13] and were required to indicate the figure of a pair they liked better by pressing a response button. The pairs (Fig. 3) were arranged vertically and presented either to the left or the right side of the fixation point in the tachistoscope with an exposure time of 150 ms. Thus, the figure pairs were projected either to the left visual field (projecting to the right hemisphere) or

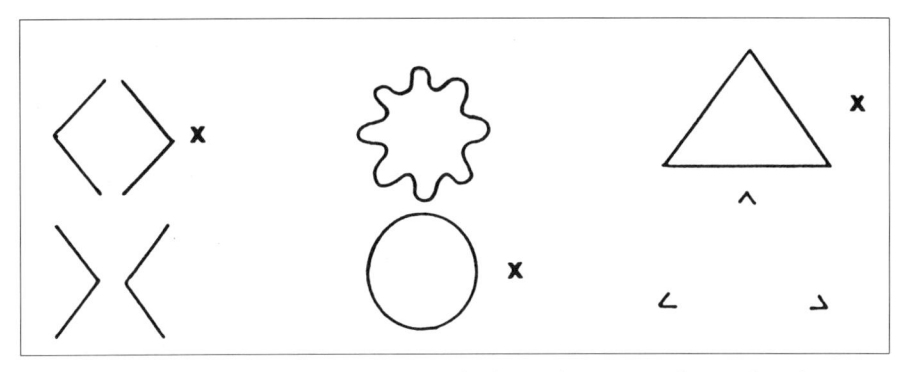

Fig. 3. Examples of the Breskin figure pairs. X indicates the *prägnant* figure of a pair.

to the right visual field (projecting to the left hemisphere). According to Breskin, one figure of each pair obeyed the gestalt law of *Prägnanz* (the tendency toward meaning, simplicity, and completeness). We measured the number of *prägnant* figures chosen (PP = *Prägnanz* preference) as well as the response latencies to stimulations of the right and the left visual fields.

We found that the *prägnant* figure was significantly preferred when presented to the right visual field (the left cerebral hemisphere) ($P = 0.004$). We also found a significant association between the judgements according to the visual field stimulated and the sex of the perceiver ($P = 0.001$). Men preferred the non-*prägnant* figure of a pair more often when presented to the right hemisphere, whereas women showed a nonsignificant trend in the opposite direction (Fig. 4).

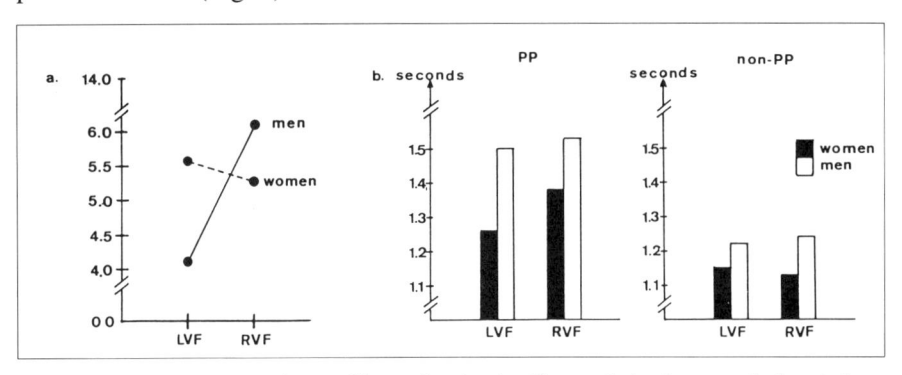

Fig. 4.a) Mean *Prägnanz* preference illustrating the significant relation between the hemisphere stimulated and the sex of the perceiver in making an affective choice. Men preferred the non-*prägnant* figure of the pair more often when it was presented to the right hemisphere (left visual field). Women showed a nonsignificant trend in the opposite direction. Fig. 4.b) Mean response latencies illustrating the significantly slower decisions when chosing a *prägnant* over a non-*prägnant* figure

This result may indicate not only that each half of our brain has different preferences, even on the level of a simple gestalt figure, but also that men and women perceive things differently. Numerous tachistoscopic recognition experiments showed that men react as a group homogeneously, whereas the results from women are often quite heterogeneous. The connection between hormones and hemispheric function may be responsible for these kinds of sex differences[6]. Hampson and Kimura[14] demonstrated that hemispheric processing in women fluctuates during the menstrual cycle. Furthermore, we found that response latencies, irrespective of the visual field of presentation, were significantly longer when subjects chose the *prägnant* figure than when they chose the non-*prägnant* figure ($P < 0.001$). This result suggests a general effect of gestalt criteria upon affective processing (Fig. 4).

The conclusions derived from this experiment are threefold:

1. Affective (aesthetic) and not only cognitive selections, as usually reported in the literature, are performed differently by the two cerebral hemispheres, implying two different systems dealing with aesthetic judgements.
2. Stimulation of the right or left hemisphere resulted in different aesthetic judgements in men than in women.
3. The stimulus quality (i.e., the "figural goodness," such as completeness, simplicity, and meaningfulness according to gestalt laws) influences not only perception but also aesthetic preference.

Affective Choices after Subconscious Perception of Faces

Since the right hemisphere is believed to process visual information faster and more globally than the left hemisphere[15] and often without verbal awareness[9], this hemisphere may also be superior in processing stimuli presented very briefly. We, therefore, designed a series of experiments applying Kunst-Wilson and Zajonc's paradigm[12], presenting a separate stimulus to each hemisphere to investigate whether a right-hemispheric "dominance" for subliminal perception really exists. Twenty subjects were initially presented a photographed face stripped of its attributes (hair and ears), a stimulus predominately processed by the right hemisphere, simultaneously with a photograph of the surface of a potato for 1 ms, an exposure duration too brief to identify the stimulus or even the side of presentation (Fig 5a). The face randomly appeared in the left or in the right visual field (projecting to the right or left hemisphere, respectively), with the potato on the opposite side. Subsequently, subjects were presented with two faces, one of which had been pre-

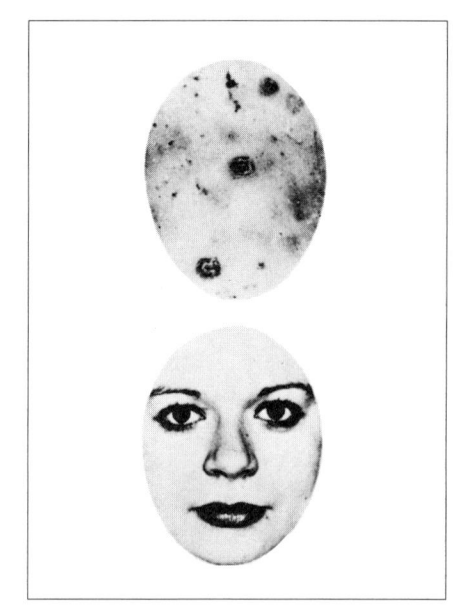

Fig. 5.a) Example of a stimulus pair with the face in the right visual field (projecting to the left cerebral hemisphere) and the distractor (potato) in the left visual field (projecting to the right cerebral hemisphere)

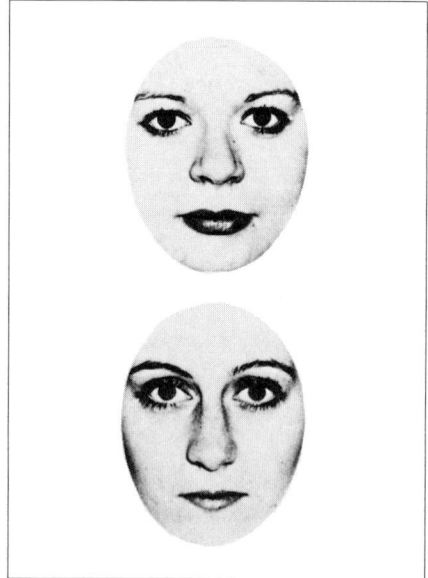

Fig. 5.b) Example of two faces presented in midline position. The *upper face* was previously presented to the left hemisphere; the *lower face* is new. There were two tasks, one a recognition task and the other, an affective judgement task.

viously presented and the other hitherto unknown (Fig. 5b) in the midline position for 1 s. Two tasks were given – one a recognition task ("Which face have you seen before?") and the other, an affective judgement ("Which face do you like better?").

In accordance with the results reported by Kunst-Wilson and Zajonc[12], we found that only the affective judgement and not recognition was influenced by subliminal face presentation. Affective judgements significantly differed with presentations to each visual field ($P = 0.015$). Faces subliminally presented to the right visual field (processed primarily in the left hemisphere) were preferred, and faces presented to the left visual field (right hemisphere) were disliked, i.e., the new face of a pair was preferred. To control the effect, two identical experiments with different subjects were conducted, one at an exposure time of 3 – 5 ms (liminal), a duration permitting the discrimination between face and potato but not an identification of the individual face, and one at the exposure time of 20 ms, allowing clear recognition of the stimulus face. When presented at threshold exposure (liminal), neither subsequent preference nor recognition was significantly influenced. When the faces were presented at recognition level (supraliminal), we found the well-known right-hemispheric superiority in face recognition ($P = 0.02$) with no discernable influence on preference (Fig. 6).

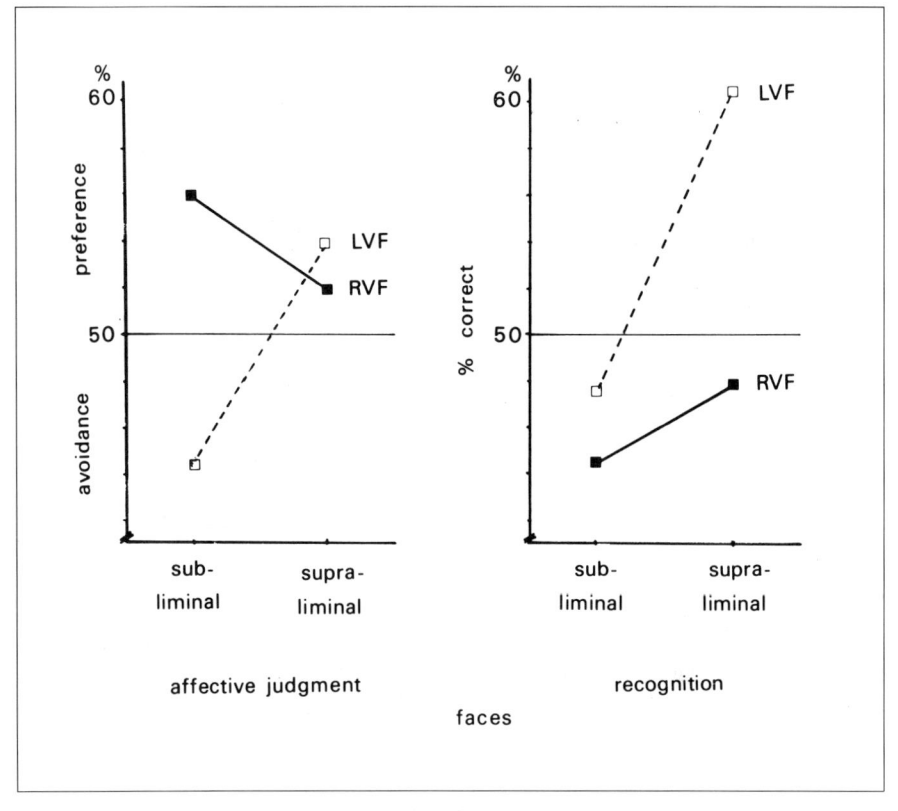

Fig. 6. Results of subliminal and supraliminal face presentations on affective judgement and recognition. *Left side*: only when faces were presented subliminally did they yield hemispheric differences in the affective judgement. The inverse result is demonstrated on the *right side*, showing that supraliminal presentation resulted in hemispheric differences in the recognition task only.

In summary, subconscious perception of faces (subliminal presentation) influenced subsequent affective choices, while recognition was not influenced. Conscious perception (supraliminal presentation), however, influenced recognition, while affective choices were unaffected. These results suggest that affective judgements and recognition may be competing processes, since only one or the other but never both together differed significantly.

Whereas a face is better recognized by the right hemisphere when consciously seen, affective judgements seem to involve both hemispheres, at least when subjects are uncertain, as in the subliminal condition. The left hemisphere prefers the known; the right hemisphere prefers the novel and unusual, a behavior also labelled avoidance. These hemispheric differences in aesthetic preference may reflect such personality traits as "curiosity" or "conservatism," traits that may conflict in a person and may be altered by mere exposure – a phenomenon sometimes known as "fashion" or "familiarity."

Hemispheric Differences in the Interpretation of Ambiguous Stimuli

Stimuli without a clear structure may permit different interpretations, a fact already discussed by Leonardo da Vinci in his *Trattato della Pittura*. In order to assess hemispheric differences in the perceptual structuring of ambiguous stimuli, we used the Rorschach inkblot plates[16] (Fig. 7). The Rorschach plates are commonly used as a projective personality test. It is assumed that subjects'

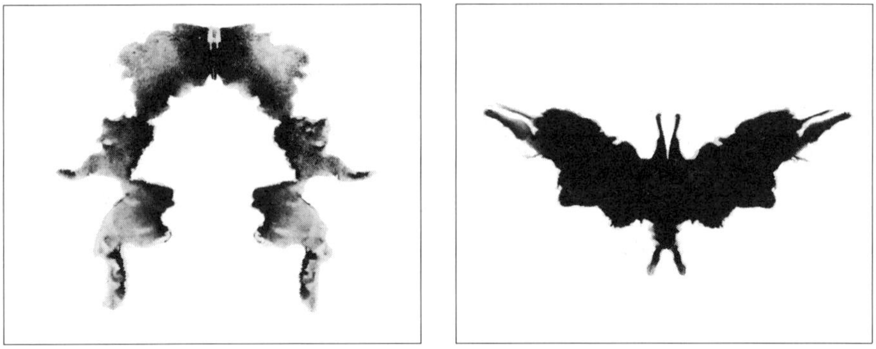

Fig. 7. Two achromatic examples of the Rorschach inkblot plates (reprinted by permission of H. Huber Verlag, Bern)

interpretations of the inkblots are influenced by their unique previous experiences. We randomly presented the ten inkblot plates to each hemisphere of 24 subjects for 150 ms.

After each stimulation, the interpretation was protocoled. As in the non-tachistoscopic Rorschach test, each response was then coded with respect to quality and kind of form, color, shading, content, and presentation of response. These quantified responses were then interpreted and conclusions drawn about a person's perceptual skills, affect management, social behavior, etc. To describe the behavior of each hemisphere separately, the protocols were first labelled with a code by a Rorschach specialist without knowledge of the hemisphere stimulated. Then the mean of all variables per visual field was computed, which enabled us to produce "psychograms," one for each visual field, as if each were a separate person.

We found that 57% of the interpretations differed when the same inkblot was presented to the left visual field or the right visual field, e.g., "dark evil man with big feet" or "frog." Twenty-seven percent of the responses were similar but differently verbalized, e.g., "dark evil man with big feet" or "black giant." Only 16% of the responses were completely identical in both visual fields. The coded responses were grouped, according to the conventional Rorschach interpretations, in a so-called mode of approach, i.e.: responses referring to the whole plates or a detail in the so-called determinants; responses determined predominately by form, color, movement, or their combinations; and miscellaneous variables, such as the content of a response (human, object, animal, etc.); and response delay. A trend analysis revealed that most subjects differed significantly in their responses determined by form, color, or movement determinants to right or left visual field stimulation.

The mode of approach differed little – that is, most answers referred to the whole plate, a result expected with fast tachistoscopic presentation. Despite the many common factors, the two psychograms resulted in unique "personality" profiles for the two hemispheres. The right cerebral hemisphere (left visual field) appears better able to combine and synthesize, although sometimes at the price of missing a comprehensive view of the whole. It grasps better what is near and immediately given, even when the "given" is not the whole. It evaluates the shapes somewhat more precisely. The percepts are more original in spite of less form: one may infer more intuitive than purely intellectual capabilities. The right hemisphere also has more fantasy. Despite the relatively good affective adjustment, this hemisphere is sometimes at risk due to its emotional responsiveness, which may lead to creativity, but also makes it more suggestible. The left cerebral hemisphere (right visual field) grasps the essential of a situation but possesses little combinatory ability. This "subject" was found to be more controlled, to censure affective impulses, and to have little emotional responsiveness. It appears somewhat dry and unstimulating, although fairly well adjusted.[17]

These findings coincide strikingly with affective peculiarities described in patients whose hemispheres have been separated, i.e., the notion of two personalities in split-brain patients.[7] As Galin[18] suspected, the healthy right hemisphere may possess a more spontaneous, unreflective reactive system, whereas the left hemisphere attempts to organize input and output to gain emotional control. The visual field differences found in our experiment contained more variables related to emotional management and fewer in the perceptual mode.

This leads us to conclude that what we see and what we like depends partly on which cerebral hemisphere is stimulated. Coinciding with previous studies reported, each hemisphere reacts affectively differently to the visual environment, indicating that each has a different aesthetic experience. However, since our two hemispheres are connected, our preferences and avoidances are probably either dominated by a more abstract, intellectual approach or by a more emotional approach.

Discussion

Aesthetics has been studied with respect to cerebral laterality only recently. Howard Gardner[19] and Jerry Levy[20] (chapter 9) were the first to investigate visual aesthetic preference and functional brain laterality. Whether one studies judgements of art (Gardner), landscapes (Levy), or other visual material, the evidence gathered suggests an interdependence between affective and perceptual mechanisms and the two hemispheres.

Our own studies show that the aesthetic choice between a stimulus which obeys the laws of gestalt and one which does not depends upon which cerebral hemisphere is stimulated and upon the sex of the perceiver. In the first study, men preferred the stimulus which did not obey gestalt laws when presented to the right hemisphere; women apparently do not differentiate. Both men and women make a quicker preference selection when the figure does not correspond to the law of *Prägnanz*. These results lead us to conclude that men are more strongly lateralized than women – for aesthetic judgements as well as for cognitive decisions. The results also indicate that there is no cerebral "dominance" in making aesthetic judgements. Moreover, the two hemispheres may differ in their preference. The results of our second experiment support this idea by the finding of a visual field difference in the affective judgement of subliminally presented faces. The very brief presentations had no influence on subsequent recognition. The inverse result was found with supraliminal presentation. Under this condition, a right-hemispheric advantage was found for the recognition of the faces. No effect on affective judgements could be observed. These results not only suggest that aesthetic and cognitive selections may be competing processes; they also suggest, as Zajonc[10] postulated, that emotional judgements may, indeed, precede recognition, i.e., cognitive processes. Preferences may be based on unconscious perceptions that involve both hemispheres, albeit differently. The left hemisphere apparently depends more on familiarity with the stimulus and the right hemisphere, more on stimulus novelty. After a face has been consciously perceived, however, aesthetic preference becomes random, and cognitive selection reveals a predominance of the right cerebral hemisphere. A biological explanation for these results is not available, although one could speculate that the arousal system in the brain stem first activates the limbic system, which is known to be of core importance in processing emotions, and only later reaches the two hemispheres, which are responsible for higher cognitive processing.[21]

In the third study, in which the Rorschach plates were briefly presented, we used an approach different from that of the other two studies on hemisphere-dependent, aesthetic preferences. Instead of a forced-choice selection, an active perceptual process was required to organize the ambiguous inkblots into a gestalt. We found that the interpretations of the inkblots differed according to the hemisphere stimulated and assume that they reflect hemispheric differences in affective-visual processing. Since the differences were mainly in the manner in which the two hemispheres dealt with the emotional trigger in the inkblots, shape recognition differed little. Some patients whose corpus callosum (which connects the two hemispheres) had been severed have been described as if they had two personalities. Our results suggest that in healthy people, also, each hemisphere has a different "personality." Since the two hemispheres are connected, conflicts can only be avoided if one postulates a functional hemispheric mechanism allowing one hemisphere to gain control over the other. This idea was put forward more than a century ago by A.L. Wigan.[22] Our study, therefore, supports the notion that aesthetic perception may be in the eye of the beholder; however, the "subject" in question is not just a single entity but a composition of a left and a right cerebral hemisphere. Aesthetic perception, therefore, differs between the two halves of the eye of the beholder.

Nevertheless, prerated stimulus qualities are important. For example, in our study with the Breskin figures, the figure which obeyed the gestalt law of *Prägnanz* and the non-*prägnant* figure yielded different preferences. Another factor that influences our aesthetic perceptions is the presence or absence of verbal awareness of the stimulus.

Functional brain laterality and its effect on aesthetic judgements is one possible way to gain insight into the complex relationships of affective processes and the human brain. We may eventually conclude that an aesthetic judgement is nothing but the affective labelling of events in the environment. This would be comparable to verbal labelling, i.e., words we have available for things we see – a library believed to be located in our left hemisphere. Words, however, are often not precise enough to reflect an aesthetic experience and, moreover, may sometimes even provide misinformation about a perceived event.[8,9] The present results suggest that "emotional knowledge" may constitute a world of experience as complex as that of verbal knowledge.[23] We certainly have to learn much more about the "grammar" of emotional communication to better understand aesthetic experience.

Acknowledgements

This paper was prepared with the help of the Swiss National Science Foundation, Grant No. 3.884.0.83.

We thank J. Casey, L. Christen, R. Graves, E. Häsler, and A. Müller for their help.

References

1. Beaumont JG (ed) (1982) Divided visual-field studies of cerebral organization. Academic, London
2. Heilman KM, Satz P (eds) (1983) Neuropsychology of human emotion. Guilford, New York
3. Kanizsa G (1979) Organization in vision. Essays on Gestalt perception. Praeger, New York
4. Landis T, Lehmann D, Mita T, Skrandies W (1984) Evoked potential correlates of figure and ground. Int J Psychophysiol 1:345–348
5. von der Heydt R, Peterhans E, Baumgartner G (1984) Illusory contours and neuron responses. Science 224: 1260–1261
6. Geschwind N, Galaburda AM (1985) Cerebral lateralization. Biological mechanisms, associations, and pathology: I. A hypothesis and a program for research. Arch Neurol 42:428–459
7. Bogen J (1973) The other side of the brain: An appositional mind. In: Ornstein RE (ed) The nature of human consciousness. Freeman, San Francisco, pp 101–125
8. Nisbett RE, Wilson TD (1977) Telling more than we can know: Verbal reports on mental processes. Psychol Rev 84:231–259
9. Landis T, Graves R, Goodglass H (1981) Dissociated verbal awareness of manual performance in two visual associative tasks: "Spit–brain" phenomenon in normal subjects? Cortex 17:435–440
10. Zajonc RB (1980) Feeling and thinking: Preferences need no inferences. Amer Psychol 35:151–175
11. Dixon N (1981) Preconscious processing. J Wiley, New York
12. Kunst-Wilson WR, Zajonc RB (1980) Affective discrimination of stimuli that can not be recognized. Science 207:557–558
13. Breskin S (1968) Measurement of rigidity, a non-verbal test. Perc and Mot Skills 27:1203–1206
14. Hampson E, Kimura P (1987) Variations in cognitive and motor skills across the menstrual cycle. J Clin Exp Neuropsychol 9:274
15. Sergent J (1982) Theoretical and methodological consequences of variations in exposure duration in visual laterality studies. Perception and Psychophysics 31:451–461
16. Rorschach H (1975) Psychodiagnostics. Huber, Bern
17. Regard M, Landis T (1988) Persönlichkeit und Lateralität. In: Oepen G (ed) Neuropsychologie in der Psychiatrie. Lateralität und Psychopathologie. Dtsch Aerzteverband, Köln
18. Galin D (1974) Implications for psychiatry of left and right cerebral specialization. Arch Gen Psychiat 31:572–583

19. Gardner H (1982) Artistry following damage to the human brain. In: Ellis AW (ed) Normality and pathology in cognitive functions. Academic, New York, pp 299–323
20. Levy J (1976) Lateral dominance and aesthetic preference. Neuropsych 14:431–445
21. Doane BK, Livingston KE (eds) (1986) The limbic system. Raven, New York
22. Wigan AL (1844) Duality of mind. Longman, London. Reprinted (1985) J Simon, Malibu, California
23. Scheler M (1928) Nature et formes de la sympathie. Contribution à l'étude des lois de la vie émotionelle. (Traduit de l'allemand) Payot, Paris, p 230

Cerebral Lateralization and Some Implications for Art, Aesthetic Perception, and Artistic Creativity*

Otto-Joachim Grüsser, Thomas Selke, and Barbara Zynda
*Department of Physiology, Freie Universität Berlin, Arnimallee 22,
1000 Berlin 33, Federal Republic of Germany*

Nature and Nurture in Brain Development

The functional left-right asymmetry of the human brain (Table 1) appears to be determined, at least in part, by genetic factors. Hemispheric laterality found in some birds and subhuman primates[1,2], statistics on structural asymmetry of cerebral hemispheres in human neonates[3], the well-documented clinical studies on functional asymmetries as revealed by localized brain lesions[4-8], and the findings on congenital left-handedness correlated with speech dominance of the right hemisphere provide the main evidence supporting this premise (see chapter 9). The following considerations ensue from these ideas. Before we discuss the possible effects of left-right brain asymmetry on aesthetic performance in the second part of this paper, we shall present some thoughts on potential environmental factors in the development of left-right asymmetry in the human brain, which are believed to modify the genetically controlled postnatal brain development.[9]

The influence of signals from the environment on brain development are thought to be especially effective during the so-called sensitive periods (imprinting periods), when the development and/or differentiation of synaptic connections within a given brain region is particularly active as compared to any other period of postnatal life. We know that such sensitive periods also exist during the postnatal development of the central nervous system in higher mammals (including man). The most carefully examined sensory system in

---

*   Dedicated to Sir John Eccles, Contra, Switzerland, on the occasion of his 85th birthday

Table 1. Lateralization and dominance distribution of neocortical brain function (right-handed subjects)

Left Hemisphere	Right Hemisphere
Spoken language	Metaphorical meaning of language
Reading	Sense of humor
Writing	Emotional modification of language
Verbal thought	
Meter of prose and poems	Melody of spoken language (prosody)
Rhythm of music	
Color naming	Tonality, timbre, and harmony of music
Color classification and categories	Spatial concepts and thoughts, stereovision, spatial rotation
Calculus	
Right segment of extrapersonal space	Space coordinates, general spatial orientation
Interpretation of gestures and mimic expression	Geometry/chess playing
	Gestalt perception
	Left and right segments of extrapersonal space
	Recognition of gestures and mimic expression
	Recognition of faces
	Emotional responses

this respect is the central visual system, in particular the primary visual cortex, where the induction of experimental amblyopia[10] by unilateral eyelid closure (monocular pattern deprivation) during the "sensitive period" was the paradigm most frequently applied.[11] Similarly, the multimodal integration properties of area 7 of the parietal cortex, a part of the cortical system essential for the recognition of extrapersonal space, depend on polysensory input early in life. Monkeys raised with binocularly deprived eyes for about one year lose their ability to orient themselves in extrapersonal space by means of visual cues, even when normal visual input is provided from the second year of life onwards. The primary visual cortex (area V1) of such monkeys functions more or less normally, but the input to area 7 from higher-order visual cortices never develops after the eyelids have been opened.[12] These observations provide a neurobiological explanation for findings in humans who were born with an opaqueness of the optic system of both eyes and had no pattern vision until late in life, when the binocular corneal turbidity or congenital cataract was treated surgically. These patients failed to achieve normal visual recognition of objects which they knew in detail by touch.[13] Such observations provide the answer to the question of the Irish scientist, William Molineux (1656–1698), raised in a letter to John Locke:[14]

"Suppose a man born blind, and now adult, and taught by his touch to distinguish between a cube and a sphere of the same metal, and nighly of the same bigness, so as to tell, when he felt one and the other, which is the cube, which is the sphere. Suppose then the cube and sphere placed on a table and the blind man to be made to see: quaere, whether by his sight, before he touched them, he could now distinguish and tell which is the globe, which the cube?"

Molineux correctly supposed that the man would not be able to solve the problem.

Many of the connections between nerve cells of the neocortical structures of the brain, even when present at birth due to growth mechanisms controlled by the genetic code, have to be reinforced by experience, at least during the sensitive periods of the growing organism. If such reinforcement does not occur, the connections will not be maintained functionally. Such rules could also apply to the differentiation of brain structures important for aesthetic evaluation, emotional response, and artistic creativity. Such "higher-order," specifically human functions might, at least in part, also depend on brain mechanisms formed during "sensitive" periods prior to or during adolescence. Consequently, our aesthetic decisions and preferences might depend not only on the type of aesthetic and artistic training impinging upon us, but also on whether it occurred during especially sensitive periods.

The Erasmus Darwin Hypothesis

The development of aesthetic perception and activity in man is usually attributed to educational periods beyond the phases of early childhood. In general, we support this view. We also find it worthwhile, however, to consider the very first months of life as periods during which sensory experience might contribute to the development of elementary perceptual categories that form the basis of later, more sophisticated aesthetic responses. The possible relation between the content of aesthetic products and the early experiences of their creators was first discussed many generations before Freud and before art theoreticians began to apply psychoanalytic doctrine in their work. Erasmus Darwin expressed this idea in his *Zoonomia*. He was a physician and natural scientist who lived from 1738 to 1802 and the grandfather of the more famous Charles Darwin. In his book, Erasmus Darwin wrote one chapter on instinct, in which he also tried to demonstrate the effect of early childhood experience on the development of elementary aesthetic categories:

"When the babe soon after it is born into this cold world, is applied to its mother's bosom; its sense of perceiving warmth is first agreeably affected; next its sense of smell is delighted with the odour of her milk; then its taste is gratified by the flavour of it; afterwards the appetites of hunger and of thirst afford pleasure by the possession of their objects, and by the subsequent digestion of the aliment; and, lastly, the sense of touch is delighted by the softness and smoothness of the milky fountain, the source of such variety of happiness.

All these various kinds of pleasure at length become associated with the form of the mother's breast; which the infant embraces with its hands, presses with its lips, and watches with his eyes and thus acquires more accurate ideas of the form of its mother's bosom, than of the odour and flavour or warmth, which it perceives by its other senses. And hence at our maturer years, when any object of vision is presented to us, which by its waving spiral lines bears any similitude to the form of the female bosom whether it be found in a landscape with soft gradations of rising and descending surface or in the forms of some antique vases, or in other works of the pencil or the chisel, we feel a general glow of delight, which seems to influence all our senses; and, if the object be not too large, we experience attraction to embrace it with our arms and to salute it with our lips, as we did in our early infancy the bosom of our mother, and thus we find, according to the ingenious idea of Hogarth, that the waving lines of beauty were originally taken from the temple of Venus."[15]

On Functional Brain Asymmetry and Development

In the following we will try to apply Erasmus Darwin's hypothesis to selected aspects of "neuroaesthetic" tasks, i.e., problems that involve very elementary neurobiological mechanisms for aesthetic appreciation. Before we discuss the possible impact of functional brain asymmetry on aesthetics, we will present some observations and thoughts on ontogeny, i.e., on postnatal individual development over and above the schematic summary presented in Table 1.

First Spatial Stimulus Asymmetries in the World of the Newborn (Tactile, Vestibular, and Auditory Signals)

During the final weeks of fetal life, the inner ear receptors and the mechanoreceptors of the body surface are the exteroceptive sense organs of the growing organism that transmit the most information to the developing brain. The states of activity of the mechano- and thermoreceptors of the fetus' skin and vestibular receptors depend on movements of both mother and fetus and on the intrauterine milieu. The walking pace of a woman in advanced pregnancy is reduced from between 0.7 and 1.0 double steps per second to between about 0.45 and 0.55 per second, an approximate decrease from tempo andante to largo, inducing a vestibular stimulation of the unborn child in a basic frequency range of 0.45–0.55 Hz. This frequency range is also very effective in sedating a baby and was, therefore, unconsciously aspired to by craftsmen building cradles.

Intestinal noise, speaking, laughing, crying, or coughing on the part of the mother are transmitted to the middle ear of the fetus, as the acoustic impedance (resistance) of the media between sound source and ear is small. One auditory rhythm in particular continuously activates the fetal receptors of the inner ear and, at least during the last weeks of fetal life, the infant's auditory brain as well: the 60–75 per minute double heartbeat sounds of the mother. Since the fetus alters its position frequently in utero up until the last weeks of gestation, it is improbable that its central nervous system receives any distinct asymmetric stimuli from the mechanoreceptors of the inner ears or the body surface before the head is fixed in the birth canal. Should this be the case, however, a behavioral left-right asymmetry is revealed: more babies are born in the left occipito-anterior position than in all others – a phenomenon that is due perhaps to an asymmetric statistical distribution of the turning tendency of the baby and a slight asymmetry in the anatomy of the birth channel.

The sensory signals reaching the baby's brain change dramatically after birth. The auditory signals vary considerably, as does the stimulation of mechano- and thermoreceptors of the skin. As a rule, the baby's visual surround is textured and provides, in addition, extended spatial luminance gradients across the visual field as well as periodic (diurnal) changes in the average luminance. An undoubtedly important left-right asymmetry in the stimulation of sense organs is generated by the interaction between baby and mother from the first days of life. Observations in different cultures have shown that in the mother-child holding pattern a significant left-sided preference exists, i.e., the baby rests more frequently on the left side of the mother's bosom with its head and body on her left arm than on the right side. When the mother wishes to pacify a restless baby, she unconsciously presses the child to the left side of her chest. Thus the baby can hear the mother's heartbeat, which most likely has a calming effect. A 65%–70% preference for the left side, as opposed to 30%–35% for the right side has been found in European mothers. Similar percentages have been observed in other cultures: the United States, different Indian tribes in North and South America[16,17], rural communities of Sri Lanka (E. Brüser 1980, personal communication) and the neolithic Eipo tribe living in the West-Irian mountains of New Guinea (W. Schiefenhövel 1980, personal communication).

We also have good evidence that this left-sided preference is not recently acquired trait of modern mothers. Our argument stems from a study of mother-child holding patterns depicted in works of art. During the last 15 years, one of us collected data from a large number of paintings and sculptures depicting a mother holding her child.[18,19] From these data, it is evident that the left-sided preference found in Western art (including ancient Egyptian art) is 2000–3900 years old. From 103 mother-child sculptures produced between 1900 B.C. and 0 B.C., we found that 99 of them depicted the baby on the left side and only four on the right. The oldest sculpture of this type stems from the late Neolithic or Bronze Age and is shown in Fig.1a. These findings, together with transcultural data, support the opinion that the left-sided preference in the mother-child holding pattern is not a result of present-day cultural development in man and may, in itself, be dependent on genetic factors. It could, for example, be related to the dominance of the right hand in right-handed mothers. When the baby is held on the left side, the right hand is free for other work, and yet left-handed mothers also show a preference for holding their babies on the left side.[16] For holding any other objects except small pets, however, female subjects seem to prefer to use the right hand or arm. Male subjects show no partiality when holding babies and are less skilled than women when doing so. The mother's preference for holding the baby on the left side might be supported by a right-sided turning tendency of the baby or indirectly by a general left-sided preference of the mothers for close bodily social interaction.

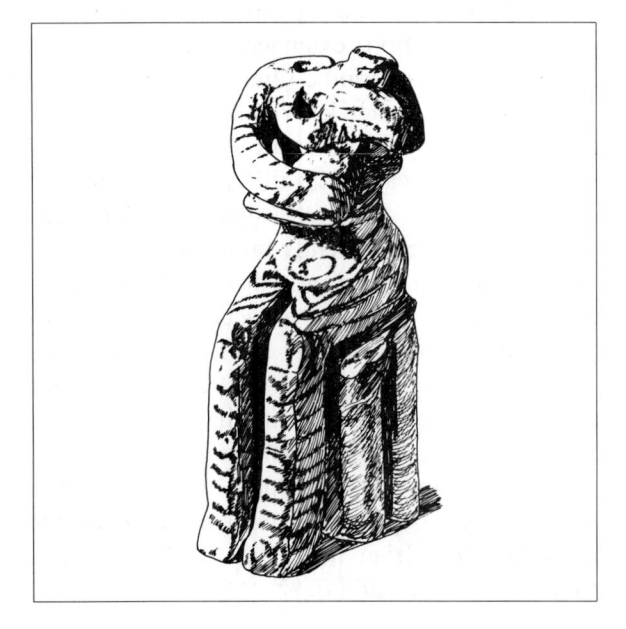

Fig. 1.a) Painted terracotta *(kovrotrophos)* from the Bronze Age, ca. 1900 B.C.[20]

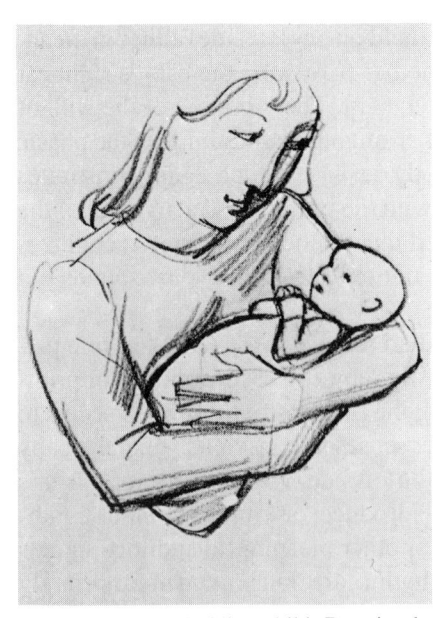

Fig. 1.b) Mother holding child. Drawing by M. Winzer 1982

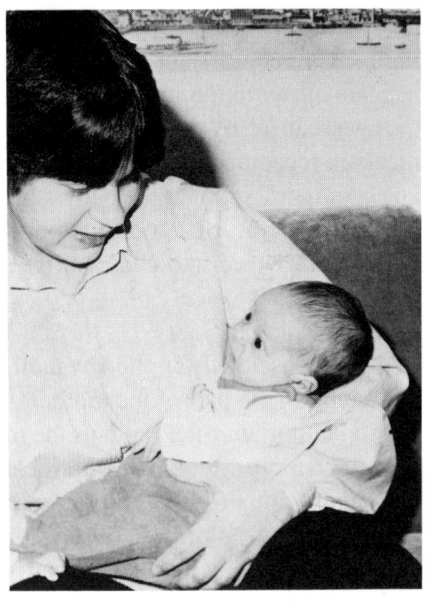

c) Eye-to-eye contact between mother and baby (from the family photographs of Drs. P. and H. Höhne)

The typical mother-child holding pattern (Fig.1b) brings the baby's right side in considerably closer contact with the mother than the left side. In such a situation, many babies have a tendency to turn their bodies towards the right. When the mother presses the baby closely to her bosom, it is very likely that the baby feels the low-frequency components of the mother's heartbeat on its right side. A similar left-right acoustic asymmetry is induced when the baby turns its head toward the mother's chest – it will hear the mother's heartbeat in its right and not in its left ear. Considering the 65%–70%, left-sided preference in mother-child holding patterns together with the asymmetry of auditory and tactile input, one can accept the hypothesis that a considerable part of the baby's early social life (when it is not asleep) is characterized by a left-right asymmetric otolithic (vestibular receptors for head position) input activation and by a stronger auditory and tactile input to the left cerebral hemisphere than to the right. This becomes even more important when one considers the fact that the auditory/tactile input of the mother's heartbeat is most likely a signal to which the baby has been conditioned during the last months of fetal life. Thus it is not surprising to learn from systematic observations that the 72-beat-per-minute heart rhythm, when transmitted to babies via loudspeakers, has a better calming and sleep-producing effect than any other rhythmic auditory stimuli, including lullabies.[16,21–23]

When the mother speaks to the baby (held on her left side) either in meaningful words or in typical, nonsensical mother-baby talk, the baby's right ear is again closer to the mother's body than the left. The vibration of the wall of the chest caused by the mother's speaking or singing could stimulate the phasic mechanoreceptors of the baby's right body surface, which again constitutes an asymmetric input to the baby's brain, with the preferential activation of the left hemisphere. It has been demonstrated that the newborn baby recognizes its mother's voice and can distinguish it not only from nonvoice sounds but also from other voices.[24-26]

According to Salk[16,21,22], the left-sided preference in the child-holding pattern is unconsciously applied by mothers, whereby an early learning or imprinting factor on the part of the mother during the first postpartum week seems to play an important role. Perhaps the mother senses unconsciously that the baby is pacified more effectively when held on the left side. Whatever the reason, this left-sided, mother-child holding pattern introduces asymmetric input conditions to the baby's brain. Speech signals or other meaningful auditory signals from the mother, including her heartbeat rhythm, are transmitted more strongly to the left hemisphere of the baby's brain than to the right.

In summary, there appear to exist genetic factors that govern the asymmetric specialization of the two hemispheres and condition a left-sided holding bias in mothers; such a bias introduces experiential asymmetries in the early months of the baby's life. Thus, the functional lateralization of the two hemispheres is reinforced by asymmetries which are, at least in part, caused by the asymmetric behavior of the mother and her left-sided heart position.

Mother-Child Holding Pattern and Visuospatial Input Asymmetries

When the baby rests on the mother's left arm, turns its body slightly to the right, and then wants to make visual contact with the mother, it must turn its head somewhat towards the left (relative to its body axis) to look into her face. We know that eye-to-eye contact and imitative babbling, laughing, or smiling are important behavioral patterns for the interaction between baby and mother and the development of the baby-mother dyad. During the first weeks of life, the mother's face is certainly the most important social signal for the baby. With the left-sided dominance in child-holding, it is shifted more often to the left side of the baby's field of gaze.

Another important spatial asymmetry also appears in partner interaction during early childhood as a result of the left-sided holding dominance. When the mother turns her head to the left and downwards to the baby resting on her left arm, the illumination of her face is generally uneven. With diffuse illumination of the scene, the right side of her face (which is then slanted upwards) will be somewhat brighter than the left. Thus, from the baby's position, the mother's face is not only shifted more towards the left side of its field of gaze, it is also brighter on the left side more frequently than on the right (left-right seen from the baby).

When mother and child are sitting in a garden on a sunny day, the mother automatically turns so that the light of the sun does not fall directly onto the baby's face. When the baby rests in the mother's left arm, the sun will then probably be on the left side of the baby's extrapersonal space. If the sun is on the right side, however, the mother will sit in relation to the sun so that her body provides a large shadow for the baby. It is most likely that the mother's behavior more frequently causes a luminance gradient with more light on the left side of the baby's extrapersonal space than on the right.

Development of Face Perception in Early Childhood

Facial expression is the most important social signal in everyday life after spoken language; facial structure is the most characteristic pattern of man's social individuality in the majority of societies. There are some exceptions to this rule. Female faces are hidden by a veil in some Arabic societies, while partial or total masking of faces is practiced not only by bank robbers but also in some military and police organizations. Masks with exaggerated expressions are worn in some societies during religious ceremonies or festivities and also during the European carnival. Some types of facial expression seem to be transcultural and are universally understood, indicating a rudimentary genetic basis for the neuronal mechanisms controlling facial expression and its recognition.

Specialized cortical regions exist in the primate brain that are important for face recognition and detection of mimic expression. In man, presumably both hemispheres are involved in these tasks, but the right hemisphere seems to predominate over the left.[27] Essential properties of these "face-specific cortical areas" are also developed in nonhuman primates[28-31], but evoked-potential studies corroborate the clinical findings of face-specific areas in the human brain, located in the basal occipito-temporal region and perhaps also in the limbic system of the deep temporal lobe and the gyrus cinguli (Bötzel, to be published).[32]

During the first months of life, babies respond to a face with a smile whenever they are in a good mood. For the first few weeks, a fairly "schematic" face is sufficient to arouse this smiling response. Movement of the face stimulus can enhance the baby's reaction, but eyes and mouth seem to be the most important components to arouse smiling.[33-35] We have mentioned that the very first face important for the baby, that of the mother, is frequently shifted somewhat to the left of the baby's field of gaze when the baby lies turned slightly to the right and close to its mother's left breast. When the mother makes cheek-to-cheek contact with her baby – a behavioral pattern enjoyed by both mother and baby – she usually touches the left cheek of the baby on her left arm with her left cheek. Thus, with respect to emotional face-to-face contacts early in life, the left part of the face (and consequently the sensory cortex of the right cerebral hemisphere) is more frequently stimulated than the right.

We do not know whether the gaze movement patterns of the child during the first months of life exhibit a lateral bias, but such a bias is present later in life. When adults view a face, a photograph of a face, or a face in a movie or on television, they tend to look at the right half more frequently than the left, i.e. they direct their center of gaze more often towards the left part of their field of gaze than to the right. This left-right asymmetry can be studied quantitatively when one records eye movements during brief viewings of faces or photo portraits. A typical recording is shown in Fig. 2. The first saccade usually moves the center of gaze to the left side and is directed most frequently to the right eye of the partner's face. Then the second saccade moves the center of gaze customarily to the left eye of the partner and the third, towards the

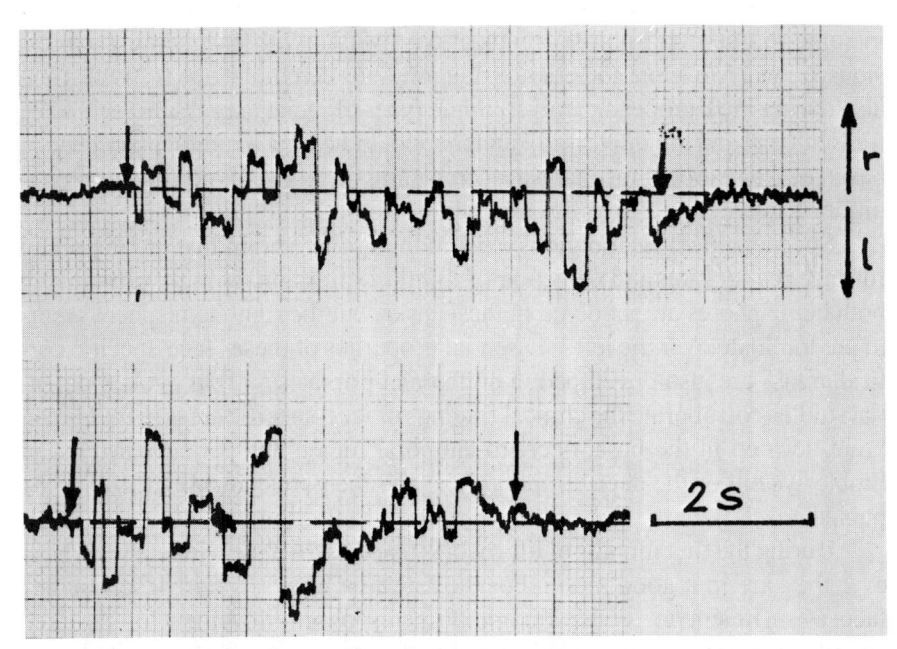

Fig. 2. Eye movement recordings (horizontal DC-electro-oculogram) during a 6-second inspection of a projected face photograph. Typically, the center of gaze is directed first to the right eye, remains on the right half of the inspected face 65%–70% of the time and on the left half 30%–35% of the time.[42]

mouth region. During a 6-second viewing period, the center of gaze is 65%–70% of the time in the left half of the field of gaze, i.e., on the right side of the face inspected. This asymmetry is also maintained when one continuously inspects a photo portrait or an actual face. The recordings published by Yarbus[36] contain such examples. The reader may test this hypothesis: when speaking with another person, observe to which half of the partner's face you direct your center of gaze (and interest) more frequently; it is highly probable that the right half and the partner's right eye will be regarded more often than the left.

Left-Right Asymmetry in Adult Perception of Faces and Mimic Expression

Barely perceivable emotional responses are expressed more readily by the left half of the face than by the right.[37–40] This is one indication that the right cerebral hemisphere of right-handed subjects is more related to emotional experience than the left (Table 1). We have evidence, on the one hand, of a left visual-field superiority by right-handers for perceiving emotional facial expressions.[41] On the other hand, in recognizing a person's identity, the right half of the partner's face seems to be more important, as shown in experiments in which subjects were asked to judge the similarity to the normal face of photographically constructed symmetrical faces composed of the two left or two right halves (Fig.3). If no left-right bias existed for face recognition, the decisions of a large group of subjects would be distributed symmetrically around a 50-percent mean. The distribution of the responses was asymmetric, however, (Fig.4) and "double-right faces" were judged to be similar to the normal face more frequently than "double-left faces." Some of the left-handed subjects showed a reversed side-preference. Thus, the "normal" right-handed

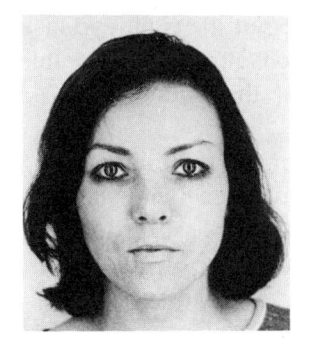

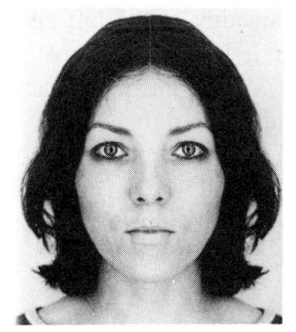

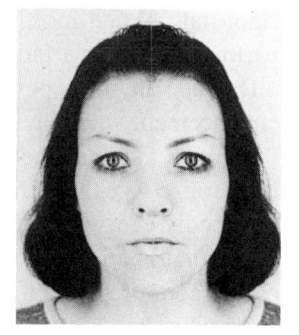

Fig. 3. Example of a test slide with a normal face *(left)* and two artificial faces composed from double-right halves *(middle)* and double-left halves *(right)*. The subjects had to judge which of the two artifical faces resembles the normal face most. For this particular combination, more than 90% of the 180 medical students shown this slide during a lecture chose the double-right face *(middle)*.

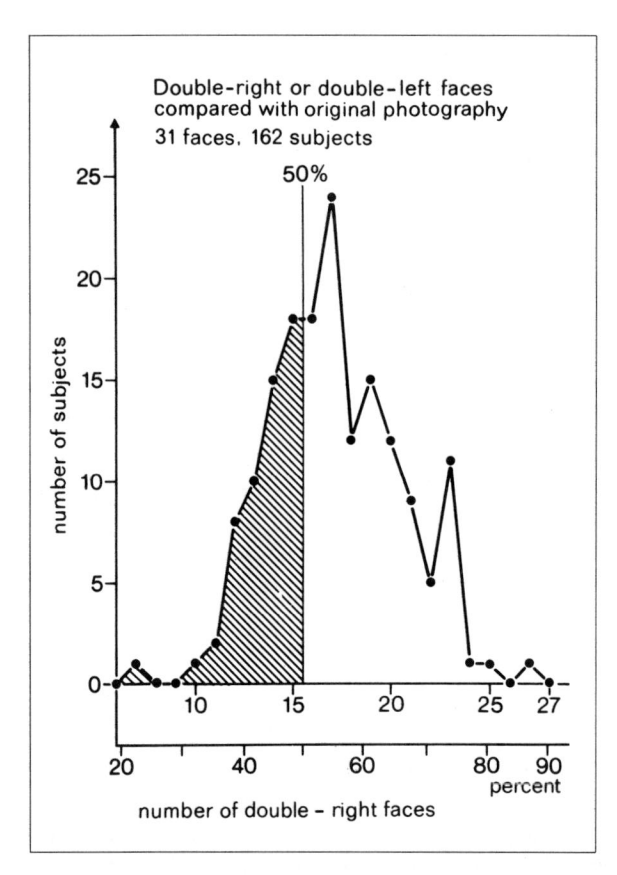

Fig. 4. Statistical results obtained in a lecture hall experiment (1978) with 31 slides of the type shown in Fig. 3 and 180 subjects. The three-face slides were shown for 6 seconds each, with a pause of 6 seconds in between. The subjects had to decide whether the double-right or double-left face looked more similar to the normal face. They were not informed of how the different faces were constructed. The figure shows the frequency distribution of the preference for double-right faces.[42]

subjects and at least half of the left-handers exhibit a "double" asymmetry with respect to face perception – emotion is expressed and perceived more readily in the left half of the face, whereas a person's identity is related more to the right half. When looking steadily at the left and then at the right eye of a partner's face (or a face on a TV screen), most persons note a considerable difference in their perception of the preciseness of the face, namely an enhancement when one fixates the right eye.

Since the introduction of artificial mirrors to human civilization during the Bronze Age or later, nearly all women and men have seen their own faces repeatedly every day. Due to the asymmetries mentioned, we regard the left (emotional) half of our face as our "public face," while for our social partners, our person is represented more by the right half of our face. Most readers will remember their surprise when seeing their own face for the first time or after an interval of some years in a double mirror or as a large portrait photograph. The interaction between self and face in a mirror may be an important component in the training and development of our face and mimic recognition system. Girls between the ages of 10 and 20 probably spend at least twice as much time in front of a mirror as boys (as observed by the senior author in his children – although we do not know of any quantitative studies on this matter). This different behavioral pattern could be one of the reasons why female subjects perform better than their male counterparts in most of the "normal" face recognition tests.[42–45]

The Ontogenetic Development of Emotional and Aesthetic Qualitites in the Perception of Faces as Compared to Other Objects

Although we have emphasized early childhood experience in the development of basic perceptual and aesthetic categories, we do not want to overemphasize the impact of the early years of life on the development of aesthetic preferences and judgements. We agree with probably the majority of art teachers that the elementary and high school years are more important than the first years in the development of aesthetic taste and, for artists, in the shaping of artistic creativity. In particular, the joyful experience of games pleasing to the eye, active performance in music and dance, and early crea-

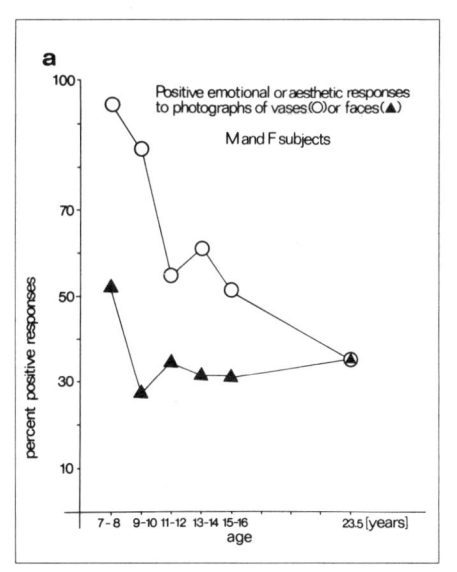

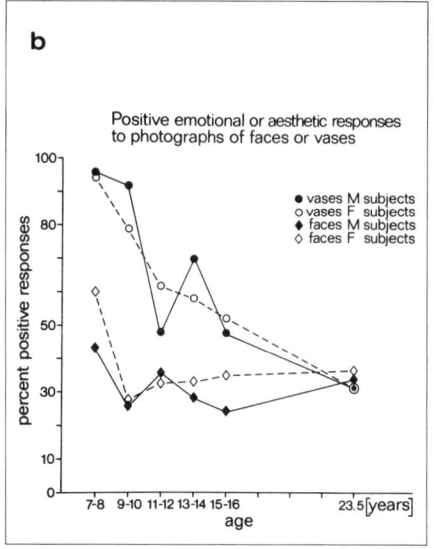

Fig. 5.a) Positive emotional or aesthetic responses to photographs of vases *(circles)* or adult faces *(triangles)* in subjects of different ages. Age groups over a 2-year period were formed. Data from male and female subjects were pooled. Note that in the same subjects the positive aesthetic responses to photographs of art nouveau vases decline with increasing age, while for faces, the positive response ("pleasant") remains at about the same level beyond the age group 9–10 years. (b) Same data as in (a), but data obtained in male and female subjects are plotted separately. Data plotted at *average* age 23.5 years were obtained in 126 medical students.[47]

tive activity in drawing and painting form the personal predilection important for later aesthetic experience. Comparing the performance of left-handed and right-handed painters, Jung[46] came to the conclusion that for highly skilled motor behavior, like writing and drawing, asymmetry as a result of training seems more important than the genetically determined left-right asymmetry. This training asymmetry, as a rule, appears only after the child has learned to write.

During a study of the ability of children and adolescents to remember and recognize photographs of faces as opposed to photographs of vases, we collected material indicating a separate development of emotional and aesthetic responses to faces and to objects of art.[45] Our subjects were school children between 7 and 17 years of age and medical students with an average age of 23.5 years. In the first inspection series, subjects saw black and white slides of a face or a vase projected for a period of 6 seconds onto a reflecting tangent screen. Within 6 seconds following this inspection period, subjects had to judge whether they liked or disliked the face or vase. Then, the next item was shown for another 6 seconds, etc. One hour later and 1 week later, the faces or vases had to be identified in a forced two-choice task. The data obtained for the emotional/aesthetic responses in the inspection series are pertinent to our discussion here (Fig.5). It is evident that positive emotional or aesthetic responses to "everyday" faces are higher in the youngest group (7/8 years) and decline thereafter to a 30-percent level in the age group 9/10 years, to remain at this level throughout adolescence. Fairly consistently, female faces were judged emotionally as pleasant or "positive" more frequently than male faces, and female subjects beyond puberty judged faces of both sexes as "positive" more frequently than male subjects. However, the percentage of positive aesthetic/emotional responses evoked by the photographs of "Art Nouveau" vases and produced mainly during the period between 1880 and 1920 decreased continuously during childhood and adolescence. In the second and third test (recognition in a two-choice task after 1 hour or 1 week), recognition of faces was better than that of vases in all age groups.

These findings indicate that for objects of art displaying a structural symmetry similar to that of faces, aesthetic response differentiation still occurs beyond puberty, while this does not seem to be the case for faces. During childhood and adolescence, no significant correlation exists in different subjects between the percentage of positive emotional responses to faces and to vases, while a positive correlation is present between the average emotional responses to female and to male faces (Fig.6a and b). These differences again support the hypothesis that perception of faces and the emotional responses evoked by them are special cerebral functions and not simply correlated to the perception of other objects.

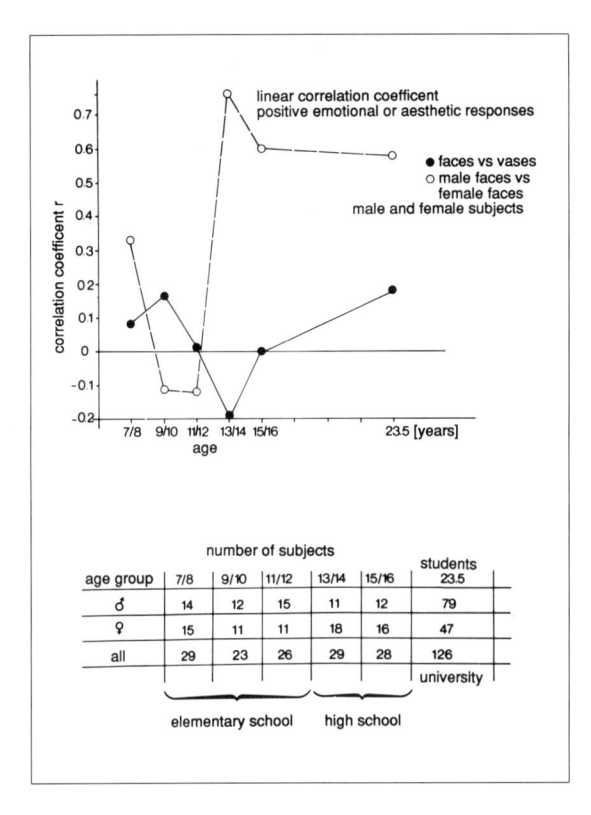

Fig. 6. Linear correlation coefficient between the percentage of positive emotional ("pleasant") or aesthetic responses. *Circles:* correlation coefficient of the responses to male faces vs female faces. *Dots:* correlation coefficient of the responses to male and female faces vs vases. In the table below the graph, the respective numbers of subjects participating in the tests from which Figs. 5 and 6 are the result are shown.[45]

Face recognition develops during the preschool period and the first years of elementary school. It reaches the adult performance level between 10 and 12 years of age. Prior to about 10 years of age, children fail to show the left-visual-field/right-hemisphere predominance present in older children and adults in recognizing "tachistoscopically" (as very short stimuli) presented, unfamiliar faces.[47] The results of face and vase recognition tests (see above) performed in children of different ages 1 hour after presentation and 1 week later support the theory that face recognition develops up until puberty (Fig.7a and b), but the ability to recognize faces matures differently from the ability to recognize simple, symmetrical objects of art.

When one looks into the development of face and human drawings by young children, the *Kopffüssler*-phase, depicting a head on two legs, is a distinct level reached at about age four and is considered to be a transcultural phenomenon.[48,49] *Kopffüssler* appear in the art of many cultures, in the drawings of adult schizophrenic patients, and in paintings of modern artists (e.g., Klee, Picasso, Miro, Antes). We maintain that the face recognition level, as expressed by the *Kopffüssler* drawn by 3- to 4-year-old children, indicates that

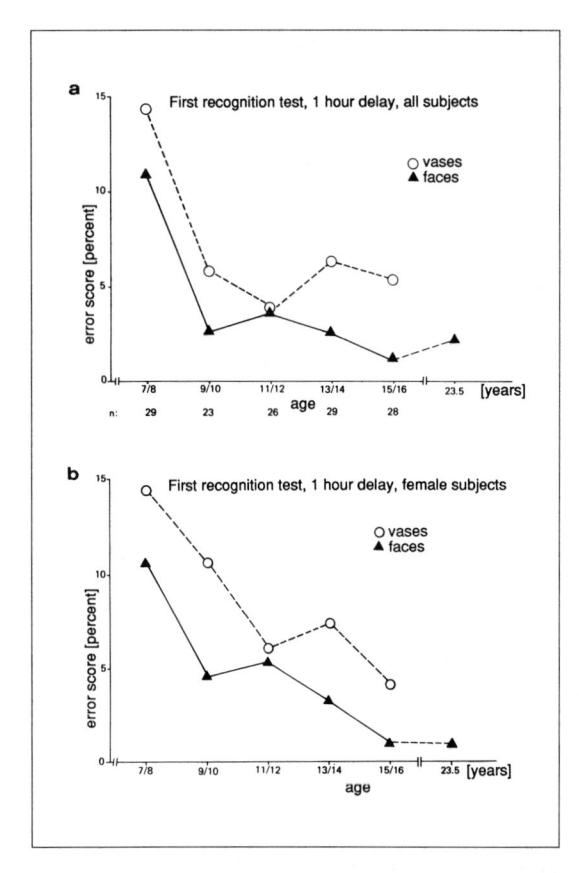

Fig. 7.a) and b) First recognition test performed 1 h after inspection series. a) Error score (percent, *ordinate*) plotted as a function of the age of the subjects *(abscissa)* for vases and faces. Data from male and female subjects averaged b) Same relationship as in a), but separate scores for female subjects

a fairly schematic face and person perception dominates the social interaction between the young child and persons in his surroundings.

Another observation supporting the impact of schematic faces on social interaction is the preference of 4- to 8-year-old children for puppet theater and the appearance of chalk facial caricatures on the blackboards of classrooms or on walls during the first 2–3 years of elementary school. Here, some components (especially mouth, teeth, and eyes) are exaggerated to express aggressive or friendly intentions. The ritual masks used in many cultures[50], which are frequently very colorful but fairly schematic facial representations (including *Fastnachts*-masks of the Middle European carnival), may be regarded as signs of a special cultural adaptation, modification, and ritualization of this activity begun "spontaneously" in childhood. Moreover, when a child has reached the age of 4–5 years, he particularly enjoys the emotional effects aroused by different types of masks.

The assumption that the perception of faces has special components not comparable to other objects is corroborated by the frequency with which faces or facial components are perceived in rather vague visual patterns, such as random dot structures or more or less symmetrical inkspots.[51,52] This tendency is also found in elementary school children and may exist in preschoolers as well. The frequent perception of faces reported by subjects when they observe the *Eigengrau* (visual sensations that belong to the *phantastische Gesichtserscheinungen* as described by Johannes Müller in 1826[53]) of their visual field shortly before falling asleep may also be an indication of a specialized brain function related to face perception.

Perception of Faces and Mimic Expression in Schizophrenia

It should be mentioned that schizophrenia leads to a considerable reduction in the ability to perceive and remember faces, facial expression, and gestures.[54-56] A peculiar disturbance in the perception of faces and mimic expression occurs frequently in schizophrenic children, i.e., at an age at which the face recognition mechanisms normally mature to the adult level. Dewdney[57] described 30 such children, who reported fairly uniform alterations in face perception. When they observed a face (real or drawn) for several seconds, it seemed to change its expression dramatically: the eyes widened; the pupils dilated; the nose extended; the mouth opened and exposed large teeth, especially canines; and the whole appearance of the face was that of a "vampire," "devil," "monster," or "werewolf," a perception increasing the psychotic anxiety. We have also observed this symptom in adolescent and young adult schizophrenic patients and called it paraprosopia (misperception of faces).[58] It also occurs in older schizophrenics (e.g., the self-report of Schreber[59]), but certainly less frequently than in children. Alterations in face perception are evident in drawings and paintings of faces produced by schizophrenic artists, as seen in the publications of the Prinzhorn collection.[60] Western paintings produced in the past 500 years teach us that the deformation of faces in drawings, paintings, or sculptures is not necessarily a sign of increased anxiety or altered facial perception on the part of the artist. When, however, the deformed face and the facial expression of anxiety and fear predominate, such as in the paintings of James Ensor (1860–1949), one wonders whether this is a manifestation of some psychological borderline situation. Especially impressive in this regard are Ensor's famous paintings "L'intrigue" in the Flemish museum in Antwerp and "The entry of Christ into Brüssels" in the J. Paul Getty Museum in Malibu (Fig.8). Ensor was also obsessed by masks, a number of which can still be seen in the Ensor Museum in Ostende.

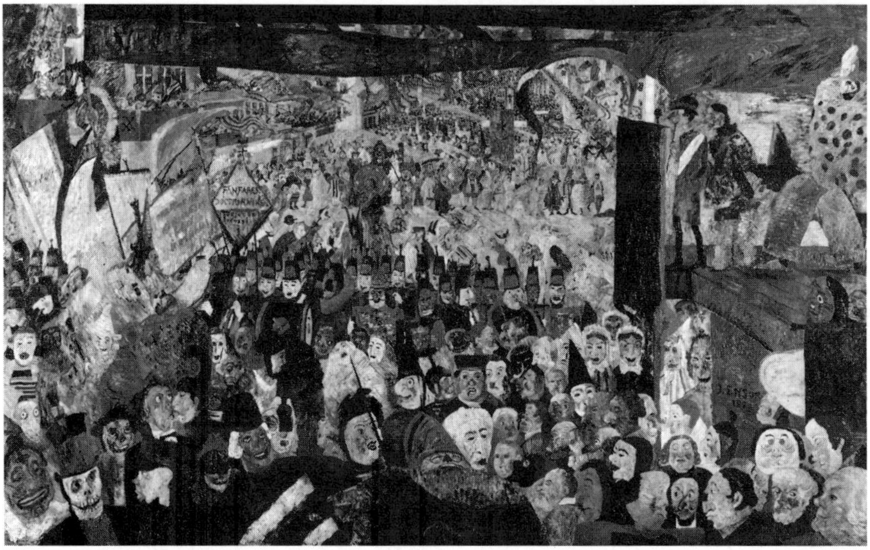

Fig. 8. "The Entry of Christ into Brussels" by James Ensor (1888, The J. Paul Getty Museum, Oil on canvas, 260 × 430,5 cm. Reproduced with permission)

Left-Right Brain Asymmetries and the Perception and Reproduction of Rhythm and Music

Musical composition can be characterized basically by rhythm, intonation, timbre, and harmony, elementary properties underlying the concept and formal structures of a larger piece of music (see chapter 4). For the production and perception of rhythm, the left hemisphere of right-handers seems to be dominant, whereas the tonal quality involves particular functions of the right hemisphere. Perception and production of rhythm seems to be correlated with language functions. We have tested more than 60 aphasic patients (women and men who had lost the power to speak and/or to understand spoken or written language due to a circumscribed lesion of the left cortical hemisphere) and explored their ability to repeat simple rhythms tapped on a table or heard as tape recordings. We found that whenever amnesic, sensory, or motor aphasia was present, perception and production of rhythm was impaired (O.-J. Grüsser, F. Reischies 1978–1980, unpublished work).

In further regard to the perception of rhythm, it is possible that the genetically determined left-right asymmetry is also reinforced by early mother-child holding patterns. As mentioned above, the baby cradled in the left arm of the mother more frequently than in the right has a better chance of hearing the rhythmic heartbeat of the mother with the right ear or feeling it with the right side of the body. It will also hear the speech sounds from its mother more clearly with its right than with its left ear. It is, therefore, reasonable to discuss possible asymmetric imprinting effects for rhythmic and auditory input signals during the first weeks of life. Due to the asymmetric auditory input, the left hemisphere of the baby is imprinted more intensely by rhythmic auditory and speech signals than the right.

In addition, observations of patients with brain lesions indicate that a lesion of the left hemisphere leads to severe disturbances in the perception and reproduction of simple musical rhythms much more frequently than a lesion of the right. As mentioned, all aphasic patients tested had considerable difficulty in reproducing simple rhythms in a standardized rhythm test. In contrast, patients with left-sided brain lesions without aphasia (including those with cortical dysarthria) and patients with right-sided brain lesions showed no severe impairment in the rhythm test. We assume, therefore, that the left-hemispheric speech regions play a more important role in the perception and processing of auditory rhythms than the homologous areas of the right hemisphere.

This left-right disparity is also seen in patients suffering from amusia caused by lesions of the right hemisphere. Amusia is an impairment in perception and recognition of tonality and harmony in music, usually associated with the inability to intonate correctly when singing. As an illustration, we shall describe some observations made in a professional singer who had suffered a cerebral hemorrhage in his right hemisphere. The main neurological symptoms were left hemiplegia, left hemihypesthesia, left-sided spatial neglect, and tonal amusia. After recovery from the acute symptoms, the patient recommenced singing. He sang the lieder or opera arias perfectly as far as rhythm and text were concerned, but always on the same note. The patient could not perceive his mistakes at all, but later recognized that something must be wrong with his singing. We tested the patient some months after the hemorrhage and found no impairment in pitch discrimination; an audiogram for the left and right ear was adequate for his age. The patient rehearsed consistently to regain his previous standard in singing. His intonation slowly improved and continues to do so, but still today, after nearly 10 years of endeavour, a severe impairment in intonation exists, while his rhythmic performance is good. Interestingly, the musical tastes of this patient have also changed. Prior to his stroke, he preferred bel canto, Romantic, and late nineteenth-century music, especially operas. After the stroke, his preference shifted to Baroque orchestral music, although he still enjoys the lieder of the Romantic composers. The patient is also able to recognize the sounds of all instruments in the orchestra, some of which are unknown to the average music listener. We tested this ability using special records with solo instrumentals. A corollary of the intonation difficulties while singing can be seen in the changes in the patient's speech prosody. He is inclined to speak with a strained, somewhat high-pitched voice and with a definite tendency to a slightly agitated monotony (O.-J. Grüsser, A. Lüchtrath 1980, Observations on amusia in a professional singer, unpublished work).

Besides chronic lesions located in the left or right hemisphere, transient inactivation of one hemisphere also indicates that the mechanisms underlying the perception and motor skills necessary for muscial tonality and harmony are located more frequently in the minor (right) hemisphere of the brain, while rhythmic performance is closely correlated with speech function, thus requiring an intact dominant (left) hemisphere. Amytal injections into the right carotid artery, for example, lead to a transitory unilateral anesthesia of the right hemisphere.[61] Patients who were required to sing during this procedure continued in a correct rhythm but lost control of pitch.[62] The close correlation between musical rhythms and language function is meaningful when one considers the meter of a poem primarily as a specialized form of the temporal structure of prose that is present in everyday speech. The intonation of a recited poem transmits emotional aspects. These signals, e.g., musical tonality and harmony, are most likely processed mainly by the right hemisphere, which is more involved in treating emotional information than the left.

Left-Right Asymmetry in Visual Art: Some "Neuroaesthetic" Considerations

To summarize some of the functional left-right asymmetries correlated with the right-left asymmetry of cerebral functions, we present a number of examples, which we believe to be of some importance in aesthetics of the visual arts.

Elementary Left-Right Asymmetries in Paintings and Drawings

Heinrich Wölfflin[63] was probably the first to discuss the significance of the left-right asymmetry when viewing paintings. He suggested that the observer begin at the lower left side and proceed to the right side, where the "more important" content in many paintings of the Renaissance, Baroque, and nineteenth-century periods is displayed. This left-right asymmetry in picture scanning is supported by eye-movement recordings. When subjects are asked to inspect slides of paintings or landscapes, the center of gaze is initially directed to the left side and then proceeds toward the right (M. Jeannerod 1980, personal communication). Gaffron[64] indicated that the "glance curve" usually begins in the left foreground, moves upward and to the background, and from there to the right foreground. It is still unclear, however, whether this asymmetry in scanning preference is related to the formal structure or to the content of the paintings. In addition, one probable cause is an asymmetric gaze motor command due primarily to cerebral left-right asymmetries. The artists may have unconsciously adapted their paintings to their own perceptual left-right asymmetries. The fact that the right hemisphere of a right-hander is more involved in spatial tasks than the left may determine the onset of the scanning function mentioned; thus the center of gaze shifts first to the left side of the painting. Pöppel and Sütterlin (1981 Emotionality and Laterality of Paintings, unpublished work) studied left-right asymmetries in paintings that were scored by subjects according to their "emotional" intensity. In the majority of paintings with high emotional intensity scores, the visual center was judged by other subjects to be located on the left side of the painting, not on the right. In paintings with an especially low emotional intensity score, the visual center was usually on the right or in the center (symmetric structures). Levy's study[65] also indicates that lateral dominance in aesthetic preference not only depends on the left-right distribution of the painting structure but also on the handedness of the observer. If this is true, we could predict the handedness of the artist (or the hand used in painting) to be a further factor determining the structure of a painting.

Light in Paintings

Art historians have studied the light in paintings of different periods and have developed intricate descriptions of an admittedly complex problem.[66] In our opinion, however, very simple questions have not been explored, at least not on a quantitative basis. In the course of visits to various museums over the past 10 years, the senior author (Grüsser) collected material on the distribution of light in paintings, i.e., on the position of the main light source for the painted scene. Analysis of 2124 paintings originating between the fourteenth and twentieth centuries led to the formation of the three following simple categories:

1. Main light source falling onto the painted scene from the left side (L, left-right from the perspective of the observer)
2. Main light source coming from the right side (R)
3. Light source from the middle of the painting, several independent light sources on different sides, or diffuse light, i.e., no left-right gradient visible with respect to luminance distribution and shadows within the painting (M)

In the majority of paintings, the light sources illuminating the scenery were positioned considerably above the horizon of the painting, but the degree of elevation was not further evaluated. Data were collected in eight museums. The results indicate the development of an interesting left-right asymmetry for the position of the main light source in canvas paintings. At the beginning of modern Western art during the early Gothic period, a preference for diffuse illumination or light sources distributed around the painted scene was found (Fig.9). In a minority of paintings from the fourteenth century that show a clear light direction, a bias to the left side is present. This left-sided preference increased at the expense of diffuse or middle light sources up to the sixteenth and seventeenth centuries and declined thereafter. In the twentieth century, the diffuse or middle type of light distribution again became dominant. This change in artistic technique is correlated with the disappearance of apparent depth (illusionary perspective) and the tendency of the artists to remain in the two-dimensional plane. It should be noted that the wall paintings of Pompeii and Herculaneum[67] (earlier than the first century A.D.) also exhibit a left dominance in light direction (Fig.9), as do the Byzantine mosaics in the churches of Ravenna.

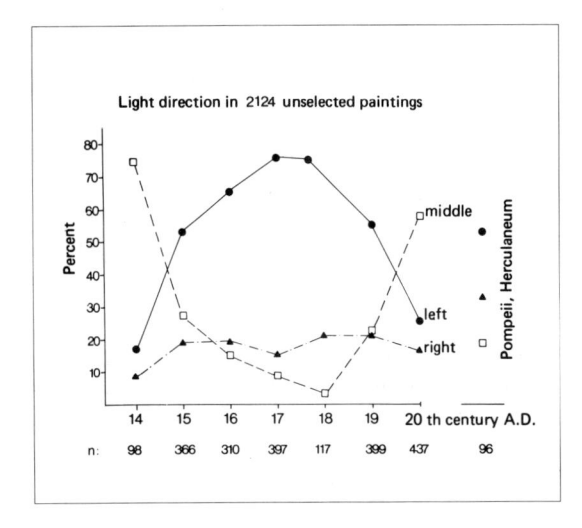

Fig. 9. Distribution of light direction (left, right, middle) in 2,124 paintings selected at random from Western art originating between the 14th and the 20th centuries. On the right, the same distribution for the wall paintings in Pompeii and Herculaneum is shown according to the figures printed in Kraus and von Matt.[67]

It is tempting to speculate whether this left-right asymmetry in light direction found in paintings of Western art could be correlated with the elementary left-right asymmetry of light distribution present during the early weeks of life and the general left-right asymmetry in space perception caused by the fact that the right hemisphere is dominant for spatial tasks. A strong left-right bias is not only present when one analyzes randomly selected paintings from the fifteenth to nineteenth centuries but also in paintings and drawings of individual artists. Such an individual analysis might shed further light on the factors leading to the left-right asymmetry. Lucas Cranach (1472–1553), a very prolific right-handed painter of the sixteenth century, exhibited a strong left-sided preference for light direction in both his paintings and drawings (Fig. 17a). The same is true for the drawings of Michelangelo. The left-handed Leonardo da Vinci, however, applied a left, middle, or right main light source with more or less equal frequency in his drawings (excluding the many drawings in which no light direction is present.[68–70] Hans Holbein the Younger (1497–1543), a dominant left-hander like Leonardo, showed a significant tendency to light directed from the right side of his drawings (Fig.18a). From such observations in the works of these two left-handed painters who painted, drew, and wrote with the left hand[46], one gains the impression that the distribution of left, middle, and right light direction in left-handed painters deviates significantly from the average distribution of light found in the paintings of other contemporary painters. It would be interesting to study the drawings and paintings of other confirmed left-handed artists, who worked exclusively with the left hand. The results of such a study could confirm or invalidate our hypothesis that light preference in paintings seems to depend on the handedness of the artist, or at least on the hand used for painting, since left-handed artists were frequently well trained to also use the right hand for painting and/or writing.

Left-Right Asymmetries in the Shading of Drawings

A right-handed artist drawing with his right hand prefers to shade with a sequence of strokes running from upper right to lower left. If he shades in the opposite direction, the regularity of the strokes changes. A left-handed artist drawing with his left hand prefers to shade in the opposite direction. Left-handed artists drawing with the right hand and right-handed artists probably shade in a similar way.[46] Nonetheless, up until the last century, left-handed painters usually wrote with the right hand (Leonardo da Vinci is a famous exception), but most of them drew and painted with the left hand. Vertical stroke shadings are more frequent in left-handers than in right-handers.[46] In comparing left-handed drawing and right-handed writing in left-handers and the fairly rare drawing of left-handers with the right hand, Jung[46] pointed out that, with respect to the "quality" of drawing and writing (i.e. the motor skill visible), training and learning are more important than inborn cerebral lateral dominance. Figure 10 shows examples of drawings with the right and left hand of two right-handers and one left-hander. One can easily recognize not only the differences in drawing quality, but also the changes in shading that characterize the use of the left or the right hand.

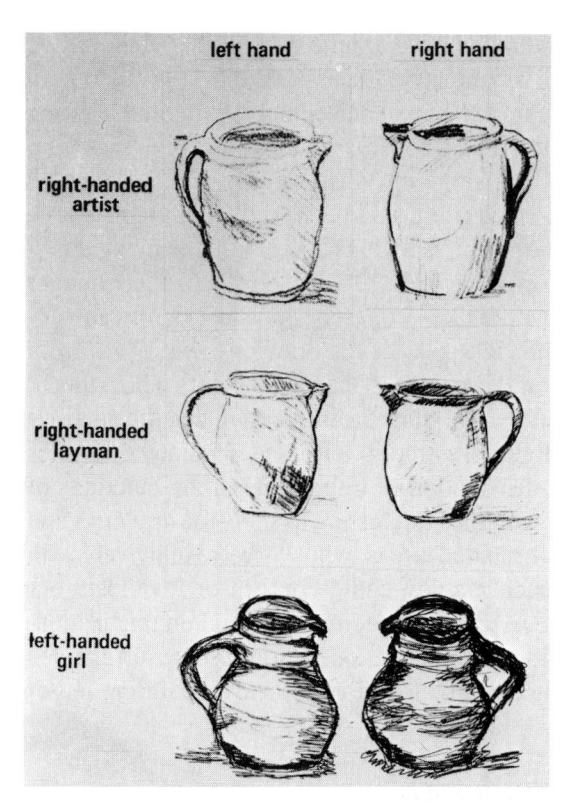

Fig. 10. Drawings of a jar (reduced in size) by a right-handed artist and a right-handed layman and of another jar by the left-handed, 18-year-old daughter of the latter. The drawings were performed with the left (L) and the right hand (R). The girl writes and draws normally with her left hand. Note the differences in strokes and type of shading between left-hander and right-hander drawings and between the drawings performed with the left and the right hand.

Asymmetries in Portrait Paintings

A detailed structural analysis of portrait paintings is a complex task and involves specific information on the historical background of painter and portrayed subject, on the one hand, and a thorough knowledge of the basic rules of physiognomy perception on the other. Gombrich[71] has presented a masterful study on this matter. Restricting ourselves again to very simple and "concrete" properties of portrait paintings – light, head position, and gender of the portrait face – we will explore how these components are interdependent and, in addition, related to the historical development of Western art. As mentioned, the left half of the face seems to be the more emotional half, whereas the right half is our more official face. During visits to museums in central Europe, one of the authors (Grüsser) analyzed 933 canvas or panel portrait paintings from the fifteenth to the twentieth centuries. The light distribution was classified according to the categories described above. The head position relative to the observer (left, middle, or right) was also noted, i.e., head left (L) meant that the subject's head was turned more or less toward his right side and thus showed more of the left half of his face to the observer than the right. Only paintings produced with the definite intention of depicting a particular person were analyzed.

From the beginning of modern Western painting, the direction of the light to illuminate the face portrayed used by the artist shows a strong preference for the left side. It is only in the twentieth century that many portrait paintings exhibit a diffuse light illumination (M). Thus, the distribution of the light direction in portrait paintings more or less follows the general rules found for nonportrait paintings (Fig.11a), but the left-sided bias is somewhat stronger in portrait paintings. The data in Fig.11b reveal a second considerable left-right bias in portrait paintings: the head positioned to the left from the perspective of the observer is preferred during the beginning of Western portrait painting in the fifteenth and sixteenth centuries and changes slowly with time. Gender does not affect the direction of light falling onto the portrayed subject (Fig. 12) but is clearly a factor for head position. Female subjects present the left half of their face to the observer (or the painter) more frequently than male subjects (Fig.13). When one analyzes the female portraits of the fifteenth to the seventeenth centuries showing more of the right half of the face, one finds that these were frequently official portraits, i.e., the female subject was a sovereign or someone of similarly high social rank. The strong correlation between gender and head position becomes obvious when one averages the data over the six centuries of Western portrait paintings, while only a slight correlation exists between light direction and head position and none between gender and light direction (Figs.14 and 15).

The gender difference for the head position of portrayed subjects becomes more evident when the quotient of left and right position is plotted as a function of historical time (Fig. 16). It is evident from this figure that from the sixteenth century onwards, the portrayed male subjects show a slight lateral bias in head position with a tendency to display the right half of their faces more frequently. In the female portraits, however, the left preference is maintained even up to the twentieth century but, with the gradual social emancipation of women over the last three centuries, the L/R-quotient in head position decreased considerably.

A More Detailed Study of a Left-handed and a Right-handed Portrait Painter

It is worthwhile to analyze the distribution of head position and light direction in male and female portrait paintings by individual artists when enough material is available. We performed such an analysis for Lucas Cranach the Elder (1472–1553, Fig.17a–c) and Hans Holbein the Younger (1497–1543,

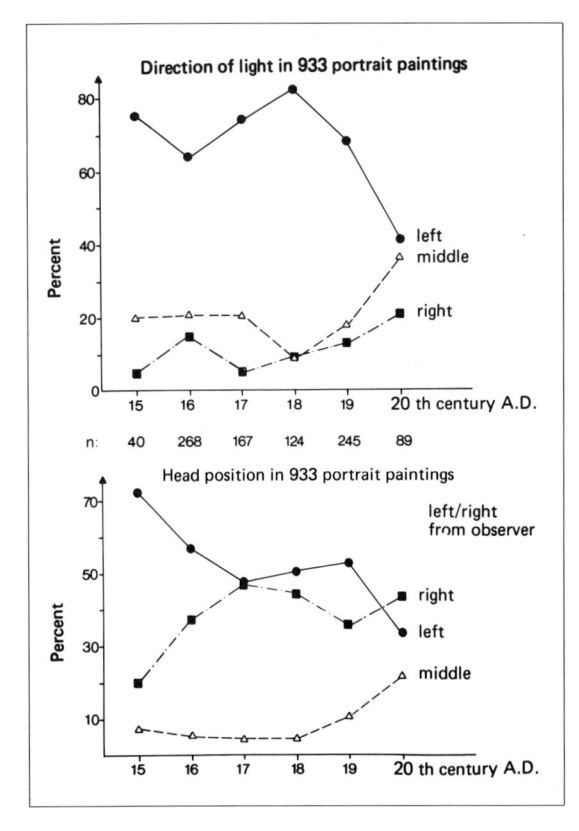

Fig. 11.a) From data pooled for each century, light distribution in 933 portrait paintings originating between the 15th and 20th centuries is plotted for the 6 different centuries. (b) Distribution of head position in the same portrait paintings. *Left* means that the portrayed head is turned towards the left side from the perspective of the observer, i.e., the portrayed subject has his or her head turned towards the right shoulder and shows the left half of the face to the observer more than the right half of the face. *Middle* means that the head position does not deviate visibly or deviates less than about 5 degrees from the fronto-parallel plane. *Right* means that the portrayed subject's head is turned to the left and displays more of the right half of the face to the observer.

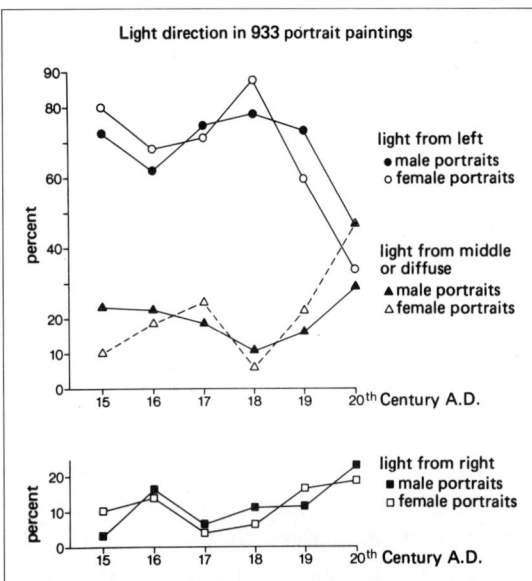

Fig. 12. Light direction in 933 portrait paintings. Same data as in Fig. 10a but separated for male and female portraits

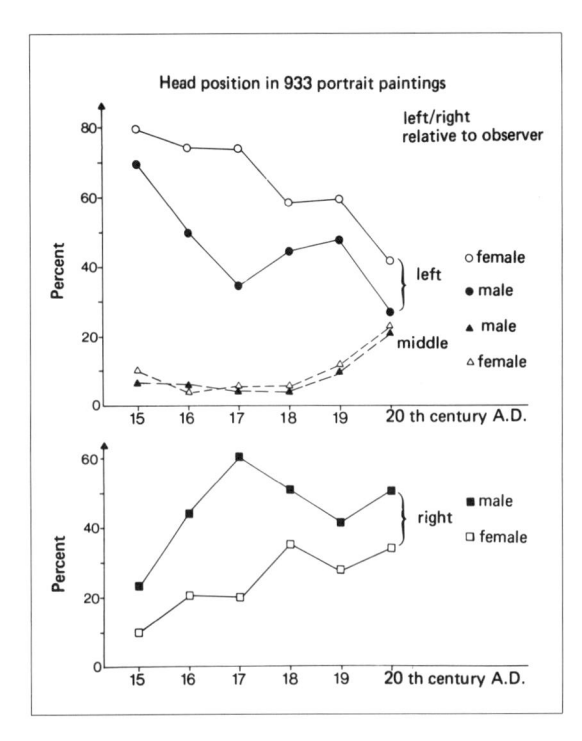

Fig. 13. Head position in 933 portrait paintings. Same data as in Fig. 10b. Separate data for male and female portraits. Note that the historical trend over 6 centuries from an initial left-sided preference to a right-sided preference is evident, but female portraits display the left facial half more often than male portraits during all centuries.

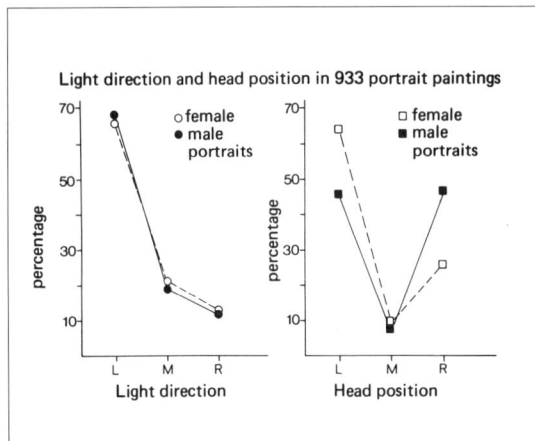

Fig. 14. Light direction and head position in portrait paintings. The data from Fig. 10 are pooled. The left-sided preference for light direction is independent of the gender of the portrayed subject, while the head position depends on the gender of the portrayed subject. In male portraits, left and right head position are about equally frequent, while in female portraits a strong left-sided dominance is found.

Fig.18a–f). In Cranach's portrait paintings, a left head-position bias is found in female portraits, a right bias in male portraits (again left and right as seen from the observer). Cranach preferred to place the light source on the side toward which the portrayed person turned his or her head.

Since we suspected that the light direction preferred by an artist could depend on the handedness (or the hand used for painting), we compared light

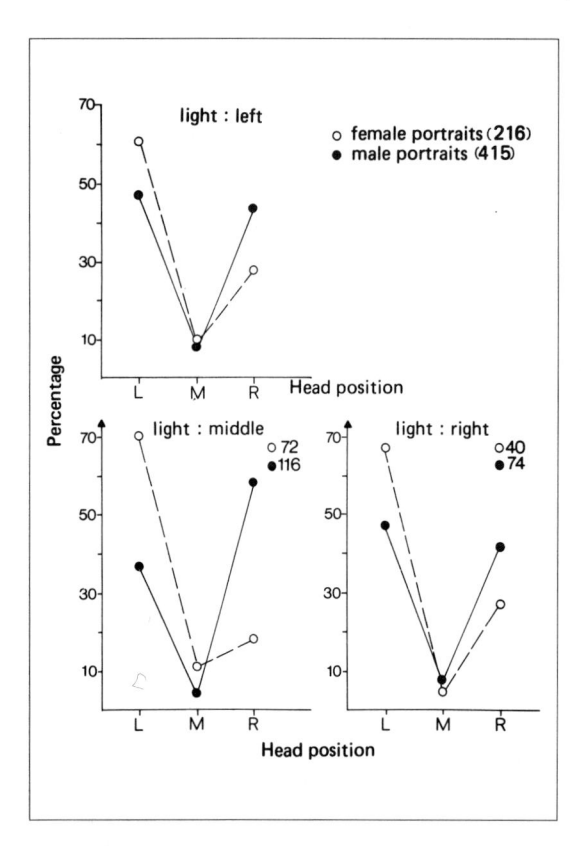

Fig. 15. Effect of light direction on the distribution of head position in male and female portrait paintings. Data of Figs. 11 and 13 are pooled.

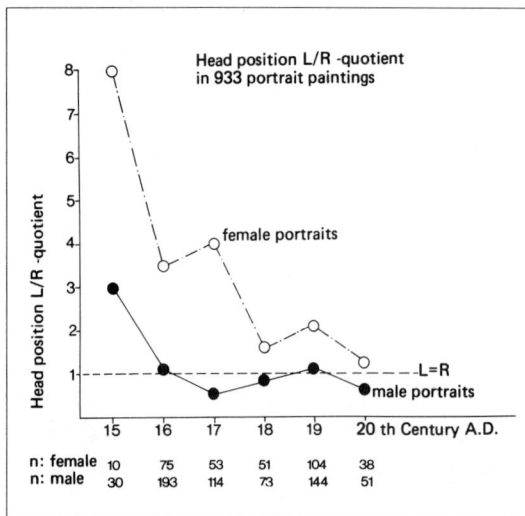

Fig. 16. Left/right quotient of head position found in 933 female and male portrait paintings is plotted as a function of time *(abscissa)*. The decline in left-sided preference with time and the difference between male and female portraits is visible. Data over three centuries show a right-sided preference in head position for male portraits while, taken over all centuries, female portraits have a left-sided preference.

direction, head position, and gender of the subject in portraits of the right-handed Lucas Cranach the Elder and the left-handed Hans Holbein the Younger, who most likely drew only with his left hand.[46,72-76] The two artists lived at about the same time, attained similar eminence, and are comparable with respect to their educational, religious, and cultural backgrounds. Figure 18 summarizes the data of light direction and head position in Holbein's general paintings and drawings, portrait paintings, and portrait drawings. A comparison of these data with the same analysis performed for Cranach's paintings revealed a statistically significant shift in light direction to the right for paintings and drawings of Hans Holbein (compare Figs. 17c and 18c), while the head position of male and female portraits painted by Holbein does not deviate considerably from the general statistical distribution of his time (compare Figs. 12 and 18b). A marked difference in the correlations of light direction and head position in the paintings of Cranach and Holbein is evident: Lucas Cranach preferred light from the direction towards which the head was turned, whereas Holbein varied the head position and light direction more freely so that the light frequently fell onto the face from the opposite side to that in which the head was turned. In addition, the fronto-parallel head position (middle), which is rare or even absent in Cranach's portrait paintings (Fig. 17b), is found in a number of the Holbein portraits. In comparing Holbein's and Cranach's works and the statistics of head position and light

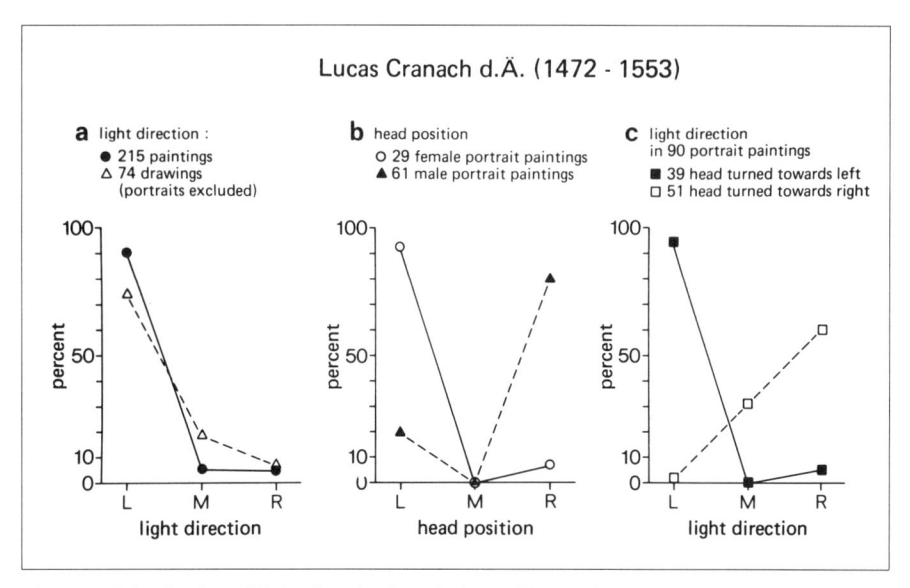

Fig. 17.a) Distribution of light direction in paintings of Lucas Cranach the Elder (b) Head position and portrait paintings of the same artist (c) Light direction in the portrait paintings related to head position

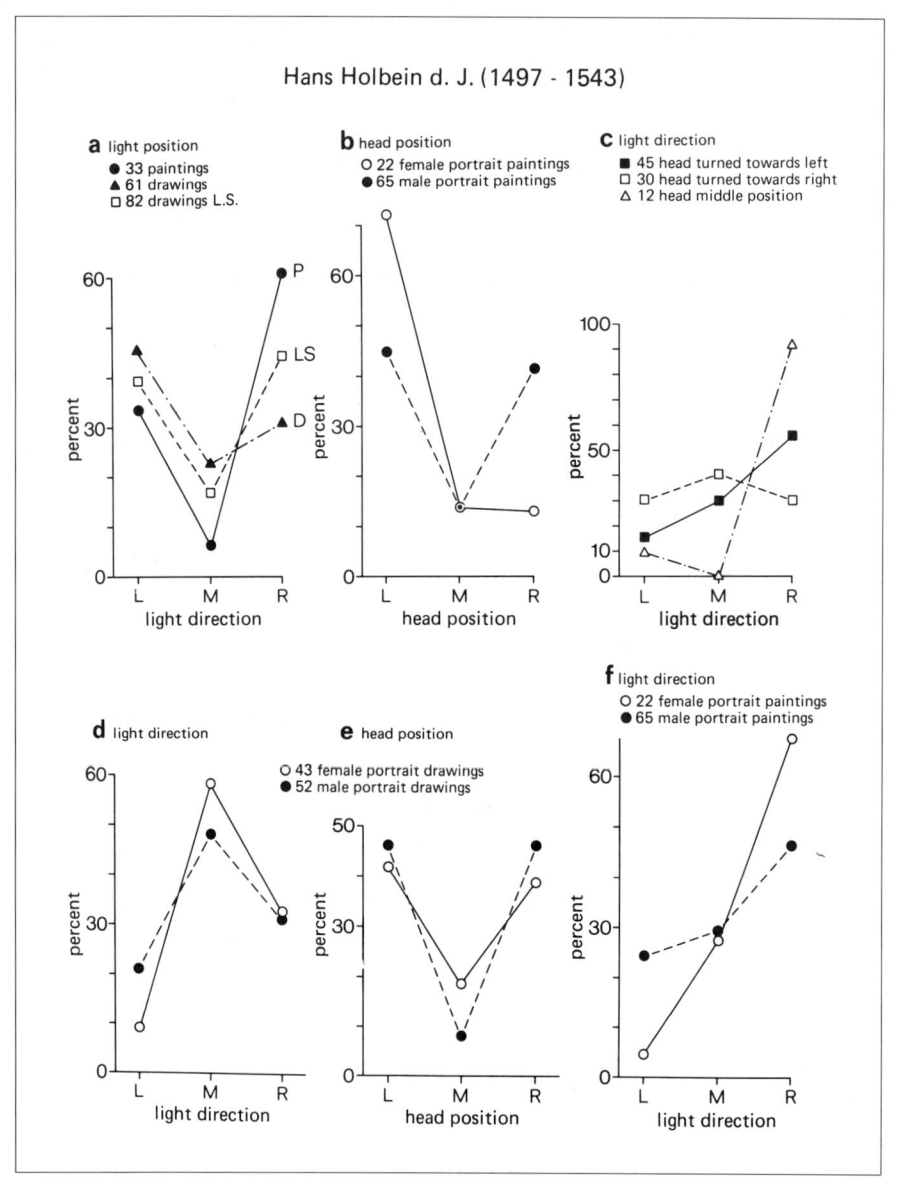

Fig. 18.a) Distribution of light direction in drawings (D) and paintings (P) of Hans Holbein the Younger; LS are the marginal drawings for the book *Laus stultitiae* of Erasmus of Rotterdam (b) Head position in male and female portrait paintings (c) Light direction as a function of head position (d) Light direction in female and male portrait drawings (e) Head position in male and female portrait drawings (f) Light direction in male and female portrait paintings. Note the difference in the distributions (a), (b), and (c) for the left-hander Hans Holbein as compared to the same distributions in the works of art of the right-hander Lucas Cranach (Fig. 17a–c). Data obtained from the reproductions in Ganz[72–74]

direction in other paintings of their time, one gains the impression that Holbein's left-handed drawings and paintings led to a significant increase in right-sided light direction. As mentioned, a similar tendency was found in the drawings of Leonardo da Vinci.

Conclusions

We have discussed some examples supporting the hypothesis that the genetically determined left-right asymmetry of the brain is functionally modified by experience. Experience may reinforce dominance, as is the case in a right-hander's writing with his right hand. Experience, however, may also counteract hemispheric dominance, as when a left-hander learns to write with his right hand. We discussed the possibility that, during the early weeks of life, a functional left-right asymmetry of the brain is modified further by the left-sided bias of the mother-child holding pattern, which again might be, in part, genetically determined. We suggest – without direct proof – that this early experience in life may also contribute to a perceptual left-right bias, which could have some influence in later years on a corresponding left-right bias in the production and perception of art.

In the visual arts, the direction of light in paintings and drawings is biased towards the left side (with respect to the observer). However, in addition to this probably biological tendency, which also depends on the handedness of the artist, a strong historical effect could be demonstrated by a statistical analysis of paintings originating in different periods of Western art. Since the probability that this historical trend is caused by some change in the genetic code is practically nil, the impact of experiential factors and (unconscious) historical tendencies becomes all the more obvious.

A further left-right bias in the visual arts appeared in the statistics regarding head position in portrait paintings. Portrait painting in Western art commenced with an overall strong preference for a left-sided head position of the subject (from the observer's perspective). During the fifteenth to seventeenth centuries, the portrayed subjects thus have a stronger tendency to show the emotional left half of his or her face to the observer (or to the painter) rather than the official right half. This left-sided preference is significantly stronger in female portraits throughout all periods of Western art and is apparently not dependent on the handedness of the artist. Nevertheless, when average data for the fifteenth to twentieth centuries were plotted as a function of time, a strong historical effect on head position was found: the left-sided preference decreased with time, which led in contemporary portrait painting to an overall right-sided preference in portraits of men (but not of women). The strong interaction of head position and gender of the portrayed subject is not paralleled by light direction and gender, although a slight relation of head position and light direction is present in the overall data. In individual painters, however, a marked head-position/light-direction correlation could be detected, leading to an apparent light-direction and gender interaction. Two examples were selected from painters of the early 16th century, one right-handed (Lucas Cranach the Elder) and the other left-handed (Hans Holbein the Younger). Significant differences were found in the paintings and drawings of both painters, who were, on the basis of their reputation at that time and the opinion of later art historians, at about the same high artistic niveau.

Another left-sided preference in paintings and sculptures, which is also based on a "biological," i.e., a genetically induced preference, indicates a strong historical influence as well:[18,19] statistical analysis of the mother-child holding patterns in Western art (sculptures and paintings) exhibited a major left-sided dominance in works from 1900 B.C. to the fourteenth century A.D.. This left-sided dominance decreased with time, and during the fifteenth and sixteenth centuries, no left-sided or right-sided dominance was present, on the average, in the pooled material, while a specific side for the child could still be preferred by a given artist or school. After the sixteenth century, however, the initial left-sided dominance reappeared. The historical trend was found to be closely parallel in paintings and sculptures and, in our opinion, depicts another historical modification of the left-right asymmetry in works of art. The increase in artistic freedom and experimentation in Western art achieved during the Renaissance was certainly a factor that modified "natural" left-right asymmetries.

For the art historian, these data on left-right asymmetries in works of art are undoubtedly elementary in comparison to the complex and sophisticated analysis usually applied and, perhaps, of relatively little interest. But in a neurobiological context, they are remarkable! For a neurologist in search of a possible neurobiological basis for elementary rules of aesthetic perception and performance, such a simple data analysis could help to explain the different contributions of the left and right hemisphere of the artist's or connoisseur's brain to the production or enjoyment of works of art.

In music as well, a functional left-right brain asymmetry seems to play an important role. Harmony, timbre, and tonality seem to be predominantly hemispheric functions, while the rhythm of music (as meter in poetry) appears to be lateralized in the left-hemispheric speech region. This functional left-right hemispheric bias may be the reason why the leading first violinists in Western orchestras are usually seated on the left side, i.e., on the side of the listeners' and conductors' extrapersonal space that is processed primarily by the right hemisphere. A more direct access to the right-hemispheric, temporal lobe regions involved in the analysis of melody and harmony is the consequence, since the left extrapersonal space is represented in the right half of the brain.

We are, of course, aware that general cultural development, tradition, and individual training during childhood and adolescence are very important factors in shaping the individual genius of an artist as well as the connoisseur's perceptual sensitivity. Although the genetically preprogrammed structural and functional asymmetry of the human brain may be modified during the early periods of life, it still forms another important determinant of human behavior. Some of these left-right brain asymmetries are reflected in such sophisticated structures as works of art and in such complex processes as the perception of art. We hope that the simple studies and hypotheses presented here may contribute to further integrative concepts and an understanding of the interplay between the human brain and the culture of mankind.

Acknowledgements

This work was supported in part by the Deutsche Forschungsgemeinschaft (Gr 161). We thank Mrs. B. Krawczynski and Mr. M. Winzer for their help in producing the figures, Mr. P. Holzner for the photographic reproductions, Mrs. B. Hauschild for careful typing of the manuscript in its different versions, and Mrs. J. Dames for her valuable assistance in the English translation. The manuscript was revised while the senior author held an Akademiestipendium of the Volkswagen Foundation.

References and Notes

1. Bradshaw JL, Nettleton NC (1981) The nature of hemispheric specialization in man. The Behavioral and Brain Sciences 4:51–91
2. Denenberg VH (1981) Hemispheric laterality in animals and the effect of early experience. Behavioral and Brain Sciences 4:1–49
3. Wada JA, Clarke R, Hamm A (1975) Cerebral hemispheric asymmetry in humans. Arch Neurol 32:239–246
4. Penfield W, Rasmussen T (1957) The cerebral cortex of man: A clinical study of localization. MacMillan, New York
5. Teuber HL (1975) Effects of focal brain injury on human behavior. In: Tower DB (ed) The nervous system. The clinical neurosciences, vol 2. Raven, New York, pp 457–480
6. Hécaen H, Albert ML (1978) Human neuropsychology. Wiley, New York
7. Springer SP, Deutsch G (1981) Left brain, right brain. W.H. Freeman, San Francisco

8. Bryden NP (1982) Laterality. Functional asymmetry in the intact brain. Academic, New York
9. Springer SP, Searleman A (1978) The ontogeny of hemispheric specialization: Evidence from dichotic listening in twins. Neuropsychology 16:269–281
10. Experimental amblyopia is a severe reduction in visual acuity and recognition ability of the temporarily deprived eye.
11. Freeman RD (ed) (1979) Developmental neurobiology of vision. Plenum, New York
12. Hyvarinen J (1982) The parietal cortex of monkey and man. Springer, Berlin
13. Gregory RL (1971) The intelligent eye. Weidenfeld and Nicolson, London
14. Molineux W (1693) Letter to J. Locke. In: Locke J (1664) An essay concerning human understanding. Book II, chapter IX, 8. Reprint in: Burtt EA (1939) The English philosophers from Bacon to Mill. Modern Library, New York, p 274
15. Darwin E (1794/1796) Zoonomia; or the laws of organic life, vol I/II. J. Johnson, London, p 568 and p 722. Reprint 1974, AMS Press, New York, pp 145–146
16. Salk L (1973) The role of the heartbeat in relation between mother and infant. Scientific American 228 (5):24–29
17. Richards JL, Finger S (1975) Mother-child holding patterns: A cross-cultural photographic survey. Child Development 46:1001–1004
18. Grüsser O-J, Grüsser-Cornehls U (1982) Mother-child holding patterns, a study of Western art. Congr Intern de Paléontologie Humaine. Résumé des Communications, 213 p
19. Grüsser O-J (1983) Mother-child holding patterns in Western art: A developmental study. Ethology and Sociobiology 4:89–94
20. Drawing of a photograph in the catalogue: Karouzou S (1982) National Museum Athens. Ekdotike Athenon, p 16
21. Salk L (1960) The effects of the normal heartbeat sound on the behavior of the newborn infant: Implications for mental health. World Mental Health 12:168–175
22. Salk L (1962) Mother's heartbeat as an imprinting stimulus. Transactions of the New York Academy of Science, ser 2, 24:753–763
23. Weiland IH (1964) Heartbeat rhythm and maternal behavior. J Amer Acad Child Psychiatry 3:161–164
24. Mehler J, Bertoncini J, Barriere N, Jassik-Gerschenfeld D (1978) Infant recognition of mother's voice. Perception 7:491–497
25. DeCasper AJ, Fifer WP (1980) Of human bonding: Newborns prefer their mothers' voices. Science 208:1174–1176
26. Alegria J, Noirot E (1981) Neonate orientation behaviour towards human voice. Intern J Behavior Develop 1:291–312
27. Hécaen H (1981) The neurophysiology of face recognition. In: Davies G, Ellis H, Shepherd J (eds) Perceiving and remembering faces. Academic, New York, p 39–54
28. Perret DJ, Rolls ET, Caan W (1982) Visual neurones responsive to faces in the temporal cortex. Exp Brain Res 47:329–342
29. Perrett DJ, Smith PAJ, Potter DB, Mistlin AJ, Head AS, Miller AG, Jeeves MA (1984) Neurones responsive to faces in the temporal cortex: Studies of functional organization, sensitivity to identity and relation to perception. Human Neurobiology 3:197–208
30. Rolls ET (1984) Neurons in the cortex of the temporal lobe and the amygdala of the monkey with responses selective for faces. Human Neurobiology 3:209–222
31. Desimone R, Albright TD, Gross C, Bruce C (1984) Stimulus selective properties of inferior temporal neurons in the macaque. J Neuroscience 4:2051–2059
32. Bötzel K, Grüsser O-J (1988) Electrical brain potentials evoked by pictures of faces and

non-faces. A search for "face-specific" EEG-potentials. Experimental Brain Research (in press)
33. Ahrens R (1954) Beitrag zur Entwicklung des Physiognomie- und Mimikerkennens. Z Exp Angew Psychol 2:412–454; 599–633
34. Spitz RA (1967) Vom Säugling zum Kleinkind. Naturgeschichte der Mutter-Kind-Beziehung im ersten Lebensjahr. Klett, Stuttgart
35. Carey S (1981) The development of face perception. In: Davies G, Ellis H, Shepherd J (eds) Perceiving and remembering faces. Academic, New York, p 9–38
36. Yarbus AL (1967) Eye movements and vision. Plenum, New York
37. Sackheim HA, Gur RC (1978) Lateral asymmetry in intensity of emotional expression. Neuropsychologia 16:473–481
38. Sackheim HA, Gur RC, Saucy MC (1978) Emotions are expressed more intensely on the left side of the face. Science 202:434–436
39. Campbell R (1978) Asymmetries in interpreting and expressing a posed facial expression. Cortex 14:327–342
40. Heller W, Levy J (1981) Perception and expression of emotion in right-handers and left-handers. Neuropsychologia 19:263–272
41. Buchtel H, Campari F, Riso C de, Rota R (1978) Hemispheric difference in the discrimination reaction time to facial expression. Ital J Psychol 5:159–169
42. Grüsser O-J (1984) Face recognition within the reach of neurobiology and beyond it. Human Neurobiology 3:183–190
43. Davies G, Ellis H, Shepherd J (eds) (1981) Perceiving and remembering faces. Academic, London, p 392
44. Zynda B (1984) Über das Wiedererkennen von Gesichtern. Thesis, Freie Universität, Berlin
45. Grüsser O-J, Selke T, Zynda B (1985) A developmental study of face recognition in children and adolescents. Human Neurobiology 4:33–39
46. Jung R (1977) Über Zeichnungen linkshändiger Künstler von Leonardo bis Klee: Linkshändermerkmale als Zuschreibungskriterien. In: "Semper attentus," Beiträge für Heinz Götze zum 8.8.1977. Springer, Berlin, p 190–218
47. Reynolds DM, Jeeves MA (1978) A developmental study of hemisphere specialization for recognition of faces in normal subjects. Cortex 14:511–520
48. Kraft H (1982) Die Kopffüßler – Psychologie und Psychopathologie der bildnerischen Gestaltung. Hippokrates, Stuttgart
49. Kraft H (1983) Kopffüßler: Ein transkulturelles Phänomen. Deutsches Ärzteblatt 80:63–66
50. Kussmaul F (1982) Ferne Völker – frühe Zeiten. Kunstwerke aus dem Linden-Museum Stuttgart. Staatliches Museum für Völkerkunde, vol I. A Bongers, Recklinghausen
51. Kerner J (1857) Kleksographien. In: Gesammelte Werke, vol I. A Weichert, Berlin
52. Rorschach H (1941) Psychodiagnostik. Methodik und Ergebnisse eines wahrnehmungsdiagnostischen Experiments (Deutenlassen von Zufallsformen), 4th edn. H.Huber, Bern
53. Müller J (1826) Über die phantastischen Gesichtserscheinungen. Eine physiologische Untersuchung mit einer physiologischen Urkunde des Aristoteles über den Traum. J.Hölscher, Coblenz
54. Berndl K, Dewitz W, Grüsser O-J, Kiefer RH (1986) A test movie to study elementary abilities in perception and recognition of mimic and gestural expression. Eur Arch Psychiatr Neurol Sci 235:276–281
55. Berndl K, Cranach M von, Grüsser O-J (1986) Impairment of perception and recogni-

tion of faces, mimic expression and gestures in schizophrenic patients. Eur Arch Psychatr Neurol Sci 235:282–291
56. Berndl K, Grüsser O-J, Martin M, Remschmidt H (1986) Comparative studies on recognition of faces, mimic and gestures in adolescent and middle-aged schizophrenic patients. Eur Arch Psychiatr Neurol Sci 236:123–130
57. Dewdney D (1973) A specific distortion of the human facial percept in childhood schizophrenia. Psychiat Quart 47:82–94
58. Berndl K, Grüsser O-J (1986) Wahrnehmungsstörungen bei Schizophrenen. Beeinträchtigung des Erkennens und Wiedererkennens von Gesichtern, Mimik und Gestik bei jugendlichen und erwachsenen Kranken. Münch Med Wochenschr 128:768–773
59. Schreber DB (1902) Denkwürdigkeit eines Nervenkranken. Reprint in: Bürgerliche Wahnwelten um Neunzehnhundert. Focus, Wiesbaden, 1972
60. Prinzhorn H (1968) Bildnerei der Geisteskranken. Springer, Berlin
61. Wada JA, Rasmussen T (1960) Intracarotid injection of sodium amytal for the lateralization of cerebral speech dominance. J Neurosurg 17:266–282
62. Borchgrevink HM (1977) Cerebral lateralization of speech and singing after intracarotid amytal injection. Neuropsychologia 15: 186–191
63. Wölfflin H (1941) Über das Rechts und Links im Bilde. In: Gedanken zur Kunstgeschichte. Schwabe, Basel, p 82–90
64. Gaffron M (1950) Left and right in pictures. Art Quarterly 13:312–331
65. Levy J (1976) Lateral dominance and aesthetic preference. Neuropsychologia 14: 431–445
66. Barash M (1978) Light and colour in Renaissance theory of art. New York University Press, New York
67. Kraus TH, Matt L von (1977) Pompeji und Herkulaneum. Dumont, Köln
68. Clark K (1969) The drawings of Leonardo da Vinci in the collection of Her Majesty the Queen at Windsor Castle, 2nd edn. Phaidon, London
69. Carlevaris P (1887) Disegni di Leonardo da Vinci della Biblioteca di Santa Maria Torino
70. Piumati G (1894–1904) Il Codice Atlantico di Leonardo da Vinci della Biblioteca Ambrosiana Milan. Milano
71. Gombrich EH (1982) The image and the eye. Further studies in the psychology of pictorial representation. Phaidon, Oxford
72. Ganz P (1910) Die Handzeichnungen Hans Holbein des Jüngeren. J.Bard, Leipzig
73. Ganz P (1912) Hans Holbein der Jüngere. Des Meisters Gemälde. Deutsche Verlagsanstalt, Stuttgart
74. Ganz P (1950) Hans Holbein der Jüngere. Phaidon, Köln
75. Friedländer MJ, Rosenberg J (1932) Die Gemälde von Lucas Cranach. Deutscher Verein für Kunstwissenschaft, Berlin
76. Rosenberg J (1960) Die Zeichnungen Lucas Cranach d.Ä. Deutscher Verein für Kunstwissenschaft, Berlin
77. After we had finished the manuscript, two publications by H.-J. Hufschmidt (see references 78 and79) came to our attention, in which extensive statistical analyses were presented, including, besides Western paintings, drawings, and sculptures, works of art of the Assyrian, Egyptian, and Sumerian cultures. Hufschmidt found a strong right-sided (left/right with respect to the observer) tendency in the turning direction of the head before the early Greek period, which he could trace back to Stone Age cave drawings. Since a preference for left profile direction had been found from the classical Greek period to modern paintings and drawings, Hufschmidt concluded that this profile shift occurred "simultaneously with an ac-

celeration of intellectual and cultural development which also influenced our present culture." As a cause for this shift, he discussed a "hypothetical change in dominance of the cerebral hemisphere for higher visual perception from the left hemisphere to the right hemisphere." In analyzing the drawings and paintings of 55 painters from the 14th to the 20th centuries (6162 portrait paintings and drawings), Hufschmidt found that 44 preferred a left-turning head position. He also noted that some of the left-handed painters tended to favor a head position towards the right. In addition, Hufschmidt remarked that head position towards the left or the right was dependent on the gender of the portrayed subject, but he did not relate the changes in the left-right tendency quantitatively to the time of origin. Another interesting finding in Hufschmidt's analyses of sketches and drawings should also be mentioned. He found that in right-handed painters a strong tendency exists to elaborate more carefully on the left side of a sketch. Furthermore, painters as well as laymen with no particular instruction in painting are very much inclined to begin a drawing or a sketch on the left side of the sheet of paper. Hufschmidt provided some evidence with regards to the left-handed Leonardo da Vinci that the reverse was true.

78. Hufschmidt HJ (1980) Das Rechts-Links-Profil im kulturhistorischen Längsschnitt. Arch Psychiatr Nervenkr 229: 17–43
79. Hufschmidt HJ (1983) Über die Linksorientierung der Zeichnung und die optische Dominanz der rechten Hirnhemisphäre. Z Kunstgesch 46: 287–294

Part V
The Essence and the Appearance

The Aesthetic Significance of Display
Some Examples from Papua New Guinea

Andrew Strathern
*University of Pittsburgh, Department of Anthropology, Pittsburgh,
Pa 15260, USA*

Introduction

Aesthetics has to do with a union of perception and feeling, biology with the nature of organisms and their survival within the environment. Why should there be a link between these apparently disparate spheres? The reason is quite straightforward: part of the process whereby organisms adapt and survive is by display, and it is in display that we find the initial lineaments of aesthetic construction and response. Materials from two societies of the Papua New Guinea Highlands, where I have been working since 1964, can be used to demonstrate this clearly. For the anthropologist, one interest in these materials lies in the unity they exhibit between meaning and function, or, to put it another way, between aesthetics and biology.

Discussions in anthropology on the relationship between culture and biology are old established. They have often taken on the mantle of political disputes, as in arguments over the "innate intelligence" of ethnic groups or the plasticity of forms of domination. These disputes are relatively unproductive because of the polarised positions they entail: that *either* nature *or* nurture is the important thing that determines how societies and individuals behave. In their efforts to carve out a legitimate domain of enquiry, anthropologists have, perhaps, been too anxious to argue for the primacy of culture over nature. But the argument is two-edged, because culture is itself a product of human evolution, and, reciprocally, human evolution has been profoundly affected by the development of cultural patterns. These patterns have, of course, meaning for the people who maintain them; they also have long-term biological significance.

An example outside of the sphere of aesthetics is provided by the Highlands societies of Papua New Guinea, where there is often a traditional rule against sexual intercourse while a mother is still breast-feeding her baby. The explanation given by the natives is that if intercourse takes place, the man's semen will spoil the mother's milk, and the child will drink this and become sickly or even die. The idea, therefore, is to protect the health of the child, thus enhancing the likelihood that it will prosper. If a child does not thrive, it is rumoured that the parents must have broken the rule of abstinence. Men contract polygamous marriages if they can, thus gaining further sexual outlets to counteract the effect of this strict postpartum taboo. There is a clear complex of culturally established practices and ideas here. The underlying biological consequences are equally apparent. The taboo actually functions to ensure the better growth of children and to enhance the probability of their survival. This example shows a parallel with the discussion on aesthetics which follows. The meaning of the postpartum taboo is intimately linked with important social values, and these values, in turn, have an obviously biological dimension.

The major context in which aesthetic judgements are made by Highlanders is the dance ceremony, during which participants are elaborately decorated. The aim of this decoration is to enhance the person, and make him or her attractive or in some respects frightening. Successful self-decoration is also a kind of sign of ancestral favour and, therefore, a guarantee of good health and fertility in the future. This is exemplified in certain cult dances, in which the men's decorations are said to be the sign of a female spirit, which is worshiped precisely because she brings fertility, the increase of pig herds, and the birth of male children to the cult celebrants' wives. The spectators who watch these ceremonies make evaluative comments, which we can recognize as "aesthetic." They criticise dancers who move awkwardly or in disharmony with the others, singing which is off-key or in bad time, and decorative plumes which are moth-eaten and dull looking.

Thus far, we might be describing a kind of disembodied artistic judgement, but such would be very far from the truth. In fact, all of these judgements add up to negative signs: the group will fail to impress others with its strength because it lacks the necessary spiritual support to do so, and any individual whose performance is particularly poor is the prime target for the magical powers of enemy groups. If there are aesthetic judgements, these are embedded firmly in issues that the people consider to be more important than the aesthetics themselves. They involve the perpetuation and successful reproduction of groups of related kinsfolk. This is the key for both the biological and the cultural significance of display.

Social Structure

The peoples I have worked with in the Highlands region of Papua New Guinea are called the Melpa (sometimes spelled Metlpa or Medlpa) and the Wiru. Their languages belong to the New Guinea Highlands stock and share some 15 % of vocabulary cognates, but they are quite distinct and mutually unintelligible. The Melpa came under European influence in 1933, the Wiru not until the 1950s. Nevertheless, the impact of change on the Wiru people was severe: they lack much more of their traditional, precolonial culture than do the Melpa. However, in both areas it is possible to understand the mainsprings of their aesthetic ideas by examining how decorations are worn and evaluated at festivals.

The Melpa number some 100,000. They are divided into a number of tribes, the largest of which contain perhaps 7,000 members and the smallest, only a few hundred. It is apparent that this great disparity in sizes is a result of patterns of warfare up to 1933, of differential access to fertile land, and of the hazards of sickness at varying altitudes. It is not possible to state the relationship between these variables with precision: let it suffice to note that the concern for successful reproduction took shape in a distinctly competitive context and that the outcomes of this competition included the unequal sizes of the basic groups in the population as a whole.

Tribes, however, are not simple unitary groups. They are extensively divided into clans, subclans, and smaller lineage-like groups. What I call the "clan" here is marked by a rule of exogamy: marriage should be with someone of a different clan, although it may be within the same tribe. Marriage ties are also of the utmost importance in defining the way the society works, for a marriage is an alliance contracted with a view to creating and maintaining friendly exchange relations between the affines. In precolonial times, marriages tended to be contracted, therefore, to secure intergroup military support. To marry into the group of one's major military enemies could create many difficulties, for example, the danger of being poisoned by one's wife and the problem of how to maintain friendship with those who might sometime be fighting against one's own clansmen. With the colonial peace, these strained relationships relaxed. Marriages and their associated exchanges became more widely dispersed, but still not randomly so.

Within the clan, the strongest solidarity is to be found in the small "men's house groups" *(manga rapa)*. It is first from within these that leaders tend to emerge. These are men of the type which has become known in the anthropological literature as "big men." Characteristically, these leaders have a forceful character, are successful in exchanges of wealth, speak well, and have more than one wife. The basis of their power is their relative control over production as well as their ability to magnify this control by the manipulation of exchange partnerships. Their daily lifestyle is not very different from that of ordinary men. During festivals, their performance as leaders is displayed, judged, and reaffirmed – or lost. The big men were not necessarily combat leaders in the past, although they inevitably influenced decisions on whether to fight or not and the plans of how to conduct a war. They were also prominent as peacemakers because of the wealth they could command. This was because the only way to make peace was by arranging exchanges in compensation for deaths sustained in fighting. The large wealth presentation known as *moka* frequently evolved from such payments.

The items used for these presentations were pigs, cooked pork, and valuable shells, especially those known as pearl shells, which have a ruddly, yellow-to-orange surface much prized by the Melpa. (These shells are often described in English as goldlip shells. The Melpa term is *ken* or *kin*.) Since the early 1970s, the shells have been replaced by money, first Australian pounds, then dollars, and, since 1975, when Papua New Guinea became independent, by the kina, whose name actually derives from the Melpa term for pearl shell. The red-coloured five-kina note also features a Melpa shell mounted on a traditional backing of tree resin to enhance its size and moonlike shape. These symbolic features have facilitated the transition from pearl shells to cash while, at the same time, masking the profound economic changes that the transition has brought about.

The position of women in the Melpa society is such that it places them, in many ways, "in between" the kin group of their fathers and their husbands. They do not lose their natal identity, but their allegiances and interests should gradually switch over to their husbands' clans. This shift of allegiance is effected by the birth and growth of children. At the same time, ties with the mother's people remain strong throughout the person's lifetime and are the basis for regular exchanges of wealth. They form a fiduciary bedrock for exchanges between the groups thus linked in alliance.

This emphasis on ties with the mother's relatives is even more predominant among the Wiru people. The Wiru number some 20,000 persons, living on a grassy plain south of Mount Ialibu in the Southern Highlands Province of Papua New Guinea. Locality is very significant: people are known as much by their location as by their clan, because the ancestral origins tend to be scattered over more than one area. In each region one may find members of several different clans, but these are usually unified by historical alliances and, sometimes, by appeal to an overall group membership, as well. In the Tunda area, for example, the dominant group name is Peri, and sections of other large groups which belong to Tunda all identify themselves at one level as Peri, also, although they recognize that they have a different origin.

Intermarriage is possible and frequently takes place within the locality complex, and accusations of sorcery may also occur within the same group. The solidarity of the local group is thus vulnerable. Furthermore, there is no avoidance of marriage into enemy territories. This makes the Wiru social structure rather different from that of the Melpa.

Exchange relations at the individual level are ideologically insulated from the level of group enmity by the imperative that payment must be made for one's body and the body of one's children to the remaining family. Hence, there are exchanges with the mother's people, whether their localities are in a hostile relationship or not. In practical terms, of course, peaceful exchange is not possible if there is fighting, and in this way the imperative to exchange must have counteracted the pressure towards warfare. At pig-killing festivals, this interplay between hostility and friendship emerges clearly in the custom of making gifts that can "kill" the recipients. These are known as *poi mokora*. Pork is cut in an unusual way and presented to a visitor. He must not let it slip when he receives it in his hands, and he must not stumble when he walks off with it. If he does, this is a sign that the gift is "heavy" *(kenda)* to him and may cause him sickness or even death. The gift symbolizes poison.

Leadership is not so strongly accentuated among the Wiru as it is among the Melpa. The big-man syndrome is certainly present: leaders tend to be polygynists, controlling more female labor than other men and engaging more prominently in exchanges. They were often, moreover, vigorous fighters in precolonial times. Oratory and verbal manipulation are less stressed by the Wiru, and the spheres of influence of big men appear to be more narrow than among the Melpa. It is difficult to assess this point accurately, however, since Wiru social and cultural life has been interrupted traumatically by the colonial and postcolonial orders. Missions banned polygyny and treated cults as dangerous manifestations of satan worship. The administration took all responsibility for judging cases or wrongdoing away from the big men and forced both men and women to work on new projects, such as road building. The power of the big men had already been weakened considerably by 1967, when I first began to work in the Wiru area, and it has never been fully restored. Some of the pressures have eased, however. For example, the demands of road work are no longer so pressing. In an effort to preserve their influence, big men have also thrown themselves into the competition for government positions of authority, especially the positions of councillor and village court magistrate.

The effect of the missions is very striking throughout the Pangia area. Everywhere there are churches, pastors, and congregations, amounting to a structural as well as a cultural overlay on the original society. In terms of decorations, women's lifestyles seem to have been most profoundly altered. Women do not decorate themselves much and almost universally desire baptism and church membership. Self-decoration is regarded as sinful. Yet imitating Europeans by wearing dresses and blouses is thought to be correct. As one woman put it, "We are always trying to be just like white women, and we forget what our own customs were."

There is, therefore, a severe gap in my understanding of women's decorations amoung the Wiru, and I possess no early photographs from which a reconstruction could be undertaken. In the case of the Melpa, not only is there a rich set of photos available from the German ethnographies that were written in the 1930s, but also more of the traditional self-decoration survives today.

Decorations and Aesthetics

Self-decoration in both societies tends to be public and ritualised. It follows established cultural norms and is worn for social occasions, when the aim is specifically to impress spectators. These spectators critically evaluate the performance, and it is in this evaluation that aesthetic judgements are embodied.

The Melpa

A description of all the items worn for decoration and their combinations would be lengthy and is unnecessary here. What is important to note is that these fall into three classes: valuable plumes obtained from birds of paradise, parrots, cockatoos, eagles, and other brightly colored birds; valuable shells, such as pearl shells, baler, green-snail, cowrie, and nassa; and facial decoration, predominantly with red, white, black, yellow, and blue paints or with oil. The oil is either obtained from pig fat or is a type of sweet-smelling tree oil traded into the Hagen area from the Southern Highlands Province. Bright leaves are also used – yellow and red crotons or chalky-white leaves of the mara tree. In addition, men wear a wig made out of human hair arranged on a framework and padded with teasles (a prickly herb whose flower head is covered with stiff hooked bracts). The most popular shape for this wig is that of a horn, and the top edges are often embellished with tufts of white feathers or pieces of cotton wool. Glass beads are also worn in loops around the neck, particularly by women. Men wear a strip of cane slats, called the *omak,* on their chest suspended from the neck (Fig. 1). The *omak* is an out-of-date status symbol. It indicates the number of times a man has participated in exchanges with the valuable pearl shell: each slat represents a set of eight or ten shells given away. Since the 1970s, these cane strips have ceased to grow in length, and they now indicate a frozen or archaic status once achieved by their wearers in an activity which is now defunct. Women also sometimes wear the *omak,* one given them by a male relative (father or brother).

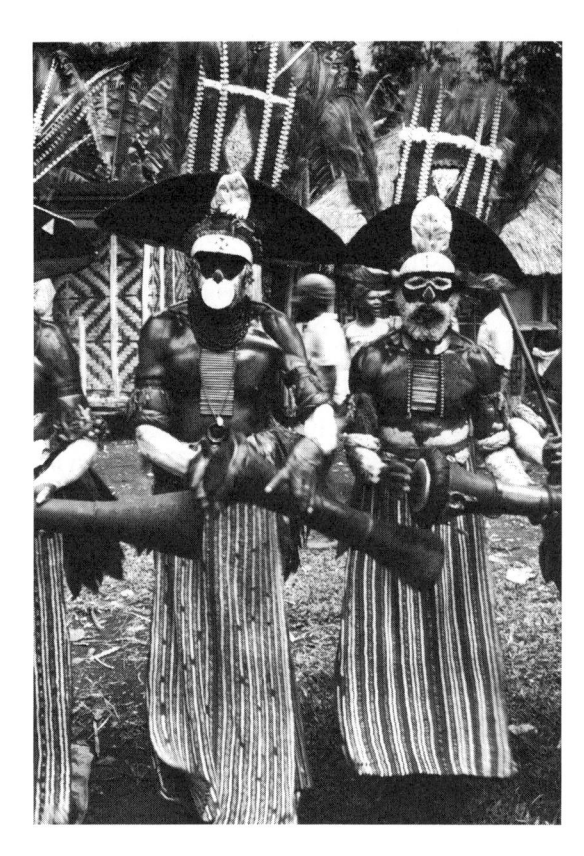

Fig. 1. Melpa dancers wearing *omaks* (strips of cane slats) suspended from their necks

Values associated with these items include the three categories of plumes, shells, and paint. One aim is that the decoration should shine and appear bright or new, another is that the wearer should appear to have "a good skin," a third is to disguise the wearer and to make him appear not bright but dark, and a fourth is to associate the wearers with the actual birds and animals whose feathers and skins are worn. The face-paint contributes both its colours to the overall design and acts as a kind of disguise for the wearers. It also acts as a gender marker. Women and girls wear a base of red face-paint, whereas men wear a base of black charcoal.

These contrasts between bright and dull, between self-display and disguise, and between red and black as colours form the dominant code, whereby decorations convey their meanings to the spectators. Let us reconsider these contrasting attributes in detail: First, bright versus dull can be applied to a set of decorations regardless of their specific colours or combinations of colours. To say that someone's decorations are dull implies an aesthetic judgement equivalent to saying that the items worn are old and worn out or appear so to the spectators. The reason is not simply that the items are literally old and faded, but rather that the ancestral ghosts have not given their proper support for the occasion, and, hence, the decorations seem dull and unworthy. The material and the symbolic intersect very strongly here. If a group is not, in fact, strong and wealthy, it simply does not obtain fine decorations and, therefore, will be said to lack the necessary ancestral support.

What we regard as material and as symbolic dimensions are not understood in this dichotomous way by the Melpa. They form an unbroken circle of influence, in which it is pointless to say that one aspect is more important than another. The specific comment which is made about men with dull decorations is that one of them will die, *ti kawa ndomba,* one will fall out of the line. This could be the effect of losing the support of the ancestors, for these also protect one against the fatal magic of enemies. Or it may be that there has been actual wrongdoing and dissension within the performing group. Their own internal conflict and anger, *popokl*, will then prevent their self-presentation as a united group from being successful, and this shows in the lack of uniformity in their headdresses, in their inability to sing and dance in time, etc. – all matters which attract swift and pointed judgements from those who watch their dance. In July 1982, I recorded a ceremonial song at a dancing ground some miles away from my home base. My own clansmen were very critical of the singing when they heard the recording, and our leader remarked, "it is like a foolish man wandering by a riverside and singing to himself," meaning that the singers were out of unison, and each seemed to be going his own way. I did not doubt his judgement, but I could not pretend that I could hear the lack of synchrony as well as the Melpa.

The assessment of performance is not limited to the decorations worn but also extends to the songs and drum beating, the dance rhythm, to the actual wealth given away to exchange partners, and to the execution of the ceremonial speeches, in which the reasons for the occasion are recited, reshaped and highlighted. Just as decorations should be bright and new, making it easy to see and evaluate them, so should the singing and drumbeating be clear. Hour-glass drums are used, and their sound is said to imitate the call of the blue bird of paradise (Prince Rudolph's bird of paradise). This is said to be loud and booming and can be heard across valleys and over hilltops. The drums likewise should be loud; they should be *oip,* and spectators should be drawn to the dancing ground by the sound of them. When a drum is hollowed out by fire, a bluebird-of-paradise feather is thrown through it by a ritual expert to make it sound like the bird itself. In this example, we see how birds of paradise serve as markers of desired qualities, and this brings us to the topic of self-display versus disguise.

Male birds of paradise display their plumage to attract females, and a single male will attempt to attract more than one female in competition with other males. Typically, they clear a space for themselves to dance in the foliage of a tree, pecking away the leaves so that they can be seen in the sunlight. The Melpa call this space the bird's ceremonial ground, comparing it to their own dancing sites, which they lay out in front of a big man's house. The birds also call out to potential mates, advertising their presence, just as the men sing in accompaniment to their dances. As this parallel between men and birds is illustrated, we can see its implication – that the male dancers are trying to attract females and, in so doing, are implicitly in competition with one another. It must be remembered, however, that the parallel represents only one metaphorical component of the meaning of the men's dance, which also carries other meanings. What it reveals is the *element* of sexual competition that enters into self-display. For this display, it is essential that the participants be recognisable as individuals, of course, but interest is also partly aroused by the fact that the decorations enhance and transform the person.

Actual courting dances often precede and run concurrently with the main public dances accompanying the transfer of wealth from one group to another. Only the unmarried boys and girls and some of the younger married men take part in these. The same categories of persons perform the secondary dances after the main dancing is over on the ceremonial ground, and in these the songs may become quite ribald and explicitly sexual, whereas the songs for the main dance are always group oriented and concerned with politics.

This counterpoint between main and secondary dances is mirrored in the contrast between disguise and display, which I mentioned above. The element of disguise is provided by the dark charcoal base that men wear on their faces. The black of the charcoal is said to cause "darkness," and they are said to look like their ancestors (*tipu rimbkö morom* "the spirit is all there"). The charcoal base was also worn in precolonial times when men went out to battle, and it has been worn in the post-independence bouts of warfare that occasionally break out. The aim is not only to disguise the wearer, but to make him look larger and, therefore, more frightening. Charcoal, then, represents two things: the anonymous solidarity of the male group and their associated aggressiveness towards outsiders. But these exhange ceremonies are also occasions for creating and reaffirming peace between groups. What are the elements that express this peacemaking? First, of course, there is the actual gift of wealth and the speeches which accompany it. But in the decorations, also the bright, glistening red, yellow, and white components stand out against the dark charcoal on the men's faces. These bright items stand both for wealth and for friendship. The term for friendship is the same as the term for porcine fat, which, when rubbed on the skin, gives it a glossy, oily look. Women wear a base of red ochre paint with bright yellow, blue, and white designs on top of it. Men have their eyes outlined in white and their noses in red or white. White

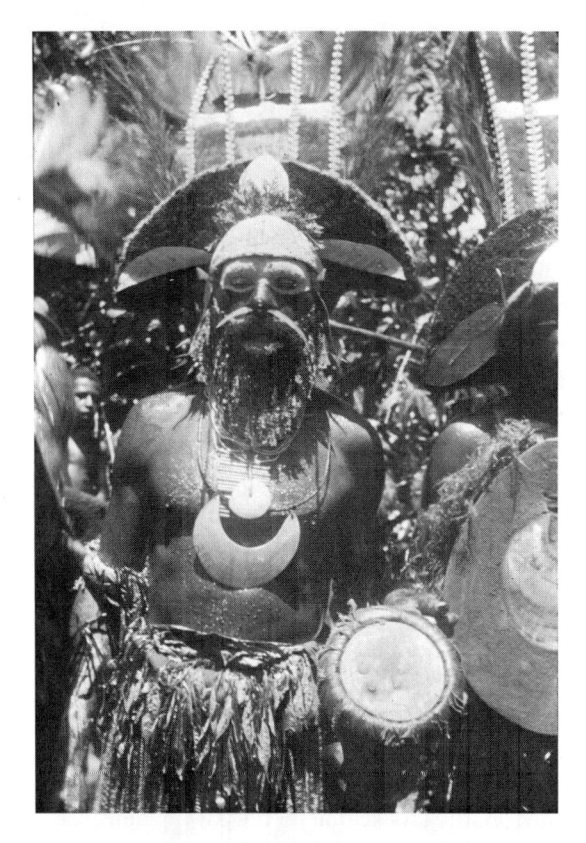

Fig. 2. Melpa dancers with *omak* and typical facial decoration (eyes and nose enhanced by white)

does not have an explicit meaning, but it is clear that it is analogous to the white of pig fat and the whitish colour of semen. It is, therefore, life giving and has to do with male fertility. All of these "signs" indicate the value of peacemaking because peace is associated with exchange, with marriage, with sexuality, and with the production of children. The group itself cannot be strong unless this aim is achieved, so the contrast between ingroup solidarity and external links is one that has to be transcended if the social system itself is to continue. The decorations are, therefore, a compact representation of values which are, at one level, contradictory but, at a higher level or organization, necessarily complementary. The successful union of these levels in a single display is what makes the display aesthetically pleasing in Melpa terms.

The Wiru

How much of this analysis of Melpa self-decoration also applies to the Wiru? We have already seen some of the similarities and differences in social structure between these two peoples. All the basic elements of display and disguise

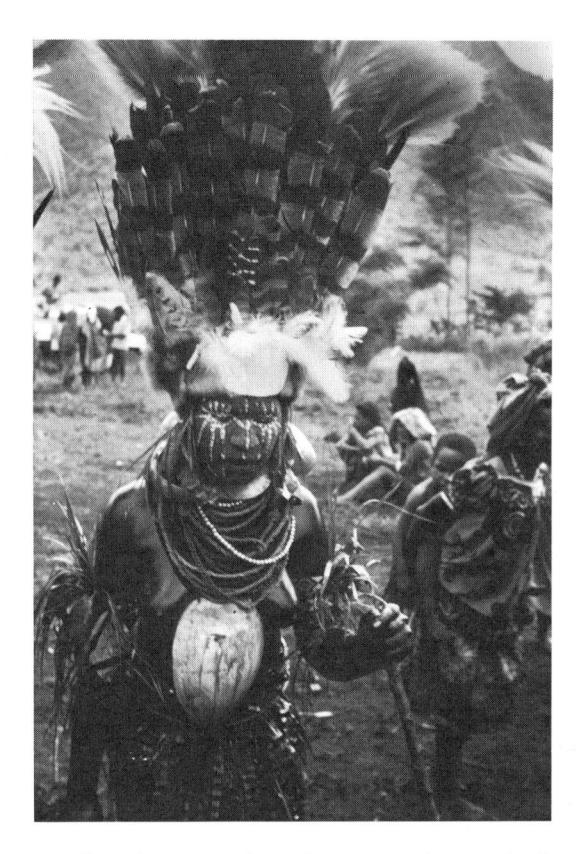

Fig. 3. Wiru woman with "teardrop" facial design and elaborate headdress

are found among the Wiru, e. g., the symbolic parallelism between men and birds, but the emphases and specific cultural meanings differ from those of the Melpa. In Melpa facial decoration, the designs have names, but these are not of particular cultural significance. They are not equated with the *persona* of the dancer. For example, one design is known as "teardrops," but wearing it does not signify that the person is sad.

In Wiru, however, facial designs are much more elaborated. Each one is given the name of a particular bird or, occasionally, a marsupial, so that the person's face as a whole resembles that of the creature in question. These are not necessarily birds of paradise, nor are these birds totemic to their wearers. Nevertheless, an explicit folk explanation is given for this use of bird names for facial decoration. Birds are said to "breed true," each generation bearing the same plumage markings as the previous generation. This reflects a concern of Wiru men – that their faces be transmitted over time within their group. Another illustration of this concern with perpetuation is the succession of names. Children of either sex may be called by names which recall those of deceased kinsfolk or periods of history, as when the group was surrounded and driven out by enemies. Predominantly, these names indicate sorrow over the deaths of relatives and a desire to take revenge for those who were killed. The continuation of the names themselves is a kind of preservation of the identities of the forebearers. Name *(imbini)* and face *(lenetimini,* literally "eye-nose") are linked together as aspects of personality. Despite the death of an individual, a part is preserved and passed on. The name of the person may be split up and altered, yet commemorated, just as the person's "face" is split up and yet passed on in the faces of descendants.

There is a male bias in this theme, since it is men who transmit names and are concerned about transmitting facial features. The transmission of resemblence is also accompanied by some ambivalence, as though too great a success in such transmission were actually dangerous. On the one hand, it is a man's aim that his individual face be preserved, and the significant parts of the face that are emphasized are the eyes (the seat of desire), and the nose (the seat of anger). One leader in the village of Tunda, who died in the late 1960s of suspected sorcery, is said to have returned many times in the faces of his grandchildren, and this is said to be a good event. He himself was cut off by hostile magic, and his own face cannot be seen anymore, but the faces of his grandchildren serve as a replacement. In this example, the reappearance of the face is in the following generation.

If the face appears too early in the next generation, it is thought that the father may die because the child has replaced him too directly. In this case, the resemblance can be regarded as bad. Nevertheless, it is the kind of bad event, which, seen from another viewpoint, realizes a cultural ideal. Birds may be thought of as realizing the same ideal on a general scale and without the associated dangers. Men's imitations of bird faces during festivals temporarily link them to that ideal, just as, among the Melpa, the wearing of plumes reenacts the courting displays of male birds of paradise. Whereas the Melpa emphasis is on competition, the Wiru emphasis here is on continuity, or, if you like, survival. These emphases, however, amount to the same thing. Melpa men seek to be polygamous and, thereby, to increase the number of their descendants. Wiru leaders are also polygynists, but all Wiru men are interested in seeing their faces reproduced. The stress is on numbers among the Melpa and on similarity of appearance among the Wiru.

Aesthetic judgements of decorated persons are really political judgements among the Wiru, just as they are among the Melpa, again with a slight shift of emphasis. Men mainly decorate themselves nowadays when they go as visiting recipients to neighbouring villages at the time of pig-killing festivals. They march in single file, a fixed distance apart so that each can be seen, and then they stand stiffly in a row until they relax and sit down, waiting for sugarcane or pork to be presented to them. Usually, men of more than one village arrive as recipients. People of the donor village and other spectators watch all these entrances with a critical eye. What they watch for is the general bearing of the visitors as well as the adequacy of their decorations. Men put charcoal or oil on their skin, hang shells from their necks, and wear cassowary feathers or bird-of-paradise plumes. These may be used to disguise the fact that their bodies are actually thin or crooked, showing that they have succumbed to the effects of hostile sorcery.

The type of sorcery involved here is called *nakene*. An enemy uses a pair of tongs or tweezers to pick up a piece of hair, clothing, or a food fragment left by an intended victim. He passes this to an expert, who places the item in the branch of a tree over a pond or in the rafters of his house. The expert chooses a branch that is sometimes underwater when it rains, or he lights a fire to subject the item to heat. The victim then wastes away as either water or fire consumes his or her relic. (Usually it is his. This kind of sorcery is used most against big men by those who are jealous of them, but it can also be used by an ex-husband angry at his wife for leaving him. The intimacy of married life, therefore, carries with it a profound danger should the marriage fail.)

Spectators try to see if one of the men entering has fallen foul of *nakene* sorcery. They also look to see if any of the visitors stumble or hesitate as they arrive. Sometimes one of the donors chooses the moment when visitors enter to kill a pig. The downward stroke of the club, accompanied by the hostile wishes of the pig killer, poses another magical threat to the soul of those entering. The man who leads a group of recipients in is often one whose father was either killed by or who, himself, killed someone in the donor village by magical means. He shows his face and dares the donors to punish him or indicates that he is not afraid to face them. The leader's bodily movements are, therefore, watched with the greatest of care. It is evident that a great deal of ritualised hostility is contained in these entrances. The hostility has to be dispelled by an invitation to sit, by the offering of food, and by the acceptance of pork fat, which the visitors must bite from in turn and thus share. Pork fat here, as among the Melpa, signifies friendship and trust, and acceptance of it is like saying, "You will not poison me, so I shall accept food from you." Life-giving food is thus counterbalanced against death-dealing sorcery.

Female decorations among the Wiru are harder to study because women and girls decorate themselves less frequently than men, largely as a result of mission teaching. One set of photographs from 1967, however, shows a feature of female body-painting that is quite unlike that of men – the practice of painting circles around leg and arm joints, the navel area, and the genitals. I do not have a folk explanation for this feature as I do for men's bird designs, but possibly it is meant to emphasize the orifices in their bodies. Women below the age of thirty find it difficult to discuss the topic in detail because their

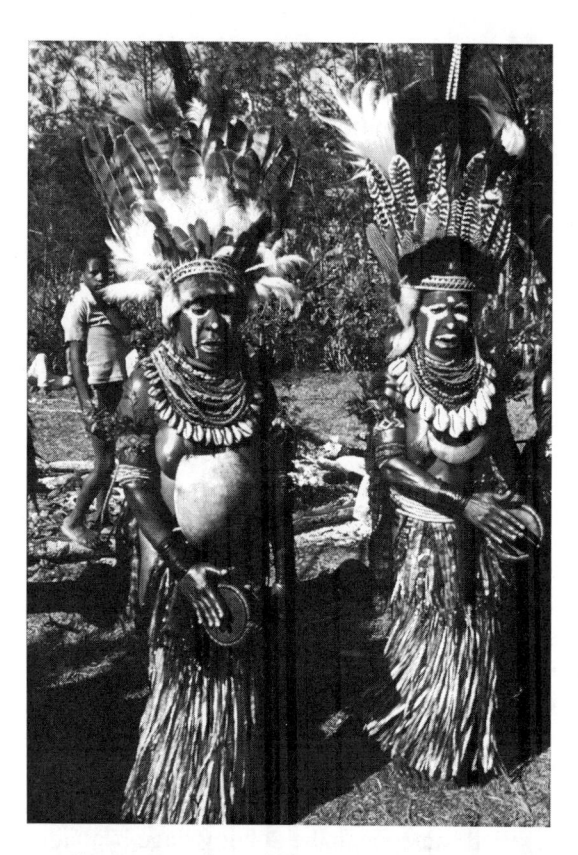

Fig. 4. Wiru dancers with shell necklaces. Bird-of-paradise plumes on left headdress

mothers stopped teaching them about these things some twenty years ago, and many of these older women are now dead. However, such encircling designs may be unconscious representations of the female womb. This would constitute the female analog of the male face representations and, similarly, indicate the desire for reproduction. Wiru women's face designs might also follow the bird motif, but, in addition, there are sun and moon designs, and the circles to which I have referred might represent, at the conscious level, these astral bodies.

Another feature of women's or girls' decorations was the practice of dressing them in men's ceremonial gear, a kind of transvestism. One woman, widowed by the death of her husband in fighting, put a man's apron on her daughter for several years until she grew up, in memory of the husband she had lost. As with the "sorrow names" to which I have referred, revenge is also intended here. Dressing a female in male clothes is done to "tread down the soul" of whoever was responsible for killing a male *(aline yomini kaurakere tokoi)*. The idea is typical of Wiru ideas of symbolic action. An unusual act can trap and kill a person's spirit and so cause his death. The act here contains a contradiction: "This is a female, but she is wearing a man's decoration." What is she, then? Such anomalous practices are also closely connected with the manipulation of power. I further suggest that they are closely connected with the aesthetic experience, in which there is recognition of something beyond what is immediately apparent. We thus find a connection between aesthetics and the expression of power.

Another contrast between the present-day Wiru and the Melpa can be adduced. The occasions when gifts of wealth are made among the Melpa are also times of great speech-making. These speeches concentrate on the political or intergroup aspect of the events and on the prominence of big men among them. Both men's and women's dance groups also sing songs that make political claims. No such thing happens among the Wiru. First, women rarely decorate themselves fully and accompany their men; they walk behind them, silently and with netbags prepared to scoop up the pork that will be given. Second, the men themselves do not sing or make speeches; they are silent. This is a recent development. Missions forbade singing and speech-making. Before 1960, both sexes decorated themselves and sang as they entered a ceremonial area as recipients. Nowadays, only individuals shout out or chant the names of the recipients when they give pork to their relatives. In these circumstances, the Wiru place great weight on nonverbal communication, e. g., the swish of a club, the stumbling of a foot, and the arrangement of men in a row. I think this also reveals a problem for the Wiru. Nonverbal communication is less flexible than verbal, and the messages regarding hostility and friendship cannot be so subtly or elaborately imparted. But, in any case, *alliance* between groups is less elaborated in the Wiru social structure than it is among the Melpa. Correspondingly, there is less to talk about at Wiru pig kills. The alliances between *individuals* are maintained by a range of very strongly sanctioned ideas about affines and maternal kinsfolk. Between groups, hostility often exists; it does not preclude exchange but lends exchange a dangerous element. This hostility is not expressed verbally but appears very clearly if we examine the meanings of nonverbal actions, particularly the *poi mokora* gifts, in which pork is cut in an unusual manner and presented, causing a dangerous "weight" to those who receive it. This "weight" can in fact cause death, the Wiru say, if the person's soul is not strong enough to bear it without flinching or stumbling.

Discussion and Conclusions

My descriptions of Melpa and Wiru ceremonial decorations demonstrate that these peoples make aesthetic judgements, but such evaluations are never only aesthetic. The realm of aesthetics is also the realm of values in which life and death, social success, fertility, and wealth are all conjoined. Dancers, however, often present some contradiction to the spectators. They display themselves, yet are disguised. They exhibit hostility, but also attractiveness and friendship. They are female and dress as male. The spectators receive two messages simultaneously, and these messages may conflict, only to be resolved at a higher level. I now suggest that this double perception and realization of contradiction is intrinsic to the aesthetic experience of the spectators, and, perhaps, of the performers as well. Logically, hostility excludes friendship. In practice, it is a matter of universal experience that relationships may alternate between these two poles. The decorations and actions at festivals among both the Melpa and the Wiru exemplify this point. The contradiction allows both groups and individuals to assess the balance between hostility and friendship as it exists between them and to alter this balance, also. Since the balance is one which is essential to their coexistence and survival (or their conflict and threat of extinction), it is obvious that such festivals serve basic social and biological purposes; and it is in this context that aesthetic experience is created, resulting in evaluations of dances as good or bad, attractive or unworthy. This kind of total evaluation contains what we would call an aesthetic element, but its meaning transcends the aesthetic itself. One of the issues I mentioned earlier is whether the concept of aesthetics is properly applicable cross culturally. To answer the question more directly: in the narrow sense, no; in the broader sense, yes. The narrow sense of the word, which I have in mind here, is the one which is associated with the supposedly disinterested and pure appreciation of beauty or form, unrelated to social and cultural functions. Such an aesthetic is foreign to the sensibility of the Melpa and the Wiru, since, for them, aesthetics is not isolated from other dimensions of experience but integral with them. For them, social facts are "total" in that they comprise political, economic, religious, and aesthetic dimensions all together.

The broader sense of the word is exemplified by Eibl-Eibesfeldt's approach, beginning with the concept of perceptual bias, which exists on a species-specific as well as on a culture-specific level (see chapter 2). Such a bias is the beginning of an aesthetic judgement. The Melpa, for example, admire relatively light skins and long noses in both sexes. They like healthy, glossy skin and bodies which are solid and strong, not thin (this again for both sexes – there is no idea that to be very slim is attractive). Men with beards which are large and, especially, long are considered attractive. Characteristics of this sort are also ones which may be enhanced by the decorations people wear for festivals, especially the appearance of the body and the beard.

Melpa displays also provoke what Eibl-Eibesfeldt has referred to as the flash of recognition. From the profusion of ornaments and paints which each person wears, there gradually emerges the realization of who the person is. To identify who this is, although decorated, is a skill which people pick up very quickly. The element of surprise is still there, for decoration truly transforms the outer person into an ideal object, an expression and amalgam of inner values. Recognition of both the ideal type and of its bearer, who embodies it for the occasion, thus contributes to the aesthetic experience.

At a further level, each individual is also able to achieve expression through this art form. While the overall impression is of uniformity, a closer look soon tells us that each individual, both out of choice and sometimes simply because of the availability of items, has made an arrangement of his or her own, particularly with the accessories, such as necklaces and armlets.

Status is also quite clearly indicated by the abundance and selection of feathers in the headdress, all of these items reflecting a certain wealth necessary to obtain them, and, finally, the total array of dancers quite clearly permits the image of the clan or wider group responsible for the occasion. I still remember the time in 1964 when I suddenly saw a group of dancers entering a ceremonial ground among the Northern Melpa. I was told that this was the Tipuka Anmbilika, an alliance of four clans of the Tipuka tribe. For some months of my fieldwork, Anmbilika had been just a name that I had heard without knowing whether it conveyed any real solidarity or if it was just a decaying classification. Then I saw the clans combined as one dancing group. The sight was moving and aesthetic, a flash of recognition. In this regard, the similarity of the men's decorations and their marching together in formation were like the ethologist's sign stimuli, indicating that these people were on their home ground and acting together. Putting this in cultural terms, one may say that the shared style of decorations also performs the ideological function of binding the participants together with a sense of their common identity.

The same is true of dance tempo. I had an interesting experience in September 1984, which brought this point home to me. Two subgroups joined together for a *mör* dance, the main men's dance associated with *moka* (wealth) exchanges. For this dance, the men stand together in a long line and bend their knees rhythmically while beating drums and singing. One of the subgroups owned clan land in the vicinity and had invited the other clan as immigrants. For the dance, they joined together. I was decorated and placed in the dance line at the intersection between the hosts and the immigrants. There I soon learned that, although both groups were performing *mör,* it was impossible to keep time with the dancers both to my left and to my right, because the immigrants on my right danced at a slightly faster pulse than the landowners. Later I found that this is well known to the dancers themselves – it was only I who was confused by it at first! The different tempo is a part of the style of the people from the mountainous area south of Hagen.

In short, Melpa dance exhibits all the features and functions mentioned by Eibl-Eibesfeldt, including that of sexual appeal. This is quite explicit and intentional. The formal dancing is followed by boisterous and often bawdy songs sung in round dances, during which girls can take the initiative and link hands with the men whom they prefer, i. e., whose decorations are good, who look lively, who perform well in the dance – all signs of vitality, which is a mark of sexual attractiveness to these people. The girls have to penetrate the men's disguise and recognize who they are, for, otherwise, they might be making advances to someone who is related to them and therefore not marriageable. There must be the correct path of action, and, even so, there is the risk that another woman (wife or girlfriend) may object. Such objections do occur and result in fights.

Melpa dances, which I have singled out for discussion and comment here, constitute only one, albeit the most salient one, of Melpa art forms, which include music and singing of other kinds, storytelling, epics, and oratory. These dances, however, are particularly suitable as topics for consideration here because they are complex and multilevel events, which attract a great deal of public notice and evaluation. They are performances that are subjected to aesthetic scrutiny. They provide aesthetic experiences for those who watch them. How can we define an aesthetic experience of this sort? Such an experience may be particularly embodied in moments when there is a shift in code or classification from one level to another, a conversion which opens up a new perspective. I further suggest that Melpa dances provide the material for such shifts in perception. For example, they present fresh statements of group unity and opposition, creatively blending in ritual those who are at other times at odds, or vice versa. They disguise the individual and then reveal him or her. They oppose the sexes, but join them. There are a number of logical operations being carried out in these dances aside from the palpable attractiveness of the bright plumes and paints which the dancers wear. It is the spectators' chance to decipher the messages which are being put forward by the vivid riot of colour and movement in the dances that also provides the opportunity for the aesthetic moment. If this is correct, the next step would be to see how well an idea of this sort can apply to art forms studied in other cultures. Our pattern-reading propensity seems to be a species-level characteristic. It becomes a matter of aesthetics when it is also pleasurable and linked to certain ideal values at the cultural level.

References

1. Strathern AJ (1971) Self-decoration in Mount Hagen. Gerald Duckworth, London
2. Strathern AJ (1981) Dress, decoration and art in New Guinea. In: Kirk M (ed) Man as art. Viking, New York, pp 15–36

Aesthetics and Cuisine: Mind over Matter

Elisabeth Rozin
500 W. Washington Avenue, Havertown, Pa 19083, USA

Cuisine is the uniquely human expression of the accumulated knowledge and traditions of the total food experience, from food procurement to preparation to serving to consumption. As with all other cultural systems, cuisine has become elaborated and individualized into a myriad of different forms, each unique but sharing at the same time certain universal characteristics.

There can be no doubt that aspects of human biology and physiology are fundamental to any consideration of cuisine, since, no matter how culturally elaborated and diverse the behavior becomes, it is ultimately involved with that most basic of behaviors – feeding.

Human beings are omnivores; like rats and cockroaches, we are capable of deriving nourishment from a wide variety of food substances – plants, animals, and varying combinations of either or both. Unlike many other more narrowly restricted animal eaters, we do not come equipped with any special mechanisms for obtaining food, except for a built-in preference for sweet and an aversion for bitter.[1] These tastes serve the omnivore well because, in the vast natural world of potential foodstuffs and particularly in the realm of plant foods, the taste of sweet generally points to a safe source of immediate energy, while the taste of bitter frequently indicates a toxic or poisonous substance.

Although the nutritional demands of the human organism can be adequately supplied by a wide variety of foods, it is clear that our basic needs are more satisfactorily fulfilled by animal foods (meat, eggs, dairy products). These foods provide an appropriate balance of all the essential amino acids and a more concentrated source of essential nutrients, including dietary fat.

Since most omnivores, including humans, are equipped with few genetically prewired abilities for selecting foods, they accomplish it primarily by learning.[1] Humans, however, are culinary animals; they are endowed with the unique inclination and ability to manipulate and process foodstuffs, thereby providing themselves with an enormously expanded set of potential foods.

Mammalian mother's milk, for example, is a maximally nutritious substance that is not available to any other mammal after weaning. Humans, however, not only collect and store it, but process it by enzyme and bacillus culturing into products like yogurt and cheese, which are digestible by the adult consumer.[2] Similarly, soybeans, which are a rich source of plant proteins, are largely useless nutritionally to humans unless they are treated by a variety of processes, including fermentation, precipitation, and heating.[3] The resulting products – soy sauce, soy curd (tofu), soy pastes (miso), soy flour, and soy milk – are nutritious foods that are unavailable to any other creature save man.

Much of human culinary practice, at least in its formative stages, can be seen as an attempt to maximize the potential food resources of any particular habitat and to overcome the limitations of human physiology by creating products that are unknown in the natural world. The culinary imperative in humans operates to enhance access to nutrients, to improve digestibility, and to lessen or remove toxic substances that may be present. Further, it seems likely that culinary practice across cultures strives, particularly with reference to plant foods, to achieve or mimic certain sensory qualities associated with animal foods.[4] Such qualities involve flavor (saltiness, meatiness), mouth feel (fattiness, fullness), texture (creaminess, chewiness), and visual appeal (reddish, bloody).

Human food behavior is, then, shaped at the very outset by the demands of our biological makeup, but seems always to elaborate itself beyond the constraints of physiology and nutrition. There are many traditional sayings that reveal what we believe the essential differences between the human and the animal eating experiences to be. "Animals eat to live; man lives to eat." "Animal eat; humans dine." Since eating, like sex, is the satisfying of an innate biological drive, animals, as well as humans, might be said to enjoy it. But it is clear that some other, rather unique pleasures enter into the human experience. The eighteenth-century gastronome, Brillat-Savarin[5], summed it up:

> "The pleasure of eating we have in common with animals; it only supposes hunger, and what is necessary to satisfy it.
> The pleasure of the table is peculiar to the human species; it supposes care bestowed beforehand on the preparations of the repast, on the choice of the palate and the assemblage of guests.
> The pleasure of eating requires, if not hunger, at least appetite; the pleasure of the table is most often independent of both."

Several things are critical in this statement. First is the perception that humans, unlike animals, can separate eating from its biological or nutritional context and take pleasure in it for other reasons, just as we can take pleasure in sex quite apart from its reproductive function. Second is the acknowledgement of that uniquely human inclination to do things to food before we eat it, in other words, to cook. The third critical concept is that of "choice." The issue of choice is essential because it removes eating and food preparation from the realm of the necessary, that is, the mere satiation of hunger, and on to an intellectual level where thought, planning, strategies, and judgements occur. Indeed, it is the enlargement of food behavior from simple food procurement and immediate consumption to food manipulation or cooking that takes us away from the direct urgency of a biological drive and into an area where aesthetics – taste, preference, palatability – come into play. The more choices we have, the more marked this tendency becomes.

For humans, two things seem to be critical for the development of culinary aesthetics: a selection, no matter how small, of appropriate foodstuffs; and a culture that informs us of how those foodstuffs are to be manipulated, served, and consumed. All people – except those reduced to a more animal-like level of existence by the special circumstances of famine, war, etc. – appear to have the ability, the inclination, and the desire for aesthetic experience. In terms of food and eating, this means that, no matter what our economic or cultural circumstances may be, we all have the potential for making judgements, having preferences, and making discriminations about the symbolic and sensory qualities of the food we eat, quite apart from any nutritional or biological concerns. We make fine judgements about flavor, aroma, appearance, and texture as qualities that are desirable and valuable in and for themselves by providing the possibility of pleasure enhancement. But the ways in which we make these judgements depend largely on the cultural and social milieu in which we operate.

In many relatively simple, traditional, nonindustrial cultures, food practices may be somewhat limited. People in such groups tend to eat the same foods at most meals and to use the same cooking techniques over and over again. Aesthetic standards are closely tied to familiar, traditional, well-liked foods and techniques; what is "good" is that which, through long custom and usage, has become entrenched and well known, with a corresponding wariness about novel or foreign elements. The American farm diet in the early 1800s, for example, had for generations consisted largely of corn and preserved pork (ham, bacon, sausage), and so strong was this tradition that the rural population was very suspicious of fresh meat and green or raw vegetables.[6]

This is the situation that exists with the fixed product and the fixed audience, characteristic of many traditional cuisines, in which the aesthetic criteria involving culinary practices remain fixed because there is little or no opportunity or motivation to expand and experiment. As the choices remain limited, so do the standards. Once new opportunities become available, however, in the form of new ingredients, new technologies, and new choices, there is a corresponding expansion of the food aesthetic.

Few cultures remain absolutely static, of course, and it seems to be a widespread human tendency to selectively accept new ideas from outside and gradually to incorporate them into the established tradition. Innovations are also frequently developed within the culture itself. Although the motivation for the acceptance or development of new ideas may depend initially on such practical concerns as improved nutritional value or greater digestibility, an equally important concern is often the enhancement of the purely aesthetic qualities of the food preparations. Each innovation provides a whole new set of choices, an ever-widening opportunity to experiment.

There is in most culinary traditions a clear tendency to develop a strong, conservative, central core and then to use selective innovations as a way of modifying or enhancing the central theme.[7] This use of theme and variation as a structural device to organize behavior is not unique to cuisine; it occurs in all forms of human culture and seems to play a particularly meaningful role in many forms of art, like music, painting, and literature.[8] It seems to function primarily as an aesthetic principle, as a way of providing relief from monotony and the pleasure of novelty or the unexpected within a familiar framework. It is one of the clearest ways that culinary traditions expand, enlarge, and elaborate themselves.

To see how the theme and variation principle operates, we can look at a cuisine that is very old and has remained very consistent. The cuisine of Mexico has, for many thousands of years, been based on a small number of core foods that were indigenous to the area and fully exploited by the aboriginal population.[9] Among these foods, the most important were the staple grain, maize, and the focal seasoning ingredient, the chile pepper. They are as essential to Mexican culinary practice today as they were for centuries before Europe discovered the New World.

But these seemingly simple, single foods are not simple or single at all. There are dozens of varieties of corn, each with a specialized use; one type is used ground for the *masa*, the dough from which tortillas are made; others are used fresh, dried, popped, or stewed, in different forms of bread or tamales, in gruels or mushes or beverages, or eaten whole off the cob. Each variety requires a different culinary technique and provides a different eating experience. The products are all made of corn, but they produce varying sensations of flavor, texture, aroma, and appearance.

Similar but even more striking is the use of the chile pepper, which exists in literally hundreds of varieties.[10] Some chiles are used raw; some are pickled; some are dried; others are roasted. Some are used chopped into fresh uncooked sauces, while others are stewed into soups or stews. Some chile peppers are stuffed and fried, while others may be eaten separately as a condiment or sprinkled directly onto cooked foods. There are subtle and not-so-subtle differences in flavor among the many varieties. There are distinguishable degrees of hotness; some are actually quite mild, while others produce different sensations of hotness or burn in different parts of the mouth. Some affect the lips and others the tongue, the palate, or the throat. Some chile burns may be immediate and short-lived; others may not occur until after the food as actually been swallowed. There is also a wide range of colors among the chile peppers, so that there is a variety of visual as well as flavor sensations. Mexican cooks deliberately exploit the variability of this single seasoning ingredient to produce flavors and taste combinations that are subtle and complex.

To say that Mexicans eat corn and chile peppers is accurate, but does not indicate the enormous variety of eating experiences that are possible within the bounds of these two foods substances. Originally, there may have been only one kind of corn and one kind of chile pepper, but the typical human desire for variations on a theme produced in Mexico an enlargement of choices and a concomitant expansion of the cuisine. Other innovations, both of ingredients and techniques, brought in when the Spanish colonized Mexico, added new varietal patterns to the central and ancient tradition.

The same kind of development based on theme and variation can be seen in almost any culinary system. It is a manipulation of the various elements of culinary structure[11] – basic foods, cooking techniques, and seasoning ingredients – for the purpose of achieving variety in food preparation and of enhancing the purely pleasurable aspects of eating. The more, however, a culture is tied to basic food procurement or food production, the less time and the less opportunity there may be for playing around with variations. The cuisine of necessity, in which one eats to fill one's stomach and nourish one's body, certainly provides aesthetic satisfactions, but the criteria for these remain relatively uncomplicated and unchanging. It is only when cultures begin to strive for the cuisine of choice that a flowering aesthetic begins to emerge. Such a striving can only occur when the limitations of any culture, in terms of resources, of ideas, and of technology, are overcome.

Initially, there may be many reasons for people to express an interest in new ideas, some of which may have to do with the cost, the rarity, or the luxuriousness of certain goods and techniques, or with the apparently widespread desire for upward social mobility. One of the clearest ways in which cuisines begin to experiment and expand is with the development of an aristocratic, prosperous, or leisure class. Privilege, in terms of economic or political power or social status, provides two distinct advantages for cultural development and expansion: first, it affords the means, the money and the labor; and second, it provides an incentive for change, the search for something "better." Almost without fail, whenever a privileged segment of the population emerges, there develops an increased interest in and commitment to an elaboration of traditional culinary practice, a deliberate widening of choices, and an increased incentive for pursuing the cuisine of choice. This desire for something better is seen by those who engage in it as a movement away from the conservative and constricting limitations of traditional practices, an expansion of culinary horizons; but, at the same time, it is almost invariably based on traditional cuisine, which serves as the thematic foundation. It can be seen as a search not only for variety (interest, novelty, unpredictability) but also as a search for quality (refinement, subtlety).

This movement toward an elaboration and refinement of traditional cuisine has two very significant aspects. First is the development of culinary specialists, and second is the movement away from private, domestic cuisine into a somewhat more public arena. One of the clearest indications of a culture's expanding culinary awareness is the emergence of a class of artisans who are professional cooks. It presupposes an interest in and a commitment to the idea that food preparation can be something better, different, and more interesting than that to which one has ordinarily been accustomed. It is clear evidence for a move away from the cuisine of necessity toward the cuisine of choice. The cook as specialist becomes the means of setting and reflecting the aesthetic values of the cultural milieu that maintains and supports him.

What happens in situations of this sort is that the culinary enterprise is removed from the routinized, predictable, and relatively rigid practices of the domestic arena into a more public domain, with a different and primarily non-familial assemblage of people. Cuisine becomes self-conscious, producing a set of heightened expectations in both the cook and the eaters. The cook, who is now a paid specialist, constantly expects judgement of the food he produces. Unlike the traditional female, who prepares food as an expected part of the daily domestic routine, the professional cook is trained and paid to provide not so much nourishment as pleasurable, interesting, varied, and memorable dining. To do this successfully, he must become deliberately experimental and innovative, for his job, his status, and very possibly his head, are at stake.

If the cook expects to the judged, the eater expects that the food, in its preparation and its service, will differ significantly from the ordinary domestic food that is eaten daily. The eater expects to judge, to criticize, and to intellectualize the eating experience, and the extent to which the circumstances and substance of the meal encourage him to do so provide some index of how far it has moved away from domestic predictable cuisine. The gastronomic experience presupposes a cognitive level that is as essential as the purely sensual.

This might lead us to conclude that traditional domestic or bourgeois cooking is aesthetically unsatisfying, and that public or festive cuisine is by definition good, or better, than ordinary fare. But this can hardly be the case. "Home" cooking has always provided its own very strong and meaningful pleasures: the savor and satisfaction of familiar and well-loved food, predictable and unassuming, associated with family or tribal warmth and security.

Which brings us to the question of what the pleasures of eating are, if the aesthetic can, in fact, be separated from other critical aspects – the satiation of hunger, the social context, the ceremonial or symbolic significance.

Clearly, the aesthetic experience is not identical for all of us since, quite independent of such variables as history, climate, resources, and so forth, we all, both as individuals and members of various social and ethnic communities, seem to seek out a rather wide range of describable pleasures. The primary aesthetic target of eating is the mouth, as the ear is the target in music, but the mouth itself affords a number of discrete and important sensations: flavor, temperature, texture, piquancy. The experience of food that coats the tongue is different from the experience of food that is chewed or licked or sucked. And what goes on in the mouth is intimately involved with what goes on in the nose, since the taste of food is inextricably linked with its aroma. In addition, the visual aspects of food – its color, arrangement, texture, size, shape, cohesiveness, its appearance on the plate and as it approaches the mouth – offer a wide range of varied and significant sensations.

We all seek from this wide range of sensations those that are most meaningful to us. We know very little about how culinary aesthetics develop on an individual level, because they are so closely tied to an individual's unique and personal history and psychology. Similarly, it is extremely difficult to say why different traditions and different cultures emphasize certain qualities of food as being more or less important. The Chinese, for example, have always been much more sensitive than other people to varieties of texture in food, and the exploitation of textural contrast and variety is central to Chinese culinary practice and a fundamental concern of Chinese gastronomy.[12]

In yet another elaborate and self-conscious tradition, we see an intense concentration on flavor as the primary aesthetic experience of food. Hindu gastronomy distinguishes between varieties and subtleties of flavor to a degree that is quite remarkable but not surprising, given India's long traditional experience with aromatic herbs and spices.[13] But even if we can legitimately say that Hindu cuisine focuses on flavor, while Chinese focuses on texture, that is surely not to say that the Chinese does not regard flavor as a critical quality, or that the Hindu is indifferent to texture, for that is clearly not the case. It is simply a question of emphasis and of the ways in which the various sensory qualities of food are perceived and appreciated.

We all make constant judgements about the aesthetic value of our food in terms of its flavor, texture, aroma, appearance, presentation, etc. These judgements and the criteria we use to make them are very largely culturally constrained. The polar Eskimo, like many western Europeans, prefers meat to other kinds of food, but not all meat tastes good to him. That which provides him with the most satisfying aesthetic experience is meat that has been allowed to putrefy, becoming soft and semiliquid in texture and "high" in flavor and aroma. He may, indeed, be disgusted by the odor and flavor of roasted fresh meat. Our response to his food, of course, is exactly the opposite, and both reactions are the result of long cultural indoctrination.

If, then, the aesthetic experience in food is so closely constrained by cultural tradition, how is it that we are able to cross over, to participate in, and sometimes to truly appreciate the unique qualities of other culinary systems? Those people who are more open to and desirous of new, different, and exotic food experiences are likely to be urban, cosmopolitan, more highly educated, and less dependent on strong ethnic or community ties. Life in multiethnic urban centers tends to broaden our outlook and to motivate us to enlarge and enrich our culinary experiences. As with any other cultural form, we must be educated, taught what to look for and what to appreciate, how to reinterpret and redefine our eating experiences in terms of new aesthetic criteria. The special qualities of Moroccan cuisine, for example, may be as complex, as strange, and as initially difficult to understand as the lines and colors of a modern abstract painting.

If the adventurous eater, the curious gastronome, is special by virtue of the time and place in which he lives and his willingness to step outside his own cultural boundaries, what about cuisines themselves and the cooks who create and produce them? Can it be said that there are some cuisines that are better, more interesting, more accessible than others, and if so, why? There are two issues here: first, the question of the cook as an individual artist and creator; and second, the question of a cuisine or a culinary tradition as a unique expression of food preparation.

In dealing with the individual artist, the cook or chef, the problem is that the culinary art, unlike most others, is both material and ephemeral. It is material in that it requires ingredients and equipment; it is ephemeral in that its products are consumed and disappear forever very shortly after they have been created. In this sense, the culinary art is perhaps closest to theater or dance than to any other art form; an individual dish or a meal is very much like a performance that can never be exactly duplicated. But cuisine, unlike dance, cannot even be recorded or preserved in the mode for which it was intended; we can make a film or a videotape of a dance but we cannot record a dish or a meal in its exact form so that it can be eaten on another occasion. Our primary preservative techniques inevitably alter the original preparation, so that the food may ultimately be almost unrecognizable. The only way we can come close to recording and preserving the individual product of a cook is through a recipe, which is, of course, an inexact kind of formula: the egg you use today can never be exactly the same as the egg you use tomorrow; Escoffier's wrist movement in beating that egg is likely to have been different from mine.

If it is impossible to retain any particular culinary performance of an artist in the same way that we can reproduce Picasso's *Guernica* or the Brahms *Requiem*, we have to base our aesthetic judgements on patterns and traditions, rather than on individual dishes or meals. There is little point in attempting to establish a hierarchy of cuisines, but it is interesting to try to discover what it is about some culinary traditions that makes them so much more widely appealing than others, both on the domestic or bourgeois level, and in their more elaborated public form. Why, for example, should the cuisine of France have attained such a widely acknowledged level of virtuosity, while many of her close neighbours have, for the most part, remained relatively undistinguished from a culinary point of view?

There is, first of all, the matter of resources. In order to experiment and to be creative, a cuisine must have available a fairly wide variety of ingredients. The greater the number of choices, in terms of different kinds of animal and plant foods, cooking oils or fats, seasonings, beverages, etc., the greater the likelihood of elaboration and a focusing of interest on the preparation of interesting food. A variety of ingredients means that you have a geographic area large and diverse enough to supply them, an area that is ecologically and climatically suitable for the production of many different foodstuffs. Theoretically, this would eliminate areas that are too cold, too hot, too arid, or too humid. The ideal environment would provide access to rivers, seas, and diverse and productive planting and farming habitats, including both temperate and warm climates. If we look at the world's great culinary traditions – in France, China, India, the Middle East – we see that they all share this feature of geographic diversity and the availability of a wide variety of food ingredients.

The second factor is a strong sense of cultural, social, or political unity, which permits an easy flow of goods and ideas between the diverse geographic areas. There may well be, and indeed often are, a number of unique and characteristic regional traditions, but there is also a strong and overriding sense of Frenchness or Chineseness that provides a general cultural framework. Moreover, cuisines of this sort, because they possess both geographic diversity and cultural unity, tend to explore and to create within the bounds of their own cultures, rather than looking to the outside world for new ideas. They tend to be insular, and their development is largely internally motivated rather than externally molded or imposed.

The third factor is a general level of cultural development, for you do not get high culinary art where you do not have as well the flowering of other art forms. A culture must have richness of resources and talent and must provide the means and the motivation for the enlargement of the artistic and creative enterprises, in whatever mode they occur.

These three factors, then, are probably necessary for the appearance of high culinary art – but they are not sufficient. For we come inevitably to that final factor, one that is ultimately unknowable and unassessable: the question of talent, of predisposition, of inclination, toward one art form rather than another. What, finally, is it that makes the Chinese and the French particularly and uniquely sensitive to and interested in the qualities of food, the pleasures of eating, the art of the kitchen? Why is it that some cultures regard food as a more important source of pleasure than others? There is no satisfactory answer, of course, just as there is no simple answer for why the Germans produce great music or the English great poetry or the ancient Greeks great sculpture, while none of these produced a cuisine of any particular distinction.

We are left only with the delicious and debatable evidence. There are some people and some cultures that are particularly tuned to the palate as an aesthetic organ, and whose history and culture have allowed them to realize more fully than others the potential of the culinary art. We recognize these traditions as superior, in the variety and creativity of the preparations, the successful exploitation of flavors and flavor combinations, in the complex structuring of food sensations within a dish and within a meal, the deliberate and ingenious interaction between flavor and texture, and in the intensity, grace, and subtlety with which ingredients and techniques are manipulated and refined.

Cuisine is the art that most surely transcends matter; the absolutely fundamental nourishment of the body becomes, in human hands, an essential nourishment of the soul. This was most eloquently summed up by Brillat-Savarin[5] 150 years ago:

"The joys of the table belong equally to all ages, conditions, countries, and times; they mix with all other pleasures, and remain the last to console us for their loss."

References

1. Rozin P (1976) The selection of food by rats, humans and other animals. In: Rosenblatt J, Hinde RA, Beer C, Shaw E (eds) Advances in the study of behavior, 6th edn. Academic, New York
2. Simoons FJ (1982) Geography and genetics as factors in the psychobiology of human food selection. In: Barker LM (ed) The psychobiology of human food selection. Avi, Westport, Conn.
3. Katz SH (1982) Food, behavior and biocultural evolution. In: Barker LM (ed) The psychobiology of human food selection. Avi, Westport, Conn.

4. Rozin E (1988) Ketchup and the collective unconscious. J Gastronomy 4 (2): 45–55
5. Brillat-Savarin JA (1970) The physiology of taste: Meditations on transcendental gastronomy. Liveright, New York
6. Cummings RO (1940) The American and his food: A history of food habits in the United States. University of Chicago Press, Chicago
7. Rozin E, Rozin P (1981) Culinary themes and variations. Natural History 90 (2): 6–14
8. Humphrey NK (1973) The illusion of beauty. Perception 2: 429–439
9. Coe MD (1962) Mexico. Praeger, New York
10. Kennedy D (1972) The cuisines of Mexico. Harper and Row, New York
11. Rozin E (1982) The structure of cuisine. In: Barker LM (ed) The psychobiology of human food selection. Avi, Westport, Conn.
12. Lin H, Lin T (1969) Chinese gastronomy. Hastings House, New York
13. Prakash O (1961) Food and drinks in ancient India. Munshi Ram Manohar Lal, Delhi

Index

A

affective choices 245–251, 253–254, 269–271, 277
abstract art 35, 203
action art 35–36, 117
adaption 37, 49, 72, 76, 171
Adorno, Theodor W. 15–17, 140
afferent neurons 174
afferent pathways 170, 183
affective object placement in drawing 236–237
altered states of consciousness 56, 59, 64, 74, 81–83, 86
ambiguous stimulus 251–253, 272
amusia 275
aphasia 223, 226, 229, 233, 274–276
anthropomorphization 39–40
apotropaic designs 34, 38–39, 44–45, 54
appeasement 37–38, 44–47, 54, 57
appetitive behavior 46, 64
aptitude 114, 229, 231–233
archetypes 63
Aristotle 15–17, 184
Arnold, Matthew 81
arousal functions 39, 56, 226–227, 272

arrows 51, 54
asymmetry, cerebral 25–26, 75, 77, 82–83, 85–87, 168, 170, 219–238, 243–254, 257–289
asymmetry, stimulus 235–237, 254, 260–267, 275, 277
atomism 183
attentional bias 235
audition 77–80, 100, 150, 162, 166, 190, 224, 226, 230–233, 261, 263, 275
auditory driving 83, 87
Augustine 20
Australian Aborigines 45, 63–64, 136
axes 52

B

Balinese culture 39, 57–60
band-pass images 193–201
Baroque style 31, 275–276
basal ganglia 177
beard 45, 48, 312
beat (music) 91, 93–114, 122, 127, 139
beauty 9, 11, 15–18, 20–26, 29, 32, 76, 85, 178, 219–220, 222, 227–228, 238, 243
Beethoven, Ludwig van 21, 91–92
Bense, Max 189
Beuys, Joseph 212

bipolar cells 153, 192
blindness 258–259, 168
bonding 37, 50–51, 56–58, 62, 139, 142, 313
Brahms, Johannes 92, 94
brain damage 25, 168–170, 176–177, 191, 224–226, 229, 232–233, 244, 257, 274–276
brain mapping 167, 190–191
brain/mind dichotomy 24–25, 166
Breskin figure pairs 246–247, 254
bright/dark symbolism 48, 61
Brillat-Savarin, Anthelme 316, 324
Burke, Edmund 16–18, 20
Bushmen 39–40, 59, 63

C

Campbell, Fergus W. 193
center of gaze 266–267, 276–277
cerebral cortex 83–84, 153, 165–166, 168, 170–179, 190–193, 227, 258, 265
chiasma opticum 246
chimeric pictures 221–222, 234–235
chimpanzee paintings 34–36

Chinese gastronomy 321, 323–324
Chomsky, Noam 24, 113
chords, musical 228, 230–232
clan 299, 300, 313
coaction 56, 58
code (see encoding)
cognition 167, 170, 227
color 48–49, 149–163, 166–167, 171, 176, 193, 210–211, 222, 229, 238, 303, 305–306, 319
color naming (lexicon) 149, 155–163, 170, 258
color vision 149–163, 170, 193
column, cortical 174–176
composition, musical 232–233
cones 151–155, 192
contrast 171–176, 211
corpus callosum 220, 228, 246, 254
Corinth, Lovis 229
cortex (see cerebral cortex)
courtship 51, 58, 62, 121, 130, 134, 141, 304–305
Craik-Cornsweet illusion 175
Cranach the Elder, Lucas 279, 281–286, 288
cubism 22, 197, 203, 205, 207–210
cuisine 315–324
culture-specific biases 29, 49–54

D

dance 11, 57–59, 86, 101, 107, 108, 117–143, 269, 298, 304–305, 312–314, 322
Darwin, Erasmus 259–260
decoration (see also: display, self-decoration) 49, 51–52, 55, 313
Delauney, Robert 207–210

Dickinson, Emily 81
disguise 303, 305–306, 309, 312–314
display 44–45, 54, 57, 142, 297–314
Doesburg, Theo van 213
dongo (finger piano) 104–105, 108, 112
Dorazio, Piero 181
dualistic position, mind/body 9
Duccio di Buoninsegna 197
dysarthria 275
divination 83–84
duration 225

E

Eccles, Sir John C. 9, 257
Ehrenfels, Christian von 183
Eigengrau 273
education 32, 76, 86–88
Einstein, Albert 190, 227
Eipo of Papua New Guinea 42, 44–45, 48, 51, 60, 62, 94, 100, 107–108, 142, 261
emotional face 280, 287
emotions 56, 59, 61, 75, 81, 86–87, 104, 178, 192, 210, 220, 223, 226–227, 232, 236–238, 243–244, 248, 252, 254, 258, 266–268, 270, 276–277
empiricism 16, 18, 183
encoding 29, 33, 50, 54, 57, 61, 64–65, 177, 182, 188–190, 192, 212, 303
endorphins 74
Ensor, James 174, 273, 274
epistemology 18–20, 182, 212
Ernst, Max 10, 17
Escher, Maurits C. 33
Eskimo cuisine 322
ethology 37, 63, 66, 118

evolution 10, 54, 61, 71, 74, 150, 160–163, 165, 188, 211–213, 220–222, 238, 297
exchange 105–106, 299–302, 304–306, 311, 313
expressionist style 117
extrapersonal space 258, 288
eye contact 38–39
eye patterns 38–39

F

facial expression (mimics) 226, 235, 258, 265, 267–269, 273
face recognition 177, 225, 249, 250, 251, 253, 258, 265, 267–269, 270–273
fashion 40–41, 251
Fechner, Gustav T. 31, 100, 183
Feininger, Lyonel 204–205
forebrain 75
free verse 87
French cuisine 323–324
form (see gestalt)

G

G/wi Bushmen 51, 94, 138, 100, 104–105, 108, 112, 138–139
Galton, Francis 32
ganglion cells 153–154, 172, 192
gemsbuck dance 125–127
gestalt 15–17, 31, 65, 137, 167, 188–189, 230, 244, 247–248, 253–254, 258
Gestalt psychology 30, 167, 170, 183, 150, 210, 244
Goethe, Johann W. von 21, 149, 154, 183

Gogh, Vincent van   17
golden section   31
Gombrich, Sir Ernst H.
   188, 207, 212, 280
Gothic style   45, 278
Gregory, Richard L.   182
grasshopper dance   132–133, 139
Graves, Robert   81
gyrus cinguli   265

H

handedness (see right- and left-handedness)
harmony   78, 274–276, 288
head position in portrait painting   280–288, 292–293
Hegel, Georg W. F.   15–16, 20
Heller, Wendy   236–237
Helmholtz, Hermann von   181, 183
Henry, Charles   210–211
Hering, Ewald   151–154, 167, 215
Hermann's contrast illusion   171, 173
Himba people   62, 130–131, 134, 139
Himou (bargain chant)   62, 103–104, 108
hindbrain   162
Hindu gastronomy   321, 323
Holbein the Younger, Hans   279, 281–286, 288
honey badger dance   101
Hopi Indians   160
hormones   248
Hottentots   40, 62
Hubel, David H.   153, 174, 211
Hume, David   9, 243
humor   226, 258
Huxley, Aldous L.   191–192

I

identity   268
idealism   16, 20, 85
ideals of beauty
 –female   40–42, 312
 –human face   41–43, 312
 –male   40, 312
illusion   25, 30, 118, 171–172, 175, 176–177, 184, 191, 231, 244
impressionism   167, 197
indoctrination   50, 61, 63–64, 322
information aesthetics   189–190
information processing, human cortical   24–25, 31–32, 37, 43–44, 72–76, 80, 84, 170–171, 176–179, 185–213, 224–225, 248
inhibition   153, 172–173, 175, 192
innate releasing mechanisms   37, 63
innate template   32, 37, 183
initiation   63–64
intonation   56, 226, 276

J

Jones, Ernest   188, 212
Jung, Carl G.   63, 270, 279

K

Kandinsky, Wassily   21, 181–182, 210
Kant, Immanuel   9, 15–20, 23–26, 178, 182–183
Kindchenschema   37, 42–43
Klee, Paul   210–211, 271
!ko Bushmen   51, 57, 94, 100–101, 104, 108, 112, 125–130, 132–133, 139
Köhler, Wolfgang   183
Koffka, Kurt   183
Kohonen, Teuvo   188, 191
Kopffüssler   271–272
Kris, Ernst   212–213
Kuhn, Thomas S.   187–188
!kung Bushmen   51

L

language   21, 32, 56, 59–63, 74–75, 77–78, 80, 87, 113, 150–151, 155–163, 184, 190, 221, 223, 225–226, 228, 258, 274–276
lateral geniculate body   152–153, 173
lateralization (see asymmetry, cerebral)
leadership, characteristics   299–301
learning   9, 32, 85, 163, 165–167, 178–179, 187, 211, 259, 270, 279, 289, 315
left cerebral hemisphere   26, 75, 77, 83, 85–87, 168, 170, 220–238, 245–255, 252, 263–264, 274–276
left-handedness   235, 257, 262, 267, 270, 279–289, 293
Legong culture   57, 59–60
Leibniz, Gottfried W. von   15–19
Leonardo da Vinci   17, 21, 167, 197, 251, 279, 285, 293
Lex, Barbara   82, 85–86
Lichtenstein, Roy   203
limbic system   178, 254, 265
liminal (threshold) stimulation   249
line, poetic   76–77, 80, 83, 87, 210
line, drawn   210–211, 223, 228
Lippe, Rudolf zur   141

Lorenz, Konrad 37, 40, 118
luminance distribution in paintings 277–279, 281–287

M

Mach, Ernst 10, 100, 215
Mahler, Gustav 94, 95
Malevich, Kazimir 181–182, 189, 192, 199, 202, 213
Marcuse, Herbert 15
Marr, David 193–194
marriage 299, 301, 306, 309
masks 38, 265, 272–273
materialism 20, 220
mechanoreceptors 260–261, 264
Medlpa (Melpa) 59, 62, 100, 105–106, 112, 299–314
melody 56–57, 230, 233, 258, 288
memory 31–32, 63, 74, 81–82, 86, 168, 219, 222, 223
metabolism 167–168, 174, 227
metaphor 59–66, 161–162, 228, 258, 305
meter, poetic 55, 71–73, 76–77, 80–90, 132, 258, 276, 288
Metzger, Wolfgang 31
Mexican cuisine 318–319
Meyer, Leonard 189
Michelangelo Buonarotti 17, 279
midbrain 162
mind 9, 18–20, 24–25, 211, 219–220, 238
mind/body dualism 9, 25
mind/body monastic position 10
missions, influence of 301, 309, 311

modern art 16–18
Moles, Abraham A. 189
Monet, Claude 190, 200, 202–203
Mondrian, Piet 21, 209–210
Morris, Desmond 35
mother-child holding pattern 261–266, 274–275, 287–288
Mozart, Wolfgang A. 92–94
Munsell color sample 155–156
Murasaki Shikibu 17, 21
music 55–57, 61, 64, 91–114, 181, 190, 228, 232–233, 258, 274–276, 288

N

nature vs nurture 43, 163, 178, 297–298, 257–289
Navari cast of Nepal 100, 102, 108
Necker cube 30, 184–185
neglect, spacial 168–169
neocortex 178, 258–259
neoimpressionism 167, 203, 210
nets 51–52
neuroaesthetics 10, 260, 276–286
neuronal networks 166–167, 170–175, 178, 191, 215
neuropsychology 167
Newton, Isaac 149, 193
Nietzsche, Friedrich 15–16, 20

O

off-center neurons 171–173, 202
on-center neurons 171–174, 202
ontology 18–20

op art (optical art) 176, 189
opponent color scheme 151–155, 160–161
optical illusions 30, 171–172, 175, 231

P

pattern recognition 30, 32, 77, 87, 184–187, 211
perceptual bias, general 29–36, 49
phallic symbol 44–45
phenomenology 118
phonemes 190
photoreceptors (see also, cones and rods) 151, 153–154, 172, 192
phylogenetic bias 49
pitch, musical 56, 78, 91, 98, 105, 228, 230j232, 275–276
plasticity of the brain 9, 178, 163
Plato 15–20
poetry 59–63, 71–90, 227, 258, 276
Poincaré, Henri 227, 238
polygamy 298, 301, 308
pop art 22, 51
Popper, Sir Karl R. 9
Prägnanz 30, 247–248, 253–254
primitive art 22, 33, 38, 63, 212, 262, 292
psychogram (personality profile) 251–252
psycholinguistics 151, 155–163
psychophysics 167, 183
public (official) face 268, 280, 287
pulse, musical 92–93, 95, 101, 104, 112, 114, 122, 127, 132, 139

Q

quantum physics 72, 213
Quechi Indians 155, 157–158

R

Räderscheidt, Anton 168–170, 229
rationalism 18–19
Ravel, Maurice 233
representational and non-representational art 182, 210–211
reality 9, 19, 85, 165, 178, 182, 185, 211–213, 226, 228, 233, 238
receptive field, visual 153, 172–175, 183, 192–194
Renaissance style 31, 94, 276, 288
retina 72, 84, 151–155, 168, 170–176, 190, 192
reward 25, 32–33, 64, 74, 76, 81, 84, 124, 137, 142, 178, 219
rhyme 11, 222
rhythm 55–56, 63, 71–73, 76–78, 82–83, 87, 91, 102, 119, 124, 134, 143, 181, 189, 228, 230, 238, 258, 261, 264, 274–276, 288
right cerebral hemisphere 26, 75, 82–83, 85–87, 168–170, 220–238, 245–255, 257, 266, 274–276
right-handedness 234–236, 221, 258, 262, 267, 270–274, 277, 279–289, 293
ritualization 43, 54, 57, 82, 85, 103, 118–119, 212–213, 272, 302
rock paintings of the Stone Age 22, 63
rods 151, 192

Rorschach inkblot 251–252, 254
rubato 95, 115
Rubin's cup 30
Romanesque style 45
Romantic style 36, 49, 275–276

S

Sabadel 168–170
saccade 266, 276
San culture 59
Schizophrenia 271, 273
Schopenhauer, Arthur 9
selection 43, 50–51, 54, 75
self-decoration 11, 298–314
sensitive periods 151, 257–259
separation, temporal 78–80, 116, 224
sequence, temporal 78–79, 116, 224
Seurat, Georges 210
sexual differences 57, 247–248, 253, 262, 268–271, 281–288, 293, 300–301, 303, 308, 311, 314
sfumato 197
Shakespeare, William 21, 73
Shannon, Claude 189
Shebalin 232–233
Sherrington, Sir Charles S. 211
sign stimuli 37, 54, 313
simultaneity 78–80
social releasers 29, 37, 61
somatosensation 166, 190–191
sorcery (magic) 298, 301, 304, 308–309
spatial neglect 168, 226, 229, 275
space-time structure 119–143

species-specific perceptual bias 29, 36–49, 85
specious present 80, 83
speech (see language)
split brain 220–223, 235, 244, 246, 252, 254
stroke direction in painting 168, 279–280
style 50j54, 192, 197, 203, 207, 211
subliminal stimulation 245, 248–251, 253
supernormal object 37–38, 42, 65
supersigns 31–32, 35, 63, 65
supraliminal stimulation 245, 249–251, 253
succession 98, 224
symbolism 33, 60–61, 63–64, 118, 186, 188–190, 212, 301, 304–307, 310

T

taboo 298
tabula rasa 18, 43
tachistoscope 221, 243–244
talent (see aptitude)
tempo 91–114, 122, 132, 134–136, 230, 238
temporal auditory perception threshold 98–100, 102, 108, 116, 224
thalamus 153, 173, 177
time measurement 96–97, 122–123
time 71, 76, 78–81, 83, 91, 99, 118, 139
tonality 230, 231, 258, 274–276, 288
totem 63–64
trance 56, 59, 82, 86, 137, 140
transcendentalism 18–21, 24–26
transactional segment 119–121

trichromatic theory 15
Trobriand Islanders 33, 54, 130
Tschaikowsky, Peter I.
turquoise 160

U

unconscious perception 245
uniforms 52

V

Vasarely, Victor 177
velocity 255
Venus, Greek 40–41
Venus of Willendorf 40–41
verbal awareness 245, 248, 254

vision 77–80, 161–179, 190–193, 220, 224, 226, 245–246, 261, 264
visiting cards 54
visual cortex 72, 93, 258, 153–154, 167, 173–178, 192–193, 204, 244–246, 258
visual defects 68, 191, 226, 229, 275
visual memory 168, 176
visual pathways 170, 172, 246
visual resolution threshold 193

W

Watanabe, Satoshi 9, 10, 184–185
Weber, Ernst 99–100

Weber Fraction 99–100, 102, 108
Wertheimer, Max 31, 181
Wiesel, Torsten N. 153, 174, 211
Wiru 299–302, 306–312
Wittgenstein, Ludwig 185
Wordsworth, William 73
Wölfflin, Heinrich 276

Y

Yanomami Indians 39–40, 54, 58, 62, 100, 103–104, 108
Young, Thomas 151

Z

Zeitgeist 243